Springer Series on **Behavior Therapy** **and Behavioral Medicine**

Series Editor: Cyril M. Franks, Ph.D.
Advisory Board: John Paul Brady, M.D., Robert P. Liberman, M.D.,
Neal E. Miller, Ph.D., and Stanley Rachman, Ph.D.

Series volumes no longer in print are listed on the following page.

Out of Print Titles

BEHAVIOR AND PERSONALITY

Psychological Behaviorism

Arthur W. Staats

 Springer Series on Behavior Therapy and Behavioral Medicine

Springer Publishing Company, Inc.
536 Broadway
New York, NY 10012-3955

Cover design by Tom Yabut and Margaret Dunin
Production Editor: Pamela Ritzer

Second Printing
97 98 99 00 / 5 4 3 2

Library of Congress Cataloging-in-Publication Data

Staats, Arthur W.
    Behavior and personality : psychological behaviorism / Arthur
W. Staats.
       p. cm.
    Includes bibliographical references and index.
    ISBN 0-8261-9311-0
    1. Behaviorism (Psychology)   2. Personality. I. Title.
BF199.S74   1996
150.19'43—dc20
                                    96-17801
                                    CIP

Printed in the United States of America

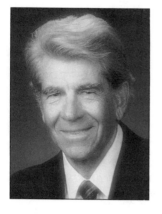

Arthur W. Staats, PhD, currently at the University of Hawaii, has also had tenured professorships at Arizona State University and the University of Wisconsin, Madison. He is a Fellow in eight APA Divisions and in the American Psychological Society and the Association for the Advancement of Science, as well as a member of the Association for the Advancement of Behavior Therapy, the Society for Experimental Social Psychology, and of the Association for Behavior Analysis. He serves on the editorial boards of various domestic and foreign journals, has authored or edited numerous journal articles, book chapters, and books. Dr. Staats has formulated a theory to unify the divided discipline of psychology and to join behaviorism and psychology. He is also known in various specialized areas for his seminal contributions, for example, in developmental psychology for his work in language acquisition, in formulating the first modern, systematic learning theory of intelligence, and in making the first behavioral analyses of early child learning, including toilet training, time out, eating, parent training, compliance, and intergenerational learning; in clinical psychology for helping to lay the foundations of behavior therapy, behavior analysis, and behavioral assessment, and the turn to language-cognitive behavior therapy, and in originating behavior modification principles and the token-reinforcer or token-economy system; in introducing the behavioral treatment of developmental disabilities, and in presenting the first systematic behavioral abnormal psychology; in personality and social psychology for his theories of personality and of social interaction and for his first experiments on attitude acquisition through language conditioning; in experimental psychology for his learning theory that interrelates classical and operant conditioning, for his theory of emotion-motivation, for his psychology of language, and for introducing experimentation to the study of language's emotional properties; in educational psychology for originating the first behavioral analysis of reading and other cognitive skills; in psycholinguistics for introducing the study of the effect of parent talk on the child's language development; and in general psychology for his philosophy of unified positivism and for formulating a unified, comprehensive theory and a new method of theory construction. Since the 1950s his theory has had various lines of influence on the development of psychology as a science.

Contents

Preface

Over four decades ago, while still a graduate student at UCLA, I began a research program that at first I did not name, then later called social behaviorism, then paradigmatic behaviorism, and now psychological behaviorism (PB). The early premises of the program were deceptively simple—that human behavior was learned; that the two most fundamental principles of learning had been established in the animal laboratory; that the preceding behaviorisms (that discovered those principles) were incompletely developed and in error in various ways; that a new behavioral approach was needed that focused on human behavior systematically and broadly; that many important human behavior phenomena had been studied already in traditional psychology; and that the theory formulated in this research had to be closely reasoned, explicit, and linked to various types of empirical work ranging from laboratory to naturalistic study.

Each of my works in the four-decade journey followed these early, sometimes implicit premises. One premise that I employed in my work long before making it explicit was that it was important to unify the psychological and the behavioral. My dissertation, for example, made a behavioral analysis of problem solving. In the mid-1950s I did a series of studies on word meaning and communication that developed into the study of the emotion-language relationship, made an analysis of the abnormal speech of a schizophrenic patient, and began an extended research project on language in general as well as another on reading and problems of reading. Each topic was a traditional psychology interest. The important point is that the research program made focal a new direction for unified research, and each study, while dealing with specific phenomena, also added to the general goal.

During this early time an interaction formed between the behaviorism I was constructing and radical behaviorism, in a mix that was to have fundamental effects on the behavioral field that was to develop. That is, when I was a student at UCLA my closest friend, Jack Michael, a physiological psychology (and statistics) graduate student, was exposed to my early PB developments, and took part in the first behavior modification treatment I arranged in the naturalistic situation. In 1955 I went to Arizona State University where I began a behavioral research and teaching program. Within a year or so Jack had become a behaviorist, adopting Skinner's radical behaviorism along with the PB human research approach (and, in return, introducing me to Skinner's works). After a couple of years I arranged for Jack (and Israel Goldiamond as well) to join the department faculty and gave Jack my teaching lab for my behavioral course, while I continued to provide the psychological behaviorism lectures for the course. The course and lab were at the center of the student program, as was Jack, a master teacher. We added additional behaviorists and later the program came to be called "Fort Skinner in the Desert," considered to be one of the primary sources beginning the field of behavior analysis. Actually, the program was as much based on psychological behaviorism as it was on radical behaviorism. In the 10 years I was at Arizona State we produced a number of students who were radical behaviorists/psychological behaviorists. Their work thus contributed to both behaviorisms in significant ways. For example, Montrose Wolf, a graduate assistant on my reading research project, with deep roots in radical behaviorism, was one of those who learned the two behaviorism traditions. Later, he used both PB and radical behaviorism in making important contributions that helped open the behavioral study of developmental disabilities. When he founded the *Journal of Applied Behavior Analysis* he asked about using the name "behavior analysis" in its title; I had introduced that term and approach in my 1963 book. This journal had a great impact on the establishment of the field of behavior analysis, publishing studies considered important not only to radical behaviorism, but to psychological behaviorism as well. Despite the fertility of this early combination of behaviorisms, the avenues of formal and systematic interaction later closed.

To continue, however, besides these specific projects of study, I also began in the 1950s to construct an overarching theory, at first in inchoate form, but with progressive systematic elaboration. In addition to formal research, I employed and developed the overarching theory in the process of analyzing all of the types of human behavior that I encountered in naturalistic situations and in my wide-ranging personal and professional reading. Such practice increases one's skill in using and developing a theory. Soon I came to see that this growing theory really applied to all human behavior and to the wide range of works in the various fields of psychology. My first book, *Complex Human Behavior* (Staats, 1963a), which I began in the late 1950s, aimed to illustrate this position.

Various of the book's analyses provided directions for the development of the new behavioral psychology (behavior therapy/modification/analysis/

assessment). In addition, however, the work in a beginning way set forth the PB framework of analyzing in terms of behavior principles phenomena that had first been described and studied in psychology. As examples, attitudes, meaning, creativity, problem solving, communication, child development, social interaction, behavior disorders, and psychotherapy were analyzed in a way that produced directions for empirical developments. And the first steps toward making a systematic analysis of personality—needs, the self-concept, intelligence, interests, values, and such—were taken. What I did not entirely recognize at first was that my program was not only making behavioral analyses of psychological topics, it was also introducing a new behaviorism that was psychological—in principle, concept, method, and content. I also did not realize at that time that in pursuing this unification I would have to contest with resistance from behaviorism as well as traditional psychology.

Because that first book was a beginning framework theory, it needed development. One needed direction involved demonstration that its beginning analyses were not empty speculations but the foundations for true theories with empirical implications. The program thus developed to include specialized theories and studies on topics such as language (Staats, 1968a), intelligence (Staats, 1971a, Staats & Burns, 1981), basic learning (Staats, 1970b), emotion (Staats, 1968b; 1975, ch. 4), and abnormal personality (Staats, 1975, ch. 8). But these and other such works, along with the works produced by others in our new behavioral psychology, provided an enriched foundation for a more advanced formulation of PB theory, called *Social behaviorism* (Staats, 1975). Importantly, the process of constructing the overarching theory itself (as in the work that follows) turns out to be a creative task. For, as the extended analysis progresses, it provides novel stimuli that have new implications for further development. (I described this process of scientific creativity in Staats, 1963a, pp. 233–257.) For example, as the 1975 book progressed the character of the overarching theory involved became more visible. By the time I did the last chapter—"Unity of science in the study of man"—I could see that what had emerged was a very broad unified theory. I also began to see that there were *levels* of study involved. For example, the behavioral sciences related in a hierarchical way that made psychology basic. But more importantly psychology's fields themselves could be seen to constitute levels of study that needed theoretical analysis and theoretical bridging with one another. In this book the theory of personality became more explicit and I began to see that a unified theory of personality was needed as the central bridge with which to unify the basic levels of study with those levels dealing with progressively more complex human behavioral phenomena. Thus, this personality theory and the method of theory construction were essential for joining behaviorism and psychology.

Unification was part of the original program and became an increasingly explicit and prominent aspect. I came to see that the central impediment to psychology's advancement was its chaotic diversity and disunity. I thus undertook the work that led to *Psychology's Crisis of Disunity* (Staats, 1983a). This project involved reading philosophy, history, and sociology of science works. This was combined with my knowledge of psychology and the conception emerged that progression from disunity to unity is fundamental in every science development. Psychology is a modern disunified science and has not yet begun to advance toward unification. Importantly, systematic consideration of what psychology is, what its grand theories are, and what the task of constructing broad unified theory in psychology must entail, provided me with an understanding of how to further construct psychological behaviorism as a unified theory.

As the reader will see, this book has several aims. One is to construct a comprehensive unified theory in psychology. Another aim is to develop, within this overarching theory, special area theories that demonstrate empirical productivity—for example, as do the theories of intelligence, emotion, reading, language, cumulative-hierarchical learning, the anxiety disorders, and verbal psychotherapy. Another aim is to develop the theories of the different levels that constitute the fields of psychology. An important position is that no special area theory, or theory of a field as well, can be constructed within a narrow range of interest. A good theory of personality, for example, must be constructed on the foundation of the levels of study below it, and must be extended to the levels of study above it. Each level (field) requires placement in the multilevel framework from which it draws and to which it contributes. (Even the index has been composed to help illustrate the structure of PB, with its interrelated theories from small to large, with multilevels within and among the theories.) Without that development a theory must remain specialized, narrow, and idiosyncratic, as can be seen with the theories in the field of personality.

The three types of theory that compose PB will serve different purposes, for professionals, researchers, and students. First, even though they are part of the larger theory, the special area theories have separate significance and should be individually compared/evaluated with respect to other such theories. The special area theories will specifically stimulate theory and research for those interested in those areas, as well as serve as general models for behavioral-psychological theory construction. Second, it should be realized that the fields of psychology each need a theory framework that distinguishes and justifies the field, establishes its goals and directions for theory and research development, and that interrelates the major specific theories and research areas within the field. The theories of the fields herein have those aims. Those interested in the fields of basic learning, human learning, developmental psychology, social psychology, personality and personality measurement, abnormal and clinical psychology will find new materials herein. Finally, the various fields and special area theories and analyses are made meaningful with respect to one another as they are part of the overarching PB theory. This theory aims to provide a broad guiding framework in various ways. It should be compared to the other theories in psychology that have general aims, such as radical behaviorism, psychoanalysis, cognitive behaviorism, or some of the cognitive theories that have been proposed. Having a general conception of human behavior or a unified theory of psychology is important for a variety of purposes, and the present work should serve such interests.

In its development the present conception first had to be extended and elaborated, which meant increasing its complexity. That process must be lasting. But part of the scientific task also involves simplification. For example, whenever common principles can be established that apply to multiple, disparate phenomena, this constitutes a simplification. Its advancements in different types of simplification help make the present work, in my opinion, the clearest characterization of the broad psychological behaviorism approach that has been made thus far—its philosophy, its overarching theory, its methodology, its construction, its findings and applications, its more specialized theories, and its new directions for the development of behaviorism and of psychology. Let me add this simplification is also valuable with respect to using the theory for didactic purposes. For example, the framework theory of basic learning/behavior in chapter 2 "renders" the great complexity of the field down to essentials. With such treatment the field can be understood more readily at the same time that the framework theory can serve heuristically in analyzing human behavior as well as in directing animal study.

The experiences and findings of the odyssey I have briefly described, and that I elaborate herein, make clear that a unified psychology can be constructed and should be constructed. But the task will be huge, demanding the theoretical, empirical, methodological, and philosophical works of many. Carrying out, and gaining a place for, those works will be a struggle, but the eventual result will be a great scientific revolution.

Acknowledgments

I would like to express appreciation to some of those who have contributed to psychological behaviorism. Let me begin with Cyril Franks, who has supported psychological behaviorism through the years. For example, he published my 1972 article on cognitive behavior therapy in his journal, *Behavior Therapy* when the rest of the field had a different view. His interest in the present book encouraged me to include a chapter on my psychological behavior therapy approach. He has also contributed much to developing psychology's interest in unification issues, as a founder and a later president of the Society for Studying Unity Issues in Psychology. I would also like to give special mention to Karl Minke, an outstanding experimental psychologist, one of my first students, who valuably contributed to early psychological behaviorism studies in the 1950s as well as in later studies, and who developed, himself, many other students (including Earl Hishinuma who has made valuable contributions in the approach). Aimee Leduc at Laval University, with prior interests in unified theory, established a group of students and associates in various universities in Quebec devoted to advancing psychological behaviorism. She and they have conducted various important studies in the framework, including several books, and Professor Leduc also founded a society for the advancement of PB as well as its journal, *Comportement Humain,* both of which disseminate psychological behaviorism to the French-speaking as well as the English-speaking communities. Rocio Fernandez-Ballesteros, already a prominent behavioral psychologist in her special field of psychological measurement, in addition to studies we did together, introduced psychological behaviorism in Spain. Jesus Carrillo and Nieves Rojo are currently conducting studies to advance the PB approach to personality and its measurement in Spain. Paolo Meazzini has taken psychological behaviorism to Italy, Carolina Bori and Geraldina Witter to Brazil, and Jean Rondal to Belgium. I have very special appreciation for the work of Leonard Burns. He began contributing to my theory of personality as a graduate student working with me on several experimental studies that added fundamental elements, and he added a valuable study on his own. Subsequently, he has published conceptual, methodological, and empirical analyses alone and with his students and others on a variety of topics in PB, especially in the anxiety disorders, reading, conduct disorder, rule-governed behavior and assessment. Elaine Heiby has also contributed valuable work—including that involving our construction of the PB theory of depression, but also in areas such as compliance and self-reinforcement. Georg Eifert and Ian Evans (1990) made an important contribution in editing *Unifying Behavior Therapy,* a compilation of PB works. Moreover, Ian Evans, whose contributions to behavior therapy have been recognized for many years—especially in child clinical psychology and in behavioral assessment— has done various works that have been based in and that have enriched PB. Georg Eifert has employed and advanced the PB theory of the anxiety disorders in addition to making other contributions. Hamid Hekmat began studies more than 25 years ago that elaborated the PB approach and has continuously added to that contribution. His works gave basic experimental evidence of the behavioral validity of "talk" therapy and thus helped provide support for PB's language (cognitive) behavior therapy approach. He continues to conduct an important experimental project in the study of pain phenomena, producing research works that are individually significant and that advance the general approach as well. Most recently, Peter Staats (an M.D.), whose major work is in the field of pain medicine, but who earlier studied psychology, combined the two in taking the leading role in constructing the new psychological behaviorism theory of pain, along with supporting experimentation, with the collaboration of Hamid Hekmat and me. That theory is a model of special-area PB theories that address an area broadly, are multileveled, but also specific and explicit and thus are heuristic for empirical as well as theoretical development.

In a work of this kind, with its roots in the behaviorism tradition, there are others I would like to acknowledge whose seminal contributions were important to me as well as generally to the beginnings of modern behavioral psychology. I have already mentioned Montrose Wolf and Jack Michael. Let me now add Signey Bijou, Teodoro Ayllon, Jack Gewirtz, Donald Baer, Nathan Azrin, Ogden Lindsley, Charles Ferster, Thomas Gilbert, Joel Greenspoon, James Holland, and Leonard Krasner, as well as Hans Eysenck, Cyril Franks, Jack Rachman, Joseph Wolpe, and Arnold Lazarus. Other behaviorists not included were important to early PB, as were many more from the broader field of psychology. The point is that a comprehensive unified theory must draw upon the works of many.

Let me acknowledge as well the institutions that have contributed. First, the American university tradition—embodied specifically in Arizona State University, the University of California at Berkeley, the University of Wisconsin, and the University of Hawaii—as well as the Federal system of underwriting basic research—embodied specifically in the Office of Naval Research, the National Institute of Mental Health, the National Science Foundation, and the U.S. Office of Education—provided indispensable opportunity and support during the years of the research program of psychological behaviorism.

I thank Pamela Ritzer for her copyediting and help in preparing the manuscript and for her forbearance in my fine-tuning the proofs, in a production process that I not only appreciated, but that surely improved this work. And, finally, let me acknowledge the friends interested in this work or in some topic in it that I described in conversation; that interest provided incentive during the long task.

CHAPTER 1

Behaviorizing Psychology and Psychologizing Behaviorism: A New Unified Approach

---

The development of psychological behaviorism was begun in the context of the second-generation behaviorisms. These behaviorisms constituted competitive schools. Each was considered to provide the basic theory and define the major positions to be taken in psychology. Most usually new behaviorists selected one or the other behaviorism within which to work. My own approach was that the second-generation behaviorisms contained important raw materials. That is, each of its different forms included some of the "pure matter"; there was a common core material in each that is "mainstream" and will continue to be part of the continuing development of behaviorism. And each also contained idiosyncratic but valuable material. But each second-generation behaviorism also contained many impurities; that is, errors, deficiencies, misdirections, and lack of development. In science developments that involve generations, part of the work of the succeeding generation is to separate the valuable material from the impurities, to reject the former and build upon the latter. The second-generation behaviorists did that with respect to the first-generation behaviorisms. Psychological behaviorism has followed four decades of continuous development, building on the core of the first- and second-generation behaviorisms, but yielding a new behaviorism.

One of the core contributions of John Watson's first-generation behaviorism (Watson, 1930) involved how he related the approach to science. He attempted to indicate what psychology had to study to be scientific, as well as how that was to be studied. In doing so Watson firmly placed behaviorism in the positivist tradition, that of applying the methods of science to the study of behavioral phenomena. His position was coincident with basic aspects of logical positivism and operationism. Building on Watson, later behaviorists elaborated this position (see Hull, 1943a; Marx, 1951; Skinner, 1948; Spence, 1944; Stevens, 1939). These works contributed importantly to those who wished to analyze psychology as a science.

In its third-generation form psychological behaviorism has developed behaviorism's nascent interest in science into a new philosophy of science as a focal interest. This philosophy of science emerged in the work of constructing a new-generation behaviorism, of advancing it within behaviorism, and of advancing it within psychology. This work revealed new considerations with respect to the nature of science, and psychology and behaviorism as areas of science. This new philosophy of science is called *unified positivism* (see Staats, 1968b, 1970a, 1981, 1983a, 1991, 1993a). Unified positivism takes the *general* characteristics of science as fundamental—that is, concerns with observation (including experimentation, measurement, naturalistic, and clinical observation) and systematic construction of theory (including concern with consistency, empirical definition, generality, parsimony, etc.). But, unlike some positivisms, it does not glorify observations as the ultimate, objective truth. And, while it is concerned with the language of science, it does not take the logical positivist position that axiomatic-mathematical statement defines scientific theory. And unified positivism does not limit theory-construction issues in psychology to operational definition and the intervening variable, the focus of second-generation behaviorism considerations (see Hull, 1943b; MacCorquodale & Meehl, 1948; Skinner, 1945; Spence, 1944; Tolman, 1936). Unified positivism recognizes that there can be subjectivity in observation as well as in theory, and that accepted science at any one time bears the mark of "social construction" and is therefore relative, not absolute. Unified positivism also recognizes, however, that such qualifications (as offered by social constructionism and hermeneutics; see Gergen, 1985) regarding the truth of science do not change the fundamental observational and theoretical nature of the science endeavor (Staats, 1983a). Philosophies that lose sight of the basic observational nature of science are misleading.

The central position of unified positivism is that, while the traditional concerns of the philosophy of science are necessary, in psychology (and like sciences) they are not sufficient. What has occurred is that the traditional philosophy of science studies sciences, especially physics, that are the most advanced because they were the earliest to begin and concern straightforward phenomena. The underlying assumption is that these sciences, because they are advanced, will serve as the model for the sciences that are less developed. But that assumption has overlooked an aspect of science—a fundamental dimension of science development. Later, advanced science is unified; but early on sciences are disunified. And the two types of science are quite different, in content, in method, and in operation (Staats, 1983a).

A science begins by individuals observing and studying interesting natural phenomena. Early in science the focus is on discovering the phenomena that come to make up the discipline. Each phenomenon appears to be different and there is no reason to believe they have any relationship. The different phenomena are studied as separate and distinct, using different methods of study. The phenomena and the findings are considered in different theory languages. This process gives rise to viewing the natural world as consisting of diverse and unrelated phenomena. Within that general view of the world, each investigator sees the particular phenomenon or phenomena he or she studies to be centrally important, and composes theory from that orientation. Since there are many such theories, each with the claim of centrality, competition and conflict result. Schools form around the focuses. No conception exists that does justice to the general field of phenomena, and there is no interest in working toward such a conception.

"[During the first half of the eighteenth century] there were almost as many views about the nature of electricity as there were important electrical experimenters. . . . [A]ll were components of real scientific theories . . . drawn from experiment and observation. . . . [However, there was general divisiveness, leading to unguided fact gathering, and this] produces a morass" (Kuhn, 1962, pp. 13–15). So, early on, physics was disunified, and the operation of physics was like that of psychology *today* with its unguided fact gathering and uncontrolled theory proliferation. Over a period of several hundreds of years physics became a unified, compact, parsimonious, largely consensual, *real* science, in products as well as operation. This does not mean that everything in physics is organized by one grand theory into a compact package of interrelated materials. There are always more facts than can be covered by one theory, and there may remain research areas that cannot be interrelated. Moreover, even in the advanced unified sciences there is not perfect consistency. There are many frontiers of research where there is disunity concerning what should be studied, what methods should be used, what principles pertain, what the phenomena mean, and what the major problems are. It is the case, however, that in each advanced natural science there are very considerable bodies of consensual knowledge—which serve as a foundation for the science. Moreover, there are expectations that the phenomena studied are related by underlying principles, and in operation the science invests part of its resources into finding the underlying unifying principles. Physics today, for example, seeks a unified theory that will interrelate the several basic forces of nature. Because the importance of these matters has not been understood, the contemporary unified sciences have not been systematically studied in their early stages *for the purpose of establishing how they advanced from the disunified state to the unified state.* Nor have the modern disunified sciences been studied in order to establish systematically their differences from the unified sciences.

Different works have dealt peripherally with aspects of the problem, but not in a manner that would provide a useful framework (see Staats, 1983a). For example, even philosophers of science who do not devote themselves to the study of psychology have been able to recognize that its fundamental features of disorganization are primitive.

> The characteristic features of *would-be disciplines* can best be illustrated. . . . [When] we turn to professional psychologists for explanations of the behavior of individual human beings . . . we find a diversity of approaches of a kind unparalleled in physics. . . . [a] split into parties, factions, or sects, which have not managed to hammer out a common set of disciplinary goals. . . . So long as a *would-be discipline* remains in this preliminary, inchoate condition, no agreed family of fundamental concepts or constellation of basic presuppositions . . . can establish itself with authority. (Toulmin, 1972, pp. 380–382, italics added)

Even without a deep understanding of what is involved, this characterization recognizes the disunity of psychology and the other behavioral sciences. Such a judgment, general in the philosophy of science, must come as a shock to those who try to make psychology a science by proliferating good experimental studies. Under the aegis of that belief, psychology has produced thousands of studies conducted with sound scientific methods and many more are added each month. Yet those who know what science is can recognize that unrelated studies do not add up to science. What is the problem? The answer lies both in psychology's state of dividedness with respect to its products, as well as in the divisiveness of psychology's mode of operation.

With respect to its products, psychology is a Babel of different theory languages. Its innumerable research works involve inconsistent and unrelated concepts, principles, and findings. Different problem areas of study use different methodologies and eschew those used by others. The studies subtract and detract from each other; the whole is thus *less* than the sum of its parts. Proliferating sophisticated studies is insufficient. Furthermore, each new but unrelated study, although it is experimentally excellent, simply contributes to the problem of disunity; the prolific nature of the modern disunified science itself becomes a handicap. For the resulting morass leads philosophers to conclude that "the preconditions do not yet apparently exist, in the fields of individual and collective behavior, for establishing a 'compact' scientific discipline, possessing a definite strategy and an authorative body of current theory" (Toulmin, 1972, p. 383). The positivistic goal of producing scientifically sound research studies is clearly not the way—or not the only way—to create a psychological science.

Thus, the content of psychology is disorganized in a way that is not scientific. Moreover, the conduct of the science is also disorganized. Psychology, only a hundred years old as an experimental science, is still in the early disunified stage, where the main thrust is to discover new phenomena, new methods, new theories, and new tests. The search for novelty is not the important thing, it is the only thing. Psychology does not yet have the goal of unification of its diverse products, and it has not developed generally tools by which to establish unification. The science does not invest a good part of its resources in unifying its products. For example, despite publishing many journals, not one journal is devoted to unification works. Other than review articles that summarize studies in some problem area, there are no attempts to formulate unifying works. Psychology's operation shows it accepts the disunified science view of the world; that the phenomena studied are fundamentally different and unrelated and that the search for unification is a silly venture (see Koch, 1981). It has not been generally recognized that a central task of the science is to organize, relate, unify, and simplify its diversity, and that the unrelatedness of its many phenomena provides an inexhaustible set of problems.

THE UNIFIED POSITIVISM PROGRAM FOR PSYCHOLOGY

The philosophy of unified positivism was born early in the development of psychological behaviorism. "The history of psychology is a history of separatism of various types, for example, learning versus cognitive approaches" (Staats, 1968b, p. 33). The disadvantage of disunity was further expanded as part of presenting an "integrated" approach to the study of attitudes.

> [I]t is incumbent upon the theory of attitudes to be stated in terms that . . . link up with conceptions concerned with man's general behavior. In this way, a unified, comprehensive theoretical structure will result. This general endeavor should range from the basic learning principles of the animal laboratory to the most significant aspects of complex human behavior. (Staats, 1968b, p. 64)

There are various schismatically arrayed endeavors in psychology that stand in the way of psychology's progress in unification, that is, progress in becoming a full science. That is part of the essential disunified nature of psychology, a nature that constitutes the science's central problem. It is necessary to understand that nature if we are to solve that problem. Part of psychology's disunified nature stems from the complexity of its subject matter.

Psychology's Range of Phenomena

Unification is especially difficult in psychology because it includes such a wide range of phenomena to study and because, as a modern science, psychology has great productivity and has isolated a great number of those phenomena. In terms of range we can see there are relatively simple phenomena—such as Pavlov's principle of classical conditioning. On the other hand, there are complex phenomena such as personality differences. Let me suggest there is a dimension that goes from the simple to the complex. Moreover, the phenomena that different psychologists study lie at different points on that dimension. That has effects on the views that are reached. For example, there are different problems of observing and measuring phenomena, depending upon where they are on the simple-to-complex dimension. On the simple side, it is possible to conduct laboratory studies that control important variables in establishing the elementary principles of animal conditioning. Thus, the terms used to describe Pavlovian conditioning are straightforwardly defined by the things that are manipulated (stimuli) and the outcomes that are observed (learned responses). A term like *intelligence*, in contrast, is much less straightforward; it is inferred from the score on a test, not directly seen. The important point here, however, is that the methods used, the ways that terms are defined, and the theories derived therefrom, are different.

Due to psychology's wide range of phenomena, and the different means of study used, separations are produced in the discipline's products. There are thus many unrelated knowledge elements. There are, of course, limitations on how many elements the individual psychologist can address, which forces most to limit interests to a few areas. The result is specialization at some point on the simple-to-complex dimension. It is difficult even to know about *one* of the large areas of study in psychology, let alone all of them. A primary concept of the present approach is that psychology is an exceedingly complex science in terms of the number of unrelated problem areas it has developed for studying and explaining human behavior. A brief description of some of the fields of psychology can be employed to illustrate the point.

There is biological study of the underpinnings of behavior—studies of the mechanisms of the brain, the organs for sensation, for motor response, for emotions, for learning, and so on. This is considered a basic level of study by many psychologists, the idea being that characteristics of human behavior, and differences in human behavior, are caused by individual differences in biological variables.

There is also a field for the laboratory study of the elementary principles of behavior—studies of the principles by which the environment, via classical and operant conditioning and other principles, affects behavior. Just as there are psychologists who look to biological study for the explanation of human behavior, there are those who look to the environment for the explanation of human behavior. Among those there are some—behaviorists— who consider the principles of animal learning to be the basic ways the environment has its effects. Radical behaviorists take the position that these fundamental principles will suffice to explain all of human behavior. In this field there are innumerable studies of animal behavior, most of them unrelated.

There is also in the field of experimental psychology the attempt to study complex human behavior in a basic way. There are many studies of problem solving, language and language development, perception, word associations, thinking, information processing, and such topics. Cognitive psychology—the study of the mind—is centered here. Another major field of study concerns social interaction, that is, how individuals affect one another. A large field of social psychology includes as its subject matter the study of social interaction phenomena, such as attitudes, leadership, communication, group cohesion, prejudice, and love. Because there are so many phenomena to be studied, and because the phenomena are studied in separate frameworks, this field also remains disconnected and amorphous, quite without any unification.

Another field or level of study concerns the phenomena of behavior development over the life span. The field of developmental psychology traditionally has taken the position that behavior develops in the child through biological maturation, although the field involves little actual study of biological maturation. The field has made many important observations of the developing behavior of the child. Without studying the causes of the behavior development, the conceptions accounting for the many types of child behavior development are generally different and independent.

There is also the field of personality theory, which concerns the description and explanation of individual differences in behavior. The field is based upon naturalistic, including clinical, observations, or on observations made through constructing psychological tests. There are many such studies, and thus many different theories—each of which infers inner personality structures or processes. These theories, for the most part, are not related to each other or to the other fields of psychology. The same holds for the field of personality measurement. Many tests have been constructed, each one as a separate entity, based on the assumption that a personality trait of some kind is being measured. There is no recognized need of the field to relate the many elements of its subject matter.

Abnormal psychology also is an explicit field of study. It is based upon the observation of categories of disordered behavior, toward the separation of different syndromes of disordered behaviors and the systematization of these observations into a classification system. Studies are also done to attempt to establish the etiology of the disorders as well as their demography, the successful avenues of treatment, and so on. There were at one time attempts to consider behavior disorders within a unified theory (psychoanalytic theory). But that was not successful and today the various disorders and the many studies of them remain generally unrelated.

Clinical psychology is the field that is concerned with the treatment of behavior disorders. It has been said that are over four hundred different psychotherapy approaches, all unrelated. Moreover, there are many studies that are unrelated. This is one of the largest fields and exhibits a corresponding disunity.

Psychology is composed of fields of study that differ with respect to the simplicity–complexity of the phenomena studied. Each field is largely conducted in an autonomous manner, producing many products—methods of study, theories, experiments, applications, philosophies, apparatuses, tests, therapies, and so on. There is a wide range of phenomena to study, with many phenomena in each field of study. This yields a multitude of elements of unrelated knowledge. These characteristics of psychology are reflected in the nature of each of the fields of psychology and, taken as a whole, the various fields contribute to a modern disunified science.

TRADITIONAL GRAND THEORY

Psychology and related fields have not yet gained understanding of how to constitute a general and unified theory. After all, there are a bewildering number of different unrelated phenomena of human behavior. How would it be possible to include them all in some manageably sized group of principles and concepts? The complex nature of the domain has forced its scientists to more delimited interests. The traditional approach has been to study in some specialized area of psychology and to obtain certain concepts and principles. Then the theorist sees that the concepts and principles could apply to phenomena outside of the immediate realm of discovery, and finally concludes that the concepts and principles have wide generality. For example, there are biologists who are sure that biology provides the explanation of human behavior and its differences (see Wilson, 1975).

Radical behaviorism is another example. Traditionally it too has been a two-level approach. That is, in the second generation of behaviorism it was thought that behaviorism's task was to compose a basic theory of animal learning, and this theory would then be sufficient to explain all human behavior (see the Preface in Hull, 1943; Skinner, 1953). It was not considered necessary to develop the basic principles through the several fields of psychology before dealing with the human behavior phenomena in the more advanced levels of study. Thus, Skinner (1950) said very pointedly that the study of behavior should take place on its own level, thus cutting out various levels, including biological study. As another example, Sigmund Freud's psychoanalytic theory was constructed on the clinical level of study. The primary source of observations involved stemmed from the statements

Freud's patients made about themselves and their lives. Finally, Jean Piaget studied how children of various ages solved types of problems that he considered to reflect their cognitive stage of development.

The general point is that each of these theorists believed that the concepts and principles (the theory) that he had formulated, on the basis of the research in one area of psychology, could be extrapolated very generally as a broad *explanation* of human behavior. This represents in each case a two-level type of theory construction. The two-level strategy of theory construction involves formulating a theory in a restricted area of the broad discipline and then generalizing that theory to other fields of psychology, or even to the whole discipline. In general, the two-level approach, by definition, rules out the possibility of yielding a comprehensive, unified theory. While pretending to be general and unified, a two-level theory only treats a small part of psychology. As such they can only gain the allegiance of a small group of psychologists (see Staats, 1993a). Let me suggest that this strategy, or methodology, contributes strongly to the fragmented, contentious state of psychology. For the scientists at each level of study know that they are working with important phenomena and that they are discovering important knowledge. They thus reject any theory that, in essence, wipes out of consideration their work and their field, which is what a two-level strategy generally does to the areas not considered. The two-level theory strategy prevents the establishment of a framework within which the scientists in the various fields can work in a way that combines and cumulates their efforts, versus being mutually antagonistic.

The fact is there are multitudes of two-level approaches that have captured attention, because they are simple, and because they promise explanations of the complex phenomena of human behavior. They die away, however, because they cannot create a research tradition that involves the various relevant levels of study, which is what is necessary for long-term, continuous development. Truncated theories are unable to deal comprehensively with human behavior and thus represent only a small proportion of psychologists and gain only a small proportion of the science's resources (see Fraley & Vargas, 1986).

Finally, let me mention another strategy that suggests it yields a grand theory but does not. That is, cognitive psychology is generally taken to compose a unified theory approach (Baars, 1984). The cognitive revolution, in this view, is unifying psychology. But that is not the case. Cognitive psychology itself is like the discipline of psychology, a confusion of separate elements of knowledge. The problem is the various elements are never brought into relationship with one another. A recent attempt to compose a real unified theory (Newell, 1990) revealed that there is no unified theory and, in fact, the steps that could be made in this direction were small and inadequate. It was demonstrated that the unified cognitive theory formulated has nothing to do with the cognitive concepts that are being used in other cognitive studies in other areas of experimental psychology or in other fields like developmental, clinical, and social psychology, and personality. Cognitive psychology simply gives license to psychologists to infer cognitive processes in whatever behavioral phenomena that are studied. But the result is an "approach" that consists of an amorphous body of multitudes of unrelated concepts, principles, theories, findings, fields, and areas of study, with no program for creating compact, consensual, organized, parsimonious science.

In conclusion, psychology in general has no strategy for constructing a unified science. The two-level strategy of theory construction may be called the part-to-whole-plus-rejectionism approach. The strategy is to study in a part of psychology, and then, by conjecture, conclude that the conception involved explains the rest of the interests of psychology. This involves, in actuality, rejection of most of the work in psychology. This is the strategy that, by definition, cannot produce broad unification. Thus none of the classic grand theories in psychology has shown that there are common underlying principles that interrelate a good portion of the phenomena in which the discipline is interested. None of these theories has rationalized the different methods employed in psychology in studying different phenomena. None of these theories has drawn upon and contributed to the different major fields of psychology, or indicated how these fields are related to each other and how they contribute in a complementary way to studying the phenomena of psychology. None of these theories has combined the many diverse and unrelated works of psychology into a more compact, parsimonious, organized body. None has had a plan and program for becoming a broad, unified theory in psychology. Therefore none of the classic grand theories has gained the support of more than a small percentage of the discipline's members.

As a science, psychology suffers grave weaknesses because it is a disunified science, does not realize this generally, does not attempt to advance toward unification, and has no goal or program for doing so. This chapter will attempt to characterize the nature of the approach that is to be presented. That nature is multifaceted, with various purposes. This approach, psychological behaviorism (PB), aims to constitute a broad, overarching, unifying theory. Unlike the traditional grand theories, PB has been constructed according to a design or plan which has become increasingly defined over the past four decades of the development of the approach. Some of the characteristics of this design can be presented here as an introduction to what follows, although other features can be described better following presentation of content of the theory. In addition to introducing the approach, these discussions are meant to suggest that psychology needs to begin systematic consideration of what its task is as a disunified science, and how that task can be accomplished.

LACK OF UNITY LEADS TO DISUNITY

John Watson, the first behaviorist, as a grand theorist also aimed at establishing a unified approach. But his aim was not unification with traditional psychology. His aim was a revolution against psychology that included rejecting psychology's concept of the mind (mentalism), methods (introspection), philosophy (dualism), and content. With revolutionary fervor his aim was to *defeat* traditional psychology and replace it with behaviorism. Watson thus generally followed the part-to-whole-plus-rejectionism strategy.

In the second generation of behaviorism there were several different approaches. Watson had said that the mind cannot be studied because it cannot be observed. Tolman (1932) sought some unity with traditional psychology by making psychology's mentalism scientifically respectable through the creation of the intervening variable strategy. His plan was to define cognitive (mental) concepts by externally observed conditioning events, on the one hand, and consequent changes in behavior. However, he later admitted failure in trying to construct a grand theory for psychology (Tolman, 1959). Hull (1943b) became enmeshed in the intervening variable strategy for defining learning, and he constructed an axiomatic-mathematic theory, a focus that produced such a complicated basic learning theory that it was an obstacle to constructing a grand unified theory of behavior (Hull, 1943a). But Hull considered his theory general to psychology. Others tried a strategy of eclectically combining psychoanalytic theory with Hull's theory (see Dollard & Miller, 1950), producing a non-heuristic incompatibility, not a grand unified theory.

Skinner, by contrast, carried forth Watson's tradition of radical behaviorism—and the rejection of psychology and mentalism—in attempting to establish a very general approach. His scientific work was restricted to animal operant conditioning, using his experimental analysis of behavior technology and methodology. His consideration of human behavior was a philosophy, not based on empirical study, and with little in the way of explicit empirical implication. Skinner's radical behaviorism did not use or include reference to works in the field of psychology, or even to other behaviorism works. Skinner did not establish a foundation for unifying behaviorism and psychology—quite the opposite.

Both Watson and Skinner, as well as other behaviorists, made an important contribution by exposing the errors in mentalism and introspective methods. But, because of behaviorism's successful criticism and its revolutionary stance, it became customary for many behaviorists to ignore psychology developments, or reject them without systematic consideration, for a variety of reasons—because the developments employ mentalistic concepts, do not use a behaviorally accepted methodology, deal with phenomena not readily interpretable in behavioral terms, and the like. A strong position today in behavior analysis is that radical behaviorism works define what should be studied and how, and that it is unnecessary to study psychology (or any other behaviorism). The strategy is to develop a science of behavior from *within,* in isolation, only treating complex phenomena when they can be considered in the concepts and methods of the approach. Fraley and Vargas' (1986) behaviorology takes this tradition of Skinner (1988) to its logical extreme, suggesting behaviorism should completely separate from psychology.

Inconsistencies in the Revolution

What is anomalous is that, while not part of a systematic program, and never formally acknowledged, each of the behaviorists did make behavioristic analyses of things that were first studied in traditional psychology. Watson (1930) made analyses of fear, talking, and thinking. Hull (1920) treated concepts and knowledge and purpose (Hull, 1930), and some Hullians attempted broader topics (Dollard & Miller, 1950). Skinner continued this tradition in his *Science and Human Behavior* (1953)—briefly describing such things as personality, psychotherapy, and thinking. However, these various analyses were conducted largely to demonstrate the weaknesses of traditional psychology. The brief analyses attempted to show that behaviorism could deal with psychology's topics better than psychology and, hence, behaviorism should be the approach to be adopted, and traditional psychology should be abandoned. The findings, analyses, and methods of traditional psychology were not presented as valuable resources—even when they yielded products that were used as the jumping-off place for behavioristic analysis. No one abstracted the important and general principle involved—that traditional psychology has begun the isolation of phenomena that, with behavioral analyses, can be valuable to behaviorism as well as to psychology. The fact is such a principle contradicts the radical behaviorism rejection of psychology, so no progress in this direction has occurred.

Traditional psychology, of course, responded in kind to behaviorism's rejection. Most psychologists, distributed over the various fields of study, in turn, reject behaviorism, are misinformed about it, and continually tilt against what they misperceive it to be. As Fraley and Vargas (1986) indicate, moreover, behaviorism's contributions to psychology are not recognized, and behaviorists do not get a good share of the resources allocated to psychology. It may be added that behaviorism has much less influence than the potential of the tradition deserves.

Disadvantages of Rejectionism

Frequently things are rejected in our discipline on a much less systematic basis than is demanded for things to be accepted. Many cognitivists, for example, reject (or ignore) behavioristic works very generally. Because they are behavioristic it is assumed they "must be" atomistic, mechanistic, anti-psychological, and simplistic. An important scientific literature is not studied, and traditional psychology lacks needed developments as a consequence. On the other side, many behaviorists reject (or ignore) anything that uses mentalistic terminology or does not employ behavioral methods, or that is part of the large (and denigrated) literature of psychology. What this means is that a vast scientific literature is unknown to radical behaviorists. Entire fields of psychology—including personality and personality measurement—are not considered. In both cases this is not good scientific practice, and it prevents construction of a comprehensive unified approach.

BREAKING THE DISUNITY HABIT: BEHAVIORIZING PSYCHOLOGY AND PSYCHOLOGIZING BEHAVIORISM

In contrast, and partly because it is a third-generation behaviorism, PB began by making behavior analyses of phenomena that had already been studied in psychology; in fact, that was PB's beginning program. To be made behavioral, several things were necessary. Psychology's mentalistic conceptions had to be set aside. The limitations of the traditional observations had to be realized—for example, that the environmental causes of the behaviors were little considered. Each phenomenon needed to be analyzed as behavior, including how that behavior was learned, in very specific terms, in order to provide implications for empirical study of a strictly behavioral nature. The intervening variable methodology had to be rejected in favor of the direct consideration of behavior, even when the behavior was internal to the subject and difficult to observe.

With these types of strictures, some of the first works of PB constituted behavioral analyses of phenomena first studied in psychology. For example, an early PB work accepted studies of human problem solving, considered in traditional psychology as an important cognitive phenomenon (see Staats, 1956). Addressing a traditional study, the PB analysis was that human problem solving involves the problem-solving objects eliciting verbal labeling responses, which then elicit learned chains of verbal responses, which, in turn, elicit the problem-solving behaviors (Staats, 1963a). This treatment, extended also to traditional psychology's interest in human purposiveness (see also Staats, 1963b), anticipated the interest in rule-governed behavior (Skinner, 1966) and is part of the PB analysis of how language behavior affects behavior (see also Burns & Staats, 1992; Staats, 1975). As another example, traditional psychology treats the concept of word meaning in a mentalistic way in analyzing language and communication. PB's behavior analysis treated the concept of word meaning as a classically conditioned response (see Staats & Staats, 1957, 1958; Staats, Staats, & Crawford, 1962). A number of studies have used PB's analysis and language conditioning method in studying language and its effects upon behavior (e.g, Berkowitz & Knurek, 1969; Early, 1968; Hekmat & Vanian, 1971; Zanna, Kiesler, & Pilkonis, 1970). PB very early made additional behavior analyses of grammatical rules, the self-concept, interests, intelligence, psychopathologies (including developmental disorders), values, communication, originality, self-determination, and many other phenomena treated in traditional psychology (Staats, 1963a).

These examples have been given to indicate that PB began with the goal of behaviorally analyzing important phenomena that had been isolated in traditional psychology studies. The analyses were explicit and lent themselves to the derivation of experimental studies to verify the principles involved.

A Systematic Method and Program

In this endeavor a general method of analyzing phenomena studied in psychology was developed in PB. Called "behaviorizing psychology" (see Staats, 1993b, 1994), the method was systematized and elaborated in PB's program to construct a general, unified theory in our science. The above examples illustrate that psychology has made preliminary studies of important behavioral phenomena, albeit under the aegis of mentalistic conceptions that generally have drawbacks. Focally, lacking analysis of its phenomena in terms of behaviors, and how those behaviors are learned, traditional psychology lacks a way of explaining those phenomena and, thus, of establishing the relationships of the phenomena to each other. For these reasons psychology's findings remain disparate and unrelated and superficial, which contributes to psychology's chaotic disunification.

Psychological behaviorism, however, has the methodological advantage that allows for behavioral analyses that indicate learning conditions. Such analyses yield the possibility of dealing with the behaviors under consideration, not just predicting them, and in this sense are explanatory. In addition, however, it is important to realize what behavioral analyses of psychological phenomena can contribute in terms of unification. Behavior principles are part of a unified set. Whatever is analyzed in terms of those principles is placed into a unified framework. For example, when attitudes, interests, values, preferences, and choice behavior are analyzed in terms of conditioning principles (see Staats, 1963a; Staats & Staats, 1958; Staats, Gross, Guay, & Carlson, 1973; Staats & Burns, 1982) the phenomena are drawn into a unified theory conception. Such behavioral analyses of psychological phenomena, moreover, are heuristic, and suggest new paths of study, as these and other works show. Psychology needs greatly (1) behavior analyses of its phenomena, (2) conduct of the research implied, and (3) systematization of the analyses into a unified theory.

What I am describing is PB's program of "behaviorizing" psychology. The goal is not that of invalidating psychology but of strengthening psychology. That is what underlies the PB methodology of retaining the traditional name whenever a phenomenon has been first studied in psychology—as in the PB analyses of attitudes, intelligence, reading, personality, and the like. There is an important difference here, in method as well as in theory, between PB and Skinner's radical behaviorism. The latter does not cite psychology materials or use psychology's names for phenomena. For example, Skinner used terms like *texting* instead of *reading* (Skinner, 1957) and *abstraction* instead of *concept formation* (Skinner, 1953), and so on, in a manner consistent with his epistemology (see Moore, 1985). His radical behaviorism aims to defeat psychology. PB's analysis of psychological phenomena, in contrast, uses the traditional names and refers to the traditional psychology works involved. Some behavior analysts superficially, without analysis of the operations by which PB defines its terms, have confused PB's use of traditional terms with the use of intervening variables or mentalistic concepts (see Plaud, 1995; Ulman, 1990). But PB's terms are behaviorally defined, strictly, closely, specifically—its methodology more stringent than in radical behaviorism concepts like abstraction, private events, rule-governed behavior, conditioned seeing, id, ego, and superego (Skinner, 1953), reflex reserve, and the like.

The brute fact is that behaviorism today is mostly cut off from the large and powerful science and profession of psychology. Behaviorism, by rejecting or ignoring the works of non-behavioral psychology, adds to that schism. Systematically ignoring psychology's interests, needs, and works simply adds to the isolation (see Coleman & Mehlman, 1992). Moreover, the result is the separation of important scientific developments, whose power is diminished because they are unrelated.

PB methodology is that all of the works in psychology may contain valuable elements. Thus, they cannot be rejected out of hand. As in the process of accepting something into science, knowledge elements can only be rejected *systematically*. Not everything in psychology—problems, methods, theories, philosophies, findings, whatever—will turn out to deserve a scientific investment. For that reason science involves "separating the wheat from the chaff." Behaviorism must expend efforts on such evaluation, for it is an important task.

Psychologizing Behaviorism: The Other Side of the Coin

The concept of behaviorizing psychology would smack of arrogance if it suggested that this method is a way of turning dross into gold. Rather, the

PB position is that traditional psychology has important things to offer our scientific discipline, as does behaviorism. Generally, rather than being in opposition, the two are complementary. This can only be seen when the necessary unifying analysis is made.

The process of behaviorizing psychology, it should be noted, is a two-way process, for it also results in psychologizing behaviorism. PB in treating such things as word meaning, attitudes, interests, values, intelligence, communication, self-concept, and defense mechanisms thereby becomes a psychological behaviorism. When PB formulates a theory of personality and of psychological tests, as a central example, this represents a critical step in the direction of being psychological as well as behavioral.

The Scientific Significance of Behaviorizing

It has been said already that when science was just beginning it was not clear at all that the phenomena of nature had any relationship to each other. It had been thought that all happenings were divinely inspired, rather than following natural law. And when scientific study began, each phenomenon appeared to be quite distinct from the others, especially since they were studied using different methods and the phenomena were discussed in different terms. As an example, in physics the laws of the oceanic tides, Galileo's law of falling objects, and Kepler's laws concerning movements of the planetary bodies were once considered to pertain to fundamentally different phenomena. Newton showed, however, that there were common principles that underlay the several dissimilar phenomena. The specific principles that had been adduced for each phenomenon were of narrow significance. The common underlying principles that Newton formulated were very general, to many different phenomena and, hence, very powerful.

It turned out that the natural events studied in physics, chemistry, biochemistry, and biology, bewildering in their number, do not each operate according to a unique principle. Were that the case understanding nature would be a monstrously complex, impossible task. Rather, what appear to be different phenomena operate according to the same fundamental principles. Thus, the many phenomena can be understood within a much smaller, knowable set of fundamental principles. Natural phenomena are characterized by their *relatedness* in terms of underlying principles.

It is the case that in the advanced sciences there has been sufficient time to establish the relatedness of events once considered to be fundamentally different. In psychology such relatedness has not been sufficiently shown or disseminated, so doubt remains. That is what Koch (1981) actually means when he says that psychology cannot be a science but is instead a number of incommensurate study areas. This says that the phenomena studied in the various problem areas are incommensurate, are different in principles, and thus cannot be interrelated.

A New Type of Unified Theory

A central point of PB's behaviorizing psychology approach is that of setting forth the general science goal of establishing the relatedness of phenomena. The disunified science of psychology lacks that goal; and it is essential in science. It is unification via common underlying principles that produces some of the most important and powerful theory, as the example of Newton indicates. Psychology as a science cannot rest content with the scientific stipulation of new phenomena. It must invest resources into establishing the underlying principles that relate the phenomena that have been stipulated. PB says that the behavioral phenomena of psychology are related because they operate according to the same set of underlying principles, just as physical events do. Moreover, PB has produced many exemplars of relatedness in behavioral phenomena, and sets forth additional cases herein.

PB's philosophy of unified science, its aim of unification of behaviorism and psychology, its methodology of behaviorizing psychology, and the psychologizing behaviorism products of this endeavor stamp PB as a new type of theory. For these characteristics result in fundamental differences in PB across the purview of its interests. One purpose of the present work is to characterize PB as a broad, overarching, unified theory.

FIELDS AND LEVELS: PB'S MULTILEVEL THEORY APPROACH

Establishing the relationships among the broad range of types of phenomena in psychology with respect to one another constitutes fundamental work for the science. However, the fields of psychology were not constructed for this purpose. Rather, they are historical developments that involve grouping into fields the study of phenomena that, on some commonsense basis, appear to have some similarity. Actually, the fields are the basis for some of psychology's disunity, for the fields themselves operate as autonomous disciplines. Scholars and researchers in one field rarely know about any of the others.

If we were to ask psychologists whether the various fields of psychology had any relationship with one another, there would be a variety of opinions. As indicated, Koch (1981) assumes that the various phenomena in psychology are different in kind. From this view there is no reason to be concerned with the relationship of the fields of psychology. However, many psychologists would no doubt assume the various fields of psychology are related in some way, without knowing what that might be, and without much interest in finding out. For example, in books on general psychology there is no attempt to relate the fields or to cumulate their knowledge into a meaningful conception. Since the fields are autonomous, the order of presentation of the different fields has little importance. The study of general psychology does not lead one to a unified conception of the discipline, but quite the contrary, as Koch's (1981) position shows so clearly, since general psychology has been his focal interest (see Koch, 1959).

If, however, a central task of psychology is progress in unification then it becomes important to consider the relationships among individual phenomena, among groups of phenomena, and among psychology's major fields. In the approach to be developed herein it will be suggested that the fields are related, not just in face value, but in terms of underlying principles. PB states that the major substantive fields of psychology are to be considered as *levels* of study, arranged on a dimension that is defined by simplicity–complexity or, perhaps, basic–advanced. That is, PB takes the view that there is a generally advancing progression, from the more basic fields to the more advanced; the basic principles and concepts at one level serve as the starting point for analyses at the next level of advancing complexity. The field of Basic Learning provides principles and concepts for use in the Human Learning level which, in turn, provides principles and concepts for the study of Child Development. The levels generally have a hierarchical relationship as depicted in Figure 1.1, with the Biological Level as the most basic (although the Basic Learning Level is the most critical for developing a comprehensive theory of human behavior).

The hierarchical relationships of the various fields (levels of study) are not simple. Although a field may provide a basic framework of principles for use at the next highest level, that is not the only type of relationship. For one thing, developments at a more advanced level may be heuristic for developments at a more basic level. Thus, as an example, those who study the biology of learning do so because it first had been observed that organisms learn. The impetus for the biological study, thus, comes from the more advanced level of study of basic learning. Thus, in Figure 1.1 the arrows between adjacent levels are bidirectional (see Staats, 1975, chap. 16; 1983). Another relationship principle is that a cumulation of knowledge is involved in the levels. For example, the child development principles add to the human learning principles which add to the basic learning principles, producing a progressively richer fund of concepts, principles, methods, and findings with which to make an analysis of personality phenomena.

The cumulative development of knowledge over the levels of study is central. However, this does not mean that the principles and concepts in one level cannot be directly applied to the analysis of phenomena in more distal (non-adjacent) levels. The basic principles of learning, for example, can be directly applied to the study of phenomena in social interaction, child development, personality and personality measurement, abnormal behavior, and clinical psychology. In fact it was the direct application of

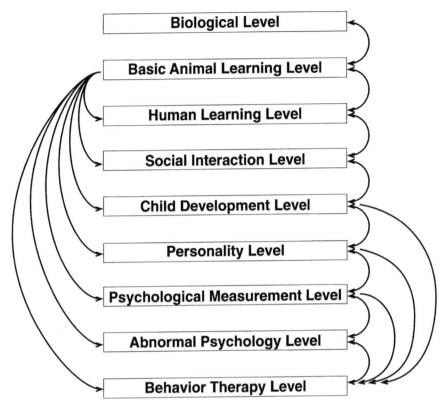

FIGURE 1.1 The multilevel conception of psychology's fields.

behavior principles by some of us that began the fields of behavior therapy, behavior modification, behavior assessment, and behavior analysis. The basic principles of learning apply to each of the levels above the Basic Learning Level. This is depicted in Figure 1.1 by the cluster of arrows going from that area to the other areas. The other areas can also have implications for the development of the basic field of learning, as will be indicated, so these arrows should be considered as bidirectional. Also, multiple fields can be basic to another field, as exemplified by the Child Development, Personality, Psychological Measurement, and Abnormal Psychology levels, each of which has applications for the Behavior Therapy Level. It should be understood that these points are relevant for each area, although Figure 1.1 does not include all the arrows that would be necessary to depict this.

Let me add that the terms *basic* and *applied* generally have been given values in our discipline, with the former having more status than the latter. This is not the PB view. The fact is, when the principles and concepts of any level are used in the next level, this may be considered an application. Each level's phenomena are explained by concepts and principles in lower levels. And each level's concepts and principles explain phenomena in more advanced levels. For example, when the basic learning principles are used to establish a theory of language (and cognition) at the Human Learning and Developmental Levels, this is an application. And, continuing, when that theory of language is used to establish a theory of intelligence, this is an application. When that theory of intelligence is used further to consider developmental disabilities in the Abnormal Psychology Level this too is an application. The present position is that each of the levels has unique methods of study to discover, unique phenomena to study, unique principles and concepts to formulate, and it has the task of relating these materials to the levels below it and to the levels above it. The study at the more advanced levels should influence the study at the more basic levels. Generally, the more basic levels need explication of what their goals of explanation are, and that must come, in part, from contact with the materials of the more advanced levels.

What is being suggested is an interdependence of the various levels. There is no room here for the elevation of one level—and its methods, findings, and theory—into a position of dominance or eliteness. This was not understood by the first- and second-generation behaviorists, who thought their basic learning theories were the *real* science, the special explanations of all behavior. This view alienated psychologists in other fields for relegating their study to a lesser role. The PB view is that different problems arise at the various levels with respect to how their phenomena are to be studied. Generally, the more complex the subject matter, the more difficult the observations, and the more difficult the general task. It can be expected, thus, that progress will be made more slowly and less directly as there is an advancement of level and complexity of phenomena.

It is not possible here to reduce the content of PB and its works to a brief summary. However, PB's range of interests—and the outline of its structure—is summarized in Table 1.1. The table indicates the levels and their relationships, in a general way, and indicates also some of the specific concerns of the levels as well as some of PB's concepts and principles for dealing with those concerns. The table provides an overview; the chapters that follow will provide a more penetrating characterization of PB. The areas which the multilevel theory addresses are presented in the left-hand column of the table. The right-hand column characterizes some of the principles, concepts, and purposes of each level.

LACK OF INTERVENING THEORY PRODUCES SCHISMS

The multilevel conception of psychology helps explain why there are seemingly irreparable schisms in psychology. The personality/behaviorism schism

TABLE 1.1 The Multilevel Theory of Psychological Behaviorism

Levels (and Content-Area examples)	Principles, Concepts, and Phenomena

1. *Biological mechanisms of learning*
  a. Sensory psychology
  b. Brain and central nervous system
  c. Response systems
  d. Evolution of learning mechanisms
	The neurophysiology of learning: The central purpose of this level of theory is to unify the biological study of organisms with behavioral study, making the two mutually heuristic, and removing the schism that separates so much of psychology along "nature–nurture" lines. The basic bridge relates the biological concepts of sensory, response, and association organs with the behavioral concepts of stimuli, responses, and learning.

2. *Basic-learning/behavior theory*
  a. Elementary study: conditioning principles
  b. Generalizing study: types of stimuli, responses, and species to which principles apply
  c. Motivation principles
	Three-function learning theory: Stimuli that elicit an emotional response will because of this be reinforcing stimuli. Both functions (emotion elicitation and reinforcement) are transferred in classical conditioning. Moreover, organisms generally learn to approach positive emotional (and reinforcing) stimuli and to avoid negative emotional (and punishing) stimuli. As a consequence, emotional stimuli direct (are incentives for) behavior. This learning theory makes the study of the various forms of the classical conditioning of emotions to be a central concern in explaining behavior, giving new directions for animal and human research.

3. *Human-learning/cognitive theory principles*
  a. Complex stimulus-response learning (e.g., response sequences, response hierarchies, and multiple controlling stimuli)
  b. Basic behavioral repertoires
  c. Cumulative-hierarchical learning principles and others unique to humans
	Complex stimulus-response mechanisms, internal responses and stimuli, basic behavioral repertoires, and cumulative-hierarchical learning: The basic theory states the behavioral principles in elemental simplicity. Human skills and general characteristics are composed of exceedingly complex combinations of the basic principles. The field of human learning must study such combinations and the manner in which these complex,

(continued)

TABLE 1.1 The Multilevel Theory of Psychological Behaviorism *(continued)*

Levels (and Content-Area Examples)	Principles, Concepts, and Phenomena
	basic behavioral repertoires are learned. Centrally complex human skills are basic repertoires that can only be acquired if the individual has already learned necessary prior repertoires (e.g., reading can only be learned after prior language repertoires are learned). Some basic behavioral repertoires constitute cognitive characteristics.
4. *The social-personality level of study* a. Attitudes and social cognition b. Interpersonal relations and group processes c. Group differences and cross-cultural psychology involve learning	*Interactions among individuals and groups:* The three-function learning principles are basic. Attitudes are emotional responses to social stimuli. Thus, such stimuli have reinforcing and incentive (directive) power, depending on their emotion elicitation. Social phenomena such as group cohesion, attraction, persuasion, prejudice, and intergroup relations function by these principles. The learning of complex human repertoires is a social interaction process and should be studied as such.
5. *Child development* a. Language-cognitive development b. Sensory-motor development, including modeling skills c. Emotional-motivational development	*Cumulative-hierarchical learning and development:* Traditional developmental psychologists have studied many aspects of the child's development. But there has been little analysis of this development in terms of its complex learning. Paradigmatic behaviorism calls for this systematic analysis, provides exemplary theoretical-empirical analyses of language-cognitive, emotional-motivational, and sensory-motor development through learning, and calls for various new types of theory and research.
6. *Personality* a. Personality concept	*Personality is composed of basic behavioral repertoires:* From birth the child begins to learn complex systems of "skills" in the three

b. The three personality systems: language-cognitive, emotional-motivational, and sensory-motor
c. Personality and environment interaction

general areas. These are learned in advancing complexity. There are subrepertoires that additional learning combines together (as language is composed of separately learned subrepertoires), and there are repertoires that are basic to the later learning of more advanced repertoires (as algebra skills rest on the prior learning of arithmetic operations). The three repertoires constitute personality. In interaction with the environment they determine the individual's experience, learning, and behavior. This theory makes many conceptual unifications possible in psychology and opens many new avenues of research.

7. *Personality measurement*
a. Theory relating behavior principles, the concept of personality, and personality measurement and behavioral assessment
b. Application of the theory to tests and their uses (clinical, etc.)
c. Applications to test construction and assessment: Paradigmatic behavioral assessment

Unifying theory for psychological behavioral psychometrics: The personality theory provides a conceptual framework within which the personality concepts, methods, and instruments of the traditional field of psychometrics can be analyzed in a manner compatible with behaviorism. Personality tests measure aspects of the basic behavioral repertoires, which accounts for their ability to predict behavior. For example, intelligence tests heavily measure language repertoires and sensory-motor skills, and interest tests measure aspects of the emotional-motivational repertoire. The theory explains why verbal tests provide knowledge of nonverbal behavior and emotional states—because the three personality repertoires are interconnected and covary—helping resolve the behaviorism/psychometrics schism. The theory is heuristic for basic research and test construction.

8. *Abnormal psychology*
a. The personality repertoires as basic determinants of abnormal behavior
b. Diagnostic categories considered as deficit and inappropriate personality repertoires

Psychological behaviorism's theory of abnormal behavior: The individual learns personality repertoires that interact with his life situation in determining his behavior. The personality repertoires may be rich or sparse, adaptive or inappropriate. Deficit or inappropriate repertoires will yield behavior that is abnormal

(continued)

TABLE 1.1 The Multilevel Theory of Psychological Behaviorism (*continued*)

Levels (and Content-Area Examples)	Principles, Concepts, and Phenomena
c. Personality and environment interaction in abnormal behavior	in certain situations. Life situations that are not normal may also produce abnormal behavior. Biological conditions can directly affect the personality repertoires and produce abnormal behavior. Using this theory, a unified analysis can be made of the various diagnostic categories. For example, schizophrenia involves disturbances especially in the language-cognitive and emotional-motivational repertoires, phobias involve only a part of the latter repertoire, and the various subtypes of depression differ in the repertoires, life events, or biological conditions involved.
9. *Clinical psychology* a. Behavior modification of simple problems, behavior therapy, and the psychodynamics/conditioning schism b. Psychological behavior therapy c. Personality change and personality measurement d. Language-cognitive methods of treatment	*Psychological behavior therapy:* The various levels of psychological behaviorism are applied to clinical problems involving various methods of treatment. The basic learning principles can be employed to directly treat simple problems. Sometimes personality or social-environmental problems are involved and assessment instruments may be needed, as well as complex social-environmental changes and learning programs. The language-cognitive level of theory indicates how behavior and personality can be changed by various verbal methods of therapy. Psychological behavior therapy has been in development since the 1950s, has yielded seminal contributions to behavior therapy, and now projects new avenues for development.

is a good example. Behaviorism's principles are drawn from the animal learning level; the principles of personality and personality measurement are drawn from study that is several levels removed on the simple-to-complex dimension. Methods of study are different, as are subjects, philosophy of science, and so on. The intervening levels of study have not been developed in a manner that connects the two. Whether potential connections might be constructed is difficult to envision because of the distance involved. That distance must be broken down by means of bridging theory; connecting the levels means that the animal conditioning principles have to be developed through intervening levels of study (Human Learning/Cognitive, Developmental, and Social Interaction) before they provide a theory structure with which to consider the phenomena in the field of personality.

Without the intervening theory development, the large gap in theory development provides no indication that basic animal conditioning studies are relevant for the analysis of personality phenomena. For this reason personality theorists look elsewhere for the explanation of personality, and are prepared to accept simplistic suggestions that personality must be determined by biological factors. For the same reason behaviorists have rejected the study of personality and its measurement; for personologists do not indicate how behavioral principles might be relevant.

The general point is that it is easier to see the relationship between principles when the levels of study are adjacent. The more distant the levels of study the more difficult it is to see the relationships of underlying principles. It is thus essential to have a conception of the fields as hierarchically related levels of study, as a guide to seek to establish the specific nature of the connections.

THE FRAMEWORK THEORY METHODOLOGY

So a unified theory must confront the numberless unrelated phenomena and groups of phenomena of psychology, as well as the unrelated fields of psychology. The size of this task is insuperable, for any one person. And this brute fact has dictated the nature of the grand theories that have been constructed. That is what accounts for the classic method of theory construction, which involves a relatively detailed development of theory in one field, with little or no consideration of other fields. Because of the great breadth of psychology's interests, even the major theorists in psychology have been specialists. Hull and Skinner, for example, were primarily animal learning psychologists, Piaget was a child developmentalist, Freud worked at the clinical psychology level, and so on. They systematically worked at one level of study and each thought the theoretical conception obtained would pertain as a general explanation of human behavior. They did not, thus, attempt to make meaningful contact with the different levels of psychology.

The "part-to-whole-plus-rejectionism" method of theory construction can be seen as a way of simplifying the enormous complexity of the subject matter, since it allowed the theorist to ignore most of the levels of study of psychology and to deal only with his or her own. The problem is, if it really is the case that a general theory for psychology can only be constructed by building connections between the various levels of study, then the part-to-whole strategy is doomed to failure. For that strategy avoids rather than confronts the task. Moreover, since the part-to-whole theories are based in different levels of study, use different methods, concepts, and problems, and construct different theory languages, they will be very different and incommensurable—thereby giving rise to disagreement and conflict, and an impression that psychology is inherently not unifiable (see Koch, 1981). That, of course, is and has been the state of psychology, as it involves hundreds of separated and usually competitive theories, large and small.

Granting that it is impossible for any one person to have an intimate grasp of everything in psychology, is there any way to make feasible the task of dealing with the various levels in constructing a general theory? Let me answer that by referring to psychological behaviorism, which, in its decades of development, has embodied another methodology, which may be called "framework theory" (Staats, 1981, 1988, 1993a). In brief description, the framework theory recognizes that it is not be possible for one theorist to construct a theory that will deal in detail with the various elements of knowledge in the various levels of study in psychology. But framework theory does not achieve simplification by means of omitting from consideration some fields of study. Rather, the approach is that it is important to address the nature of the task and its great complexity. The various major levels of study must be dealt with, analyzed with respect to the phenomena that characterize them, with respect to the goals of study of each level, and with respect to the nature of the whole. The methods of each level require characterization, in order to see their relationship to the methods of the other levels. The concepts, principles, and major findings of each level require that same consideration.

The original strategy of PB involved the concept of a dimension of progress, going from the basic to the more advanced (complex) phenomena. Phenomena were selected to be analyzed and studied within the principles and concepts of the basic principles. As this simple-to-complex strategy unfolded in successive works, I progressively realized that a general method was involved. I saw that levels of study could not be rejected in the interests of simplification. Rather, each level had to be confronted, not comprehensively, at least at first, but by sampling problems at that level. Thus, PB included studies and made analyses in each of the major levels of study. And, in each case that created a framework theory (see Staats, 1963a, 1975), not by rejection of knowledge without due process, but by dealing with psychology's complexity in a sampling manner, not all at once. The *framework theory methodology* involves constructing a theoretical *skeleton*, an open and developing theory. This includes the major fields. Some features (concepts, principles, findings) are included in the theory for a level. The aim is to sample the elements in a systematic way, first dealing with some of the fundamentally significant elements in each field for the purpose of constructing a unified, preliminary theory of the field. The goal is to demonstrate the framework theory's relevance for the field, to show that the theory should be extended more broadly (and deeply), ultimately to confront all the elements in each field. The whole framework theory of PB, then, is composed of the conception that overarches the several framework theories in the fields (levels) (see Staats, 1963a, 1975, 1988).

In psychology there is a huge amount of material produced in each field. Not all of it is of the same significance, so there is a large task of simplification, of rendering the complexity into a manageable conception. It is necessary in each complex field to pick and choose (and reject) and reconstitute elements, as well as to generate necessary elements, by which to construct a framework theory of the field. The framework theory needs to represent the essence of the level of study in each case, in order to establish the role of that level in constructing the overarching theory. Thus, in the field of animal learning there are thousands of experiments. The basic principles that can be employed in the multilevel structure have to be selected and formulated, in relation to the two aims of (1) constructing a theory for the level itself; and (2) constructing a theory that is to serve in the multilevel overarching theory.

The overarching framework theory is thus different from traditional grand theory, which is detailed in a specialized field, but undeveloped in other fields. The framework theory is more evenly developed at each of its levels. Each framework theory for a level must be a "summary" theory, a skeleton, an incomplete theory—as is the whole that is composed of the level theories. But this is done by systematic design, retaining classic theory goals. Everything in the framework theory must be made consistent with the basic principles. But those principles are elaborated as the theory task advances through the materials in the various levels treated. The framework theory is a true theory, operationally connected to the phenomena studied—and the theory in each field must show its heuristic properties for generating theory, method, and findings. The framework theory is different from the classic behaviorist theories of the second generation. These two-level theories were developed in detail at the animal learning level of study, and not developed much or at all in any of the other fields of psychology. We can see this in Skinner's theory. Psychological behaviorism, on the other hand, has a much less detailed basic theory development than does Skinner (1938; Ferster & Skinner, 1957). But PB has empirical and methodological development at each of its levels of study and is heuristic at each level.

Demand for Progressive Detail

The framework theory methodology explicitly recognizes its incompleteness, in contrast to the part-to-whole method, which hides incompleteness by rejecting that which it cannot treat. Essentially, if a theory is a framework it must be filled in. That means the program must be a systematic, long-term, continuing effort, involving many people. That recognition is one of the strengths of the framework theory, because it can be clear just how much development it needs. One dimension of progress, thus, is in multiplying the number of analyses of phenomena in each particular level of study. Another dimension is in including additional fields.

Another dimension of development concerns the movement from the simple to the complex. For example, while at the beginning of the modern behavioral development it was important to analyze simple symptoms as learned behaviors that could be replaced by more desirable behaviors (see Ayllon & Michael, 1959; Staats, 1957a), progress involves making analyses of more and more complex forms of behavior disorder. As another example, while it is significant and useful to show that the self-care behaviors of schizophrenics can be trained using reinforcement (Atthowe & Krasner, 1968), that must be considered a beginning step. Ultimately it is necessary to progress to an analysis and understanding of schizophrenia, how it is acquired, how the schizophrenic person is different from those not schizophrenic, and how this condition can be prevented and treated. That, of course, calls for a complex program of study that will yield a more profound understanding of the phenomena.

Let me add that the PB approach also involves progress in making finer and finer (more detailed) analysis of that which is confronted. This feature is related to the specificity of the concepts and principles employed in the theory. The use of vague, general terms—like modeling, shaping, establishing stimulus, augmenting, stimulus equivalence, rule-governed behavior, the private event, symbolic modeling, and so on—constitutes loose theory. Vagueness is characteristic of cognitive social learning theory, contextualism, and other theories that address human behavior (such as those in behavior therapy and behavior analysis). Psychological behaviorism methodology requires that concepts and principles be capable of clear statement, and capable of clear empirical definition. In the case of any human behavioral phenomenon, PB asks for analysis of the behavior in specific terms. And then it is the task to explain that phenomenon explicitly in terms of the principles and concepts contained in the theory. When this is done, heuristic empirical and theoretical projections are to be expected—in contrast to the case where the analysis is vague, or the concepts and principles used are vaguely specified empirically.

BRIDGING THEORY: VARIOUS SIZES, FORMS, AND USES

It has been suggested by various philosophers of science that the scientific disciplines have an order from basic to less basic. Physics is considered basic to chemistry, chemistry to biology, and biology to psychology (see Popper, 1972, p. 294). In some cases intervening disciplines have developed, like biochemistry, that establish bridges between disciplines (Darden & Maull, 1977).

The notion that psychology's fields are related emerged from PB's program of first studying simple behaviors and then moving on to the study of more complex behaviors (see Staats, 1963a, 1975, 1993a). Thus, for example, relatively simple samples of language behavior were first dealt with at the human learning level. Later those types of language were studied in the context of child development, and then these findings were applied to the study of personality, and then abnormal personality. It is suggested that the traditional fields of psychology, because they operate so autonomously, artificially break up the study of the natural phenomena of psychology. But the phenomena studied at the different levels are not fundamentally different and independent; moreover, the principles that apply at the basic level apply at the advanced levels. Adding principles through advancing levels does not vitiate the relevance of the more basic principles. This PB conception of psychology has general implications that are just beginning to be recognized (see Darden, 1993; Rappard, 1993).

Bridging Theory

The program of behaviorizing psychology that has been described may be seen as a program for constructing "bridging theory" (see Staats, 1983). Bridging theory and how to construct it needs specialized consideration, for a central aspect of science is seeing how different things are related to each other (see, for example, Feigl, 1970; Kuhn, 1977, p. 471). In a science with as much diversity as psychology, seeing underlying relationships among things that appear unrelated is perhaps the most needed skill.

Psychology requires the construction of bridging theory of various kinds, depending upon the task involved. For example, there are innumerable research areas whose studies need to be interrelated, first within groupings with other relevant studies. There are also research areas, considered to deal with unrelated phenomena, that bridging theory would prove to involve phenomena that are explained by common principles. There are theories that are considered separate and competitive that actually share common principles and concepts. Bridging theory is also needed to resolve psychology's schisms, such as the nature–nurture issue or the person-situation issue. Bridging theory must be formulated to indicate the complementarity of methods of study whose differences are the basis for separations. Thus, to a radical behaviorist the methods of longitudinal study and psychometrics are useless—while to psychologists in these fields the laboratory study of animal learning is irrelevant. In addition to these types (see Staats, 1991), bridging theory is also needed to connect the different fields (levels) of psychology to each other. The most general of bridging theory is required in composing an overarching theory. The framework theory of any level must connect to the framework theories of the adjacent levels and thus become part of the whole. Works to perform the unification of psychology's chaos of disorganization of all sizes and kinds are needed. It can be expected, as for other natural sciences, that the construction of theory bridges by which to interrelate phenomena will yield some of psychology's most important products.

THE PSYCHOLOGICAL BEHAVIORISM
THEORY STRUCTURE

Psychological behaviorism grew in its four decades of development from a beginning learning theory, with several applications to human behavior areas, to a large structure. Understanding what PB is calls for analyzing the constituents of this structure. First, there is the large overarching theory. It contains the sum total, and ties together the other developments in the theory. Second, the level theories themselves are framework theories that address the fields of psychology. These are interrelated by the overarching theory. Third, within each level theory there are subtheories that deal specifically with problem areas of psychology and behaviorism, and they are tied together by the level theories. The subtheories have differing ranges of generality. Some are more specific and may be considered analyses or minitheories. This applies to the PB analyses of such things as walking acquisition and toilet training (Staats, 1963a), or problem solving and learning to count (Staats, 1956, 1963a). Other analyses treat more general phenomena and are recognizable as formal theories, for example, the theories of language (Staats, 1968a) and emotion (Staats, 1975, Chap. 4; Staats & Eifert, 1990), in the human learning level; language development (Staats,

1971a,b), in the developmental psychology level; attitudes (see Staats, 1968b), in the social psychology level; reading (see Staats, 1975, Chap. 11), in educational psychology; intelligence (Staats, 1971a; Staats & Burns, 1981), in the personality level; and depression (Heiby & Staats, 1990; Staats & Heiby, 1985) and the anxiety disorders (Eifert, Evans, & McKendrick, 1990; Staats, 1975, Chap. 8; 1989), in the abnormal psychology level. Each theory is a framework that calls for more detailed analysis and for research.

Thus psychology as viewed through the PB lens consists of a broad range of many diverse phenomena. These phenomena need to be systematically studied. When this is done within a consistent framework of principles it is found that the phenomena can be grouped in a manner that shows their relationships. For example, walking acquisition, speech acquisition, toilet problems, reading acquisition, and writing acquisition constitute related phenomena, as can be seen when they are studied within a set of explanatory learning principles. The various fields of psychology already group phenomena, but do so as eclectic constituents that remain unrelated. When analyses within PB theory are made, however, the broad range of phenomena within a field can be treated with a smaller set of consistent principles and concepts. The result is great simplification (parsimony) as well as explanatory power.

When the phenomena within several fields have been subjected to analyses using common principles and concepts, then the relationships of the fields can be seen. As an example, there are phenomena that have been studied in the experimental psychology of language that are not employed when the phenomena of language acquisition have been traditionally studied in the field of child development. The multilevel theory methodology of PB recognizes such relationships and attempts to provide the necessary bridges.

When the several fields of psychology have been related, within a consistent set of principles and concepts, there is the basis for constructing the overarching theory. This description of the structure of PB is thus a prescription for theory construction in psychology. In PB the theory constituents are of varying sizes and at varying degrees of completion. There are also many empty spaces, of various sizes, that need to be filled in by theoretical, methodological, and empirical work. The framework theory may begin with one person, but the large and complex task demands the contributions of many—theoreticians, methodologists, basic and applied researchers, and philosophers. The task is large; for the framework is heuristic.

THE CENTRAL IMPORTANCE OF LEARNING

Progress in constructing this approach has revealed that it has characteristics that are different from those of orthodox radical behaviorism, traditional psychology, cognitivism, or cognitive social learning approaches. Some PB characteristics are methodological, some are empirical, and some are theoretical. One central example is that psychological behaviorism places basic *learning* theory in a focal position to a greater extent than in contemporary approaches, even behavioral approaches. There is a general belief, for example, that Skinner's behaviorism puts an extreme emphasis on learning (environmentalism). But Skinner never considered himself a learning theorist; his approach and his research emphasize the effects of the *present* environment on behavior, rather than the study of learning.

To illustrate, in the basic experimental analysis of behavior technology—so central to the approach—the animal is quickly trained to the response, such as pecking a key by a pigeon, or pressing a bar by a rat. The fact is the technology is designed to employ a response for which the learning is minimized; learning is not the topic of study. The study concerns how reinforcement variables affect the characteristics of the response, not how the response is acquired. As another example, Skinner's "learning" approach is frequently illustrated by reference to his "baby box." The general belief is that this box was a training device for infants. It was not. In actuality, the automated crib was for the purpose of maintaining easy, hygienic, and healthy physical care for the infant. There are very few analyses in Skinner's various works of children *learning* simple behavior, and none of the learning of complex behaviors. His *Verbal Behavior* (Skinner, 1957) illustrates this very well; certain categories of verbal behavior are described as operants. But there is little or no treatment of how, or under what conditions, those verbal operants might be learned. To illustrate, reading (texting) is described as verbal operants under the control of printed words. But Skinner never analyzed the process of learning to read—which turns out to be much more complex than the texting analysis. The field of behavior analysis has generally followed Skinner's lead in this respect, as in many others.

Psychological behaviorism, in contrast, from the beginning focused on the analysis of how complex human behavior is learned. Its whole thrust has been on composing a set of basic learning principles with which to analyze the progressively more complex types of human behavior treated. For example, when PB developed a behavioristic analysis of language behavior, the manner in which language is learned was focally treated (Staats, 1956, 1957a, 1963a, 1968a; Staats & Staats, 1957, 1958).

Radical behaviorists, when called upon to explain why individuals' behavior differs when in the same situation, fall back on the concept of the "conditioning (or learning) history" as an explanation. But that concept is left vague and unspecified (Wanchisen, 1990), because radical behaviorism has not provided the necessary learning foundation. It is not functional to say that differences in learning history determine individual differences in classroom learning, or anything else, unless that learning history is stipulated. For the concept of learning history to be explanatory the account must be explicit and have sufficient detail to serve as the basis for training or preventing the type of behavior involved. Only through detailed analysis can prediction and control of complex behavioral phenomena be obtained. And only this type of analysis provides avenues for further development, in both applications and research.

The PB position, as will be made clear, is quite different here—the study of the learning of behavior is raised to center stage. Psychological behaviorism states that it is necessary to analyze complex human behavior in a detailed manner, finer than is the contemporary radical behaviorism tradition. And PB also focuses on the *conditions* of learning, not only the general principles of conditioning. Only in this way is it possible to explain complex human behavior and the endless variations and individual differences that occur in human behavior.

THE CENTRAL IMPORTANCE OF PERSONALITY

One of the central schisms in psychology centers around personality. For one thing, the concept of personality is important in all of the traditional fields of psychology. As examples, in developmental psychology most psychologists are interested in personality development, in abnormal psychology in abnormal personality, in experimental psychology in various cognitive processes, in social psychology in attributions, attitudes, and self-esteem, and in clinical psychology in the treatment of personality disorders.

This notwithstanding, study and measurement of personality at the present time are conducted largely in isolation from the other fields of psychology. Psychoanalytic theory's approach to personality, for example, connects very little to such broad fields as experimental, child, educational, and social psychology. There is even less connection to psychology involved for the phenomenological personality theories of Carl Rogers, Abraham Maslow, and George Kelly. The radical behaviorism of Skinner establishes little relationship to psychology in general, and does not develop a theory of personality that does so. Julian Rotter (1954) set forth a social learning theory of personality derived from a Hullian-Tolmanian combination of behavior principles, but this also provides little bridging to the other fields of psychology, and there has not been further formulation to do so. The concept of self-efficacy (Bandura, 1977) is a social learning theory personality concept. But it is not a general theory of personality, and neither does it provide a foundation for connection to the various fields of psychology. Walter Mischel (1974, 1995) as well as Bandura (1978) have described general "person" events as determinants of behavior, but do not give specification regarding what those events are, how they are learned, or the principles and mechanisms by which they function. These approaches thus do not provide a foundation for connecting to the major fields of psychology.

As has been indicated, the fields of psychology operate largely as autonomous disciplines, disconnected and essentially irrelevant for each other. In the PB view personality theory should play a pivotal role in psychology in establishing the foundation for connections among the fields. For the personality theory provides one of the key bridges by which the study of basic principles—as in behaviorism—can be unified with the study of complex human behavior as it is of concern to the more advanced fields of study in traditional psychology. Thus, as an example, there is little connection between the study of language phenomena in experimental psychology, in the child's development in developmental psychology, in the phenomena of abnormal psychology, and in the clinical treatment of behavior disorders. However, when a basic theory of language learning is developed in the context of the child learning language, of individual differences in language (personality), and in how those differences in language determine individual differences in behavior, this yields a theoretical structure that makes connections among experimental psychology, developmental psychology, personality measurement, abnormal psychology, and clinical psychology.

For the large field of personality and personality measurement to be connected to the multifarious strivings of the mother psychology, a personality theory is needed that plays a pivotal bridging role. Very importantly, a primary reason that behaviorism has been isolated from traditional psychology has been because behaviorism generally rejects the concept of personality. Behaviorism, in doing so, makes itself a non-player in an area that is essential to psychology and the development of psychology.

COMPLEX BEHAVIOR REQUIRES A RICH SET OF PRINCIPLES

The model provided by the second-generation behaviorists was that a handful of conditioning principles would serve as the basic theory with which to explain human behavior generally (see Dollard & Miller, 1950; Skinner, 1953, 1957). But even a more complete set of conditioning principles really constitutes a very sparse set with which to undertake the task. Similarly, traditional psychology also takes an oversimplified approach to the various phenomena of complex human behavior. For example, various trait theorists have suggested that it will be possible to understand the various aspects of human behavior in terms of a small number of personality traits. John (1990) suggests that five traits will do the trick, as one example. In recent years success in treating certain psychological problems (like depression and anxiety) with drugs has led to the simple view that personality is determined by biochemical properties of the brain, which can be altered pharmacologically. Popular accounts suggest that "scientific insights into the brain . . . are raising the prospect of nothing less than made-to-order, off-the-shelf personalities. For good or ill, research that once mapped the frontiers of disease—identifying the brain chemistry involved in depression, paranoia and schizophrenia—is today closing in on the chemistry of normal personality" (Begley, 1994, p. 40). This simplistic approach, like that of sociobiology and others, would cut out all other levels of study in psychology.

These are all attempts to find a "cheap and easy" way of understanding and treating the complex subject matter of human behavior. The PB position is that such attempts will all fail, because their simplicity is disproportionate to the complexity of human behavior. Humans were constructed by evolution to be marvelous learning mechanisms (see Staats, 1971a). If that is the case it occurred because it was functional for humans to learn, that significant aspects of human behavior depend on learning. Learning is crucially important for humans because it is long term, cumulative, and very complex. Psychology must pay its dues in dealing with that complexity. What is not realized is that suggesting that human behavior comes about via brain structures denies the great importance of learning. Such approaches overlook the lesson that consideration of evolution provides. Human behavior can be considered in an adequate manner only by using a set of principles capable of dealing with complex learning—and that means a rich set of principles, not a handful.

CONCLUSION

Let me conclude by saying that there is a major shift in theory-construction methodology from traditional approaches to the multilevel construction approach to be developed here. With respect to human behavior there is no easy way to be found. The study of human behavior is complex, and it is not possible to restrict study to one phenomenon, one problem area, one field, or one small set of concepts and principles. There is no one level that can be studied alone to yield a full, explanatory theory of complex human behavior whose eventual purview is the broad field of psychology. The PB approach to constructing a theory of human behavior involves a systematic program; building from the basic learning level of study, through the human learning/cognitive, developmental, and social levels, to the personality and personality measurement levels of study. And the theory goes on to connect to the abnormal and clinical psychology levels of study. A behavioral

CHAPTER 2

The Basic Learning/Behavior Theory

Psychological behaviorism considers the principles of learning as basic in the acquisition of complex human behavior. The experimental psychology of learning-behavior is thus the basic field of study for PB. But that field did not arise in the context that is being proposed, that is, to provide a basic theory level for a general, overarching theory approach to psychology. The study of animal learning-behavior principles arose as an autonomous field, and generated its own goals, interests, and problem areas. Having gone on for almost a century the field has created a huge mass of empirical, methodological, technological, and theoretical products. This mass of material is too large, complex, and disorganized to serve as the foundation for a human behavior theory. It contains much that is irrelevant, and it *lacks* much that is needed. The theorist who wishes to compose a theory of human behavior based on conditioning principles has the task of first composing a basic learning theory for that purpose—because that is not done by the animal conditioning specialist. This task means sifting the grains of knowledge that have been produced in the field of animal learning, in order to abstract those principles that have central utility for the larger task. If too few principles are abstracted, then the theory is impoverished and cannot provide an adequate foundation, as with Dollard and Miller (1950), Skinner (1953), and Wolpe (1958). On the other hand, the major behaviorism theories—for example, the theories of Hull (1943) and of Skinner (see Ferster & Skinner, 1957; Skinner, 1938)—are specialized treatments addressed to animal study. Besides lacking crucial developments, they contain much irrelevant material and thus are too complex and cumbersome. Formulating a set of basic principles for use in constructing a theory of human behavior is a theory task of deleting irrelevancies, abstracting relevant parts, adding needed developments, and formulating the lot into a consistent theory framework. The human perspective is needed to guide the theory-construction task, as not realized in the first two generations.

This chapter presents a basic learning theory whose foundation lies in animal conditioning research. Even in terms of the basic principles, however, the theory has been constructed differently than were the second-generation theories. Although it is based in the first two generations of animal research on the basic principles, its perspective is human behavior. Its statement of principles has been formulated to be used in analyzing human behavior, not just for organizing the animal literature. Its central aim is to compose a nucleus of principles that can be elaborated for the detailed study of specific areas in *both* animal and human behavior. For that reason it does not address issues that are solely of concern in animal learning theory (such as radical behaviorism's excessive detail in the study of reinforcement schedules). Moreover, principles important at the human level are developed that have not been considered important at the animal level and are not present in radical behaviorism.

THE FIRST GENERATION OF BEHAVIORISM

Learning phenomena can be observed on the naturalistic level, and philosophies have included principles of learning. The philosophical methodology, however, can not provide the precise and detailed study of the principles of conditioning. But the philosophical analyses did provide the context that gave significance to two accidental discoveries in the laboratory that constituted the birth of behaviorism.

One involved the discovery by Ivan Pavlov of the principle of classical conditioning (later called respondent conditioning by Skinner). Pavlov, a Russian Nobel-prize-winning physiologist, was studying the salivary reflex. A food substance was placed in a dog's mouth and the animal automatically salivated. Pavlov later accidentally discovered that an irrelevant (non-food) stimulus, which happened to be occur just prior to the animal's receipt of the food, came also to elicit the salivary response. Things "associated" (the philosophical term) with a food stimulus would come to elicit the same response as the food stimulus itself. Pavlov studied various aspects and variations of this principle. Others studied the principles with different species, different kinds of responses (various physiological responses of internal organs), and different variations. This framework produced a huge number of studies (and still does).

Edward Thorndike, also around the turn of the century, discovered the principle of instrumental conditioning (later called operant conditioning by Skinner), the other empirical foundation of behaviorism. The principle is that motor behaviors that are followed by certain stimuli are strengthened. Such stimuli were called *satisfiers* by Thorndike, are now called *reinforcers* (of behavior), and in contemporary life are called *rewards*. (Philosophers had used related terms like satisfaction, pleasure, desire, appetite, feeling, sentiment, happiness, and good.) Like Pavlov, Thorndike himself conducted a number of studies of the principles of operant conditioning, as did many others, with various species, various responses, and variations of the various conditions involved. Different types of apparatus were constructed for this study, such as the T-Maze, straight runway, and Skinner's operant conditioning chamber that, with automation and recording, is called the experimental analysis of behavior technology.

THE SECOND GENERATION OF BEHAVIORISM

This first generation of behaviorism was momentous in establishing laboratory means for studying and specifying the two basic principles of conditioning. It was a heady prospect that psychology could be a hard, laboratory science and study the evanescent phenomena of behavior. The second-generation behaviorists (such as Tolman, Hull, and Skinner) all had the same context—that is, the philosophy of science and theory of Watson and the experimental studies and theories of the other first-generation behaviorists. The second generation concentrated on the animal laboratory as the means of establishing their theories. Each major behaviorist attempted to improve upon the experimental procedures, the experimental designs, and the theory statements that had been developed in the first generation. The goal of each was to produce *the* basic learning or behavior theory that was in the best scientific tradition and would be general for all of behavior, all of psychology. This led to the age of grand theory (Koch, 1981).

Competition among the theories was the focus of the second generation. As a consequence, behaviorism, by not abstracting its considerable consensual knowledge, presented a confusing and weak approach for other psychologists to use, as can be seen in the textbook treatments (Hilgard, 1948).

Emotion and Behavior: The Unresolved Relationship

In addition to these features, the classic learning theories had other weaknesses and errors. For example, there were various issues on which the second-generation behaviorisms differed that were not resolved. One very major issue arose because of the two research traditions established by Pavlov and Thorndike, each of which contained many studies. Although quite separate, both traditions dealt with how the environment affects the organism's behavior. The question arose whether there were one or two types of conditioning. Guthrie's (1935) solution was that there was only one kind of conditioning, that which involves association (classical conditioning). Hull (1943) took the position that there was only one kind of conditioning, that involving reinforcement (operant conditioning). Both were one-factor theories. Skinner's (1938) position was that there were two types of response. There was emotional responding, considered as an inferior type of responding, involving glands and smooth muscles, and taking place through the autonomic nervous system. (One of the problems resides in this definition of the emotional response.) This responding is reflexive and slow and unprecise. Emotional responding to a new stimulus is learned through contiguity (association) in a process he renamed respondent conditioning instead of classical conditioning.

There was also motor responding, which involves the striated skeletal muscles, and which takes place via the central nervous system. This type of responding was considered quick, precise, and of the type that is generally called voluntary, rather than reflexive. Skinner renamed these responses operants. Speech responses were also considered operants (Skinner, 1957). Operant behavior was learned via the principle of reinforcement. When an operant was followed by a reinforcing stimulus, the response was strengthened.

Skinner described these two basic types of conditioning, but he did not consider them of equal importance. In his view it was behavior that counted, which meant motor behavior. Emotional responses were really irrelevant; they were only collateral events, epiphenomena, which "have no explanatory force" with respect to behavior and operant conditioning (Skinner, 1975, p. 43). Since emotion did not affect the individual's (or animal's) behavior, classical conditioning, was something to be noted but disregarded. (His original conception of emotion [Skinner, 1938] was really vague, as will be indicated.) Thus, Skinner did not study classical conditioning, or construct methods for doing so, and did not set a foundation or program for those who followed his approach to study emotion, how it is learned, or its effects on human behavior. There is no basis in Skinner's approach for appreciating and studying the vast importance of classical conditioning and emotion for human behavior, or how emotion is learned in uniquely human ways. Contemporary radical behaviorists, who are just now becoming interested in such topics, have had to draw their interests from other sources. Thus, Skinner took a "two-factor learning" approach, that there are two types of conditioning, but that they are unrelated (Skinner, 1975).

THE PB THEORY OF LEARNING AND THE BASIC THREE-FUNCTION PRINCIPLES

One of the primary problems in the second generation of behaviorism concerns whether there are two types of conditioning and whether they are related—centrally whether emotion affects behavior. The heart of PB's basic learning theory provides a resolution of the question of whether there are two types of conditioning and, if so, how the two types are related. The position taken is quite opposite that taken by Skinner.

Emotion Fundamental: The Emotion-Reinforcer Relationship

To begin, let us first deal with definition. Skinner defines a reinforcing stimulus by its effect upon the strength (rate) of behavior. A response that is followed by a reinforcing stimulus is strengthened. This definition has been criticized as circular, because the reinforcing stimulus does not have a definition independent of its effect.

The PB three-function learning theory, in contrast, defines the reinforcing stimulus fundamentally, in terms of its elicitation of an *emotional response*. It is stimuli that elicit a positive emotional response that will also strengthen the behaviors they follow and thus serve as positive reinforcers. Reinforcers are thus defined independently of their effect on behavior. The stronger the emotional response elicited by the stimulus, the stronger that stimulus will be capable of serving as a reinforcer. The same principles apply on the negative side; there are also stimuli that elicit negative emotional responses. Such stimuli will serve as negative reinforcers (in the present terminology); that is, they will weaken the behaviors they follow.

It is the emotion-eliciting power of the stimulus that defines its reinforcing power. Definition of reinforcement power by emotion-eliciting power is fundamental and suggests various lines of inquiry. One is that unlearned emotional responses are reflex responses, built into the organism's biological structure. On a primary level that applies also to the emotion–reinforcer relationship. This has been built into organisms through biological (evolutionary) development (Staats, 1963a, 1975). Emotional responses are elicited by stimuli that are biologically important to the organism—either to obtain, like food, or to avoid, like painful stimuli. It is thus biologically important that those same stimuli will also act as reinforcers and affect the organism's behavior. That is the essential *behavioral* reason why emotions are important, because they define what will be reinforcing for the organism in the sense of affecting what behaviors the organism will acquire. Relating the emotion-eliciting value of a stimulus to its reinforcing value is basic in relating classical and operant conditioning and emotional responding and motor responding.

It was an anomaly that classical conditioning and operant conditioning could have been considered to be separate and unrelated when the same stimuli are involved in each case. Food was used by Pavlov to elicit a salivary response in classical conditioning. And food was used by Thorndike to reinforce the animal's behavior of escaping from a box. The one stimulus, thus, *functions* behaviorally in two different ways. This fundamental fact must be confronted in composing a learning theory and underlies the PB conception of the *functions* of a stimulus. The PB conception is that a stimulus can have multiple functions.

By way of example, we know that an emotion-eliciting stimulus can function to produce classical conditioning. That is, if we present a neutral stimulus along with a stimulus that already elicits an emotional response, then the neutral stimulus will also come to elicit the emotional response. So one function a stimulus can have is to elicit an emotional response which allows it to operate in classical conditioning, where it transfers this function to another stimulus. In addition, however, an emotional stimulus has a second function. It can serve as a reinforcing stimulus. When presented *after* a motor response it can strengthen or weaken that motor response (depending on whether it is a positive or negative emotional stimulus). The same stimulus thus has two functions.

The Emotion–Incentive Relationship

Emotion-eliciting stimuli are also important behaviorally because they have another, third, function. A stimulus that elicits a positive emotional response, and that can serve as a reinforcer *when presented contingent upon a behavior,* will also have an incentive function. That is, when a positive emotional stimulus appears (*is presented*), the organism will approach the stimulus. The stimulus, thus, has an eliciting function. It elicits approach behavior.

A stimulus, on the other hand, that elicits a negative emotional response, and that can serve as a reinforcer, will also have a negative incentive function. That is, the stimulus will elicit behaviors that escape from and avoid that stimulus. It is important that incentive (or *directive*) power be distinguished from reinforcing power. In reinforcement, the stimulus is presented following any motor behavior, and has a strengthening effect on the behavior for future occasions. The incentive function, in contrast, occurs when the stimulus is presented first and it then elicits or brings on a particular behavior in that situation.

The present theory states, thus, that stimuli that involve elicitation of an emotional response have three functions: (1) They elicit the emotional response, which is one function; (2) such stimuli can act as reinforcers when presented contingent on a behavior; and (3) such stimuli will act as directive (incentive) stimuli—in the positive case when presented they will attract approach behavior, and in the negative case they will bring on escape and avoidance behavior. These are the basic principles of the PB *three-function learning theory*, which will be elaborated in the following sections.

Biological Definition of Emotional/Reinforcing Stimuli

The fact that emotion-eliciting stimuli have reinforcing properties has been described as biologically based. Some stimuli will elicit an emotional response without prior learning, simply on the basis of the organism's biological structure. Food stimuli elicit a positive emotional response, for example, as do the tactual stimuli that caressingly contact the erogenous zones of the body. These different types of stimuli elicit different responses that have been considered to be emotional in nature, such as salivation in the one case, and tumescence in the other. How can both types of stimuli be considered in the same terms, as positive emotional stimuli? In the present view there is a central nervous system response to all positive emotional stimuli (see Staats, 1975, chap. 4; Staats & Eifert, 1990) as well as specific peripheral responses. Responses such as salivation and tumescence are a peripheral *part* of the *whole* emotional response. The peripheral emotional responses vary depending upon the type of stimuli involved, such as food or sexual stimulation. However, in each case there is a *common* central (brain) response. Because all positive emotional stimuli activate the emotion centers of the brain, all positive emotional stimuli have the same functions described in the three-function theory. The same is true for negative emotional stimuli. Although a painfully bright light and a painfully loud noise elicit different peripheral responses, they also share a common negative brain response and thus they have similar effects with respect to the three learning functions (see Staats, 1975, chap. 4; Staats & Eifert, 1990). Skinner's (1938, 1975) analysis thus is awry in its definition of the emotional response. That definition only addresses the peripheral responses— the responses of the smooth muscles and glands in the body. This has been a common error in psychology, as will be discussed later. A recent theory of emotion (Lang, 1995) is supportive in that it also dichotomizes emotions into positive and negative, including elaboration of the brain mechanisms involved. Lang's theory also supports other principles in the PB theory.

In the present context, in any event, stimuli that elicit an emotional response on a biological level—without prior learning—will also have reinforcement power. Without learning, an electric shock will decrease the strength of any behavior it follows. Without learning, food will increase the strength of any behavior it follows. Whether or not a stimulus elicits a central emotional response in the organism, without prior learning, determines whether or not the stimulus can function as a reinforcer without prior learning.

Three-Function (A–R–D) Learning Principles

So far I have said that some stimuli elicit an emotional response in the organism without learning, and that such stimuli will hence also be capable of functioning as reinforcers. Let me now add that these important functions of stimuli can also be learned. This is centrally important. For the number of primary biologically determined emotional/reinforcing stimuli is limited. The number that can *become* such stimuli, however, is limitless. And this is very important in understanding human behavior. It is appropriate, now, to consider in a little more detail the two types of learning that have been described, that is, classical conditioning and operant conditioning.

Classical Conditioning

Any stimulus can become an emotion-eliciting stimulus. All that has to occur is that such a neutral stimulus be paired with a stimulus that does elicit an emotional response. The contiguity of the two stimuli, over some number of trials, will produce that result. The stimulus that originally elicits the emotional response is called the unconditioned stimulus (^{UC}S). Pavlov used food powder as a ^{UC}S. The stimulus that comes to elicit the emotional response is called the conditioned stimulus (^{C}S). Pavlov is supposed to have used an auditory stimulus, a bell, as the ^{C}S. Research has shown that this principle functions very widely through the animal kingdom, with humans as well as lower species.

Many peripheral emotional responses have been conditioned such as heart rate, salivation, blood volume, vasoconstriction and vasodilation, and sweat gland and other glandular activity. These responses are peripheral in nature. It should be emphasized that it is the central emotional response that is focal in the present analysis. The peripheral responses are valuable as indices of classical conditioning in laboratory study, but the several behavioral functions of stimuli depend on the central emotional response the stimuli elicit. Classical conditioning is schematized in Figure 2.1.

Instrumental (Operant) Conditioning

When I described this type of conditioning at the beginning of this chapter, I employed Skinner's definition—that the reinforcement simply strengthens the response. That definition is too simple. Actually, when a positive reinforcer is contingent upon a particular motor response, the motor response is not strengthened in and of itself. When a rat has been reinforced for pressing a bar in an operant conditioning chamber, it does not continue to make the bar-pressing response when it is put back in its home cage where there is no bar. What the animal has learned through the conditioning is to make a particular (bar-pressing) response in the presence of

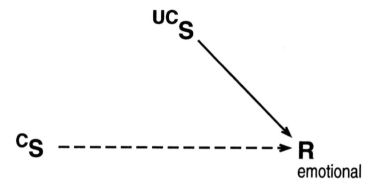

FIGURE 2.1 The classical conditioning of an emotional response (R). The ^{UC}S is a stimulus that already elicits the emotional response. The ^{C}S is a stimulus that at first does not. When the two stimuli occur together in time, the ^{C}S comes to elicit the emotional response.

particular stimuli. Responses are not somehow strengthened irrespective of some controlling (eliciting) stimulus. It would be very maladaptive if responses were independently strengthened in and of themselves.

Thus, the organism actually learns to make a response, or not to make a response, *in the situation* in which the response is or is not followed by the reinforcing stimulus. Responses are always stimulus-controlled. In the present terminology the situation (or some aspect of it) may be called the directive stimulus (^{D}S), the response (R) is the motor response, and the reinforcing stimulus can be labeled as ^{R}S, as Figure 2.2 indicates. Operant conditioning in the PB theory involves the organism learning to make a response to a stimulus, because the response is reinforced in the presence of that stimulus.

Positive and Negative Reinforcers

There are only two types of fundamental emotional response, positive and negative. (The many emotions popularly defined, as will be indicated later,

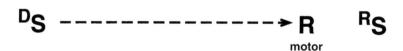

FIGURE 2.2 The operant conditioning of a motor response (R). In a particular stimulus situation (^{D}S) if a motor response occurs and is followed by a positive reinforcing stimulus (^{R}S) the stimulus situation will more strongly call out that response in the future.

differ on other secondary conditions.) And there are only two types of reinforcers, positive and negative, corresponding to positive and negative emotional responses. However, each type of reinforcer can work in two ways. That is, a reinforcing stimulus can be presented following a behavior. Or, if the reinforcing stimulus is already present, it can be withdrawn.

A positive reinforcing stimulus if presented after a motor behavior will strengthen that behavior (or maintain its strength if it is already strong). In addition, however, when a positive reinforcer that the organism already has is taken away following a motor response, this consequence (or contingency) will weaken that motor response. Thus, a positive reinforcer can be used either to strengthen or weaken behavior.

Negative reinforcers also can work in two ways. If the negative reinforcer is presented following a behavior, this will weaken that behavior in that situation. Conversely, if the organism is experiencing a negative reinforcer (such as a loud noise), and that stimulus is removed following a motor response, that response will be strengthened in that situation. That is how we learn to put our hands over our ears when a loud noise occurs, because doing so removes (actually attenuates) the noise.

Conditioned Reinforcers

One of the fundamental principles of the three-function learning theory is that a stimulus that elicits an emotional response will also be a reinforcing stimulus if applied in a response-contingent manner. It is important to understand that this pertains to conditioned stimuli as well as unconditioned stimuli. Any stimulus, on a learned or unlearned basis, that elicits an emotional response can serve as a reinforcer. Thus, when Pavlov's dog learned an emotional response to the bell, the present theory would state that the bell as a result became a potential reinforcing stimulus. If Pavlov had presented the bell contingent upon some movement of the animal, the dog would have learned that movement.

Not knowing the principle involved, Pavlov did not study this possibility. It is interesting to note, moreover, that the principle has not been studied in animal research in the systematic way that is called for. One animal study will be used in describing the principle, although it was conducted in the framework of another theory, and thus is given a different analysis. Zimmerman (1957) used rats as subjects. He presented a buzzer (the ^CS) and then gave the animals access to food (the ^{UC}S), a number of times. In the present view, as a consequence of this classical conditioning, the buzzer came to elicit a positive emotional response and, hence, to be a potential positive reinforcing stimulus. The next part of his experiment tested whether the buzzer was a reinforcer. That is, Zimmerman put the rat into a chamber that had a bar. Each time the animal pressed the bar, this was followed by the sound of the buzzer. If the buzzer was a positive reinforcing stimulus the animal should learn to press the bar, which is what happened. The animals made the response many times, when the response was followed by the buzzer. This study, as fundamental as it is when viewed in terms of the three-function learning theory, was not presented as, or recognized as, the classic study it actually is, for showing the interaction of the two types of conditioning.

Let me add that this analysis indicates that in the process of classical conditioning a stimulus is formed that is important for the operant conditioning of behavior. After all, what stimuli will be reinforcing for the individual will be a determinant of the behaviors that are later learned. Rats not exposed to Zimmerman's pairing of the buzzer and food would not learn a response because it was followed by the buzzer. What stimuli are reinforcing is a very important topic in human behavior, as we will see.

There is a similar circumstance in the study of operant conditioning. When a reinforcing stimulus such as food is presented following a response, the interest is on the extent to which the response is strengthened. What is not ordinarily considered is that the reinforcing stimulus also elicits an emotional response (including salivation), which will be conditioned to the stimuli in the situation. This classical conditioning, however, is ignored generally by those who study operant conditioning. Because they do not make a complete analysis, however, they lack the necessary principles by which to analyze many types of human behavior that appear to involve operant conditioning but that also involve classical conditioning of emotion.

This lack of study of classical conditioning in operant conditioning and of operant events in classical conditioning results from separation of the two traditions of conditioning. Let me thus indicate that in Figure 2.2 only the reinforcing function of the ^RS is depicted in the figure. It is the case, it should be noted, that the reinforcing stimulus is also a ^{UC}S; that is, the stimulus also elicits an emotional response. That emotional response will be conditioned to the stimulus situation, the ^DS.

Emotion-Controlled Instrumental Behavior: The Directive (Incentive) Stimulus

I have already generally described the principle that if a stimulus elicits an emotional response, in addition to being a reinforcer, the stimulus will also serve as a directive (incentive) stimulus to elicit either approach or avoidance behavior. This involves a very central part of the PB learning theory, and some additional specification is necessary. To begin, the relationship between emotion elicitation and reinforcing value of stimuli is determined by biology. So a stimulus that elicits an emotional response also will be a reinforcing stimulus. But the third function—that stimuli that elicit an emotional response will also elicit approach or avoidance behavior—is not built into the organism; it is learned. And the learning is a bit complicated, which calls for explication.

When a stimulus elicits a positive emotional response, if the organism happens to approach it, the organism will be reinforced by contact with the stimulus. We can see this with food, water, and sexual stimuli. To illustrate, suppose that the sight of an apple on a table elicits a positive emotional response in the hungry child. It is also the case that approaching, grasping, and biting the apple will yield reinforcement for the child.

Such experience is ubiquitous, and it produces two types of learning, one specific and one very general and important. Let us take the example of the child and the apple. Having been reinforced by contact with the apple, the child will have learned to approach the apple. This learning is specific—the child has learned a specific response to a specific stimulus. In addition, however, the emotion the child experiences on seeing the apple constitutes a stimulus. (Emotional responses, in fact most responses, have or produce stimulus properties.) When the child is reinforced for approaching the apple, the child is also being reinforced for approaching a stimulus that elicits a positive emotional response. Through this experience the child will learn an association between the stimulus of the positive emotional response and an approach behavior, as indicated in Figure 2.3.

It must be remembered that organisms, including humans, will have countless experiences in which approaching something that elicits a positive emotional response (stimulus) will be followed by positive reinforcement. As a consequence this association between the internal stimulus of a positive emotion and an approach response will become very well learned. Anything that elicits a positive emotional response will automatically tend to elicit approach behavior—*the stronger the emotional response, the stronger elicitation of the behavior.*

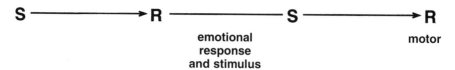

S ——————▶ **R** ——————— **S** ——————▶ **R**
                           emotional   **motor**
                           response
                       and stimulus

FIGURE 2.3   This drawing depicts how a stimulus can elicit an emotional response (R) which produces an internal stimulus that in turn elicits a motor response (R) in the subject. The individual learns approach motor responses to stimuli that elicit a positive emotional response and avoidance motor responses to stimuli that elicit a negative emotional response.

Once firmly learned this is a mechanism *that will generalize to any stimulus that elicits a positive emotional response*. That is, having learned to approach stimuli that elicit a positive emotional response, the organism will tend to approach any new stimulus that elicits a positive emotional response—even though the organism has not been reinforced for approaching that stimulus. For example, if someone names and describes a new movie to us in terms that elicit a positive emotional response in us, we will learn a positive emotional response to the movie's name. Because the movie now elicits a positive emotional response in us we will be likely to attend (approach) a theater showing that movie, although we have never in the past been reinforced for doing so. This general mechanism is enormously adaptive; it enables humans to respond without learning trials, in an anticipatory manner, to many things. Such anticipatory behavior makes traditional psychologists unable to accept that humans only *learn* their behaviors—and in one sense they are right. What is necessary, of course, is to explain how learning has been involved.

This account must be expanded in several ways. First, there are a wide number of different *approach* responses the individual will learn to emotion-eliciting stimuli—to walk toward, to reach for, to ask (for in many ways), to swim toward, to run toward, to go around obstacles for, to work for, to plead for, to do nice things for, and so on. Any stimulus that elicits a positive emotional response will, as a consequence, have tendencies to elicit this very large class of approach behaviors. It should be noted that the particular response that is called out by the positive emotional stimulus will be determined by the other features of the stimulus situation. As an example, whether the young man will walk or swim toward a young woman acquaintance who elicits a positive emotional response in him will depend on whether there is a stretch of land surface between them or a body of water.

The same things are true for the negative emotional response. We learn a large number of behaviors that have the effect of escaping and avoiding stimuli that elicit negative emotional responses in us. Any stimulus that elicits a negative emotional response will tend to elicit that class of responses, including walking away from, running away from, swimming away from, crawling away from, requesting removal of the stimulus, and so on. It also includes such responses as driving another person away by threatening, menacing, insulting, hitting, disagreeing with, voting against, telling negative stories about, and so on. With positive as well as negative emotional responses, both the class of approach behaviors and that of avoidance behaviors will include verbal responses as well as motor responses.

The important thing is that much human behavior can be described as either approach or avoidance behavior, under the control of the extent that the stimulus situation involved elicits a positive or a negative emotional response. This makes emotions and classical conditioning so important, for emotions widely govern human behavior and account for individual differences in behavior, as we will see. It may be noted here that the principles involved help explain the purposive, goal-directed nature of human behavior.

Research Stipulation of the Three Functions

The three-function learning principles are very well supported by various studies in animal learning and human learning. However, many of the studies have been conducted within the aegis of other theories. As a consequence the research has not always been as pointed as could be, and there are implications of three-function learning theory that still have not been empirically investigated.

Human Research

Research done within PB, however, has explicitly investigated the three-function learning principles. For example, Staats, Staats, and Crawford (1962) showed that an emotional response could be classically conditioned to a word stimulus and this has been replicated in later studies (Maltzman, Raskin, Gould, & Johnson, 1965; Zanna, Kiesler, & Pilkonis, 1970). And other PB studies (see Staats & Staats, 1958, 1959) have shown that words that elicit an emotional response can transfer this function to other stimuli in a human type of classical conditioning. This has been verified and extended in a large number of studies (see Bugelski & Hersen, 1966; Carriero, 1967; Coleman, 1967; Harbin & Williams, 1966; Hekmat & Vanian, 1971; Leduc, 1980a, 1980b, 1984; Sachs & Byrne, 1970).

In the three-function learning theory, if a word stimulus elicits an emotional response then it should also have the reinforcing function. This expectation has been tested (Finley & Staats, 1967; Harms & Staats, 1978) showing with human subjects the principle that emotional stimuli are also reinforcing stimuli. Silverstein (1972) later tested this PB principle with ten-month- old infants. He paired a tone with a positive emotional stimulus. After this conditioning he showed that the tone could be used to reinforce a particular motor behavior. Finally, it has been shown that a word stimulus that elicits an emotional response will control approach behavior (Staats & Burns, 1982; Staats & Warren, 1974), demonstrating the third (directive) function of emotional stimuli.

It is necessary that the principles be studied in detail with human subjects as well as animal subjects, for in the three-function learning theory classical conditioning is centrally important. With people, classical conditioning determines in large part the multitudes of stimuli that will serve as emotion-eliciting stimuli, as reinforcers (rewards and punishments), and as directive (incentive) stimuli.

THE EVOLUTIONARY–BIOLOGICAL CHARACTER OF EMOTION

One of the reasons that Skinner's basic theory did not recognize the importance of emotion and classical conditioning with respect to behavior, in the present view, is that the theory lacked an evolutionary (biological) perspective. Skinner (1966) considered that there were two types of adaptation: one was evolutionary and the other was through operant conditioning. The PB view (Staats, 1963a) was that organisms had evolved to operate according to the principles of classical and operant conditioning. When an evolutionary perspective is taken, questions arise with respect to Skinner's theory that emotion has no effect on behavior. Why, if this type of responding had no significance for the organism's adjustment (behavior), would organisms be constructed such that their emotional responding *was experienced* and also that they could learn those responses to so many different stimuli? After all, emotional responding is retained in evolution throughout the higher forms of life, over a variety of organisms. Moreover, there is considerable biological apparatus involved in the learning and experiencing of emotions. Why would such an apparatus be developed and retained if it had no behavioral (adaptive, including procreative) significance?

Paradigmatic behaviorism's basic learning theory, in contrast to Skinner's theory, puts classical conditioning and emotions into a biological framework. The theory states that organisms are constructed in such a way that emotions can be learned to many stimuli because emotions have great adaptive significance for the organism's behavior. To illustrate, when a young deer learns an emotional response to the scent of a mountain lion, on being prodded by the mother to take flight, the young deer learns a negative emotional response to that smell. And the young deer also learns flight behavior under the control of the stimulus properties of that emotion. Any stimulus that elicits that emotion in that young deer will elicit flight behavior. The behavioral mechanism is generally adaptive.

The Experience of Emotion: Central Not Collateral

Skinner (1975) accepted that emotional responses create feelings, are experienced, but he maintained that feelings have no behavioral significance. Again, it is necessary to analyze the evolutionary–biological significance of the *experience* of emotion. That analysis indicates why the experience of emotion provides the mechanism by which emotion affects operant behavior. Let me follow the question asked in the above section and ask further why emotions should have sensitive and very differentiated stimulus properties. If emotions indeed served only physiological functions, as in the way that pain stimuli prepare the organism for strenuous physical activity, this could be done automatically, without the accompaniment of the extra stimuli involved in *experiencing* the fear. There are many internal actions of organs that take place automatically, "quietly and unnoticed," that is, without producing stimuli (experience). We do not experience our changes in blood pressure, heart rate, digestion, the action of the salivary and other glands, and a host of other physiological responses. In the present view, when organisms *experience* physiological states it is because "experiencing" them is important in a behavioral (adaptive) sense.

Definitionally, it is the present position that, when an emotion is experienced—"felt"—that means that the response involved also produces a stimulus. It is that stimulus-producing function of stimuli that provides the mechanism by which emotions can affect behavior. *The reason that internal emotional responses produce stimulus feelings is so the organism can learn motor responses to those emotional stimuli.* Then any stimulus that elicits an emotional response can thereby have effects on those motor responses. The role of experienced emotions is to mediate behaviors that have been operantly conditioned to those feelings. If the adaptive behavior to be elicited by the emotions was unlearned, as it must be in lower organisms (such as insects), then experienced emotional stimulation would not be necessary. A bee can react to intruders by a buzzing attack. This is a fixed response, however, so it would not be necessary that the bee's nervous system provide a means of *experiencing* an angry emotion. The process in such a simple nervous system must occur automatically, without learning. Experienced emotions are necessary only when emotional stimuli are there so that other responses can be learned to the stimuli, in the process of producing variability in behavior.

In the present theory, fear is an adaptive behavioral process in an evolutionary sense for two reasons. First, the individual can learn a fear response to many stimuli. And second, the individual can learn avoidance responses that are elicited by the experiential stimuli produced by fear. Those avoidance responses are learned because they reduce the fear stimuli—constituting reinforcement. But those avoidance responses enable the organism to escape contact with stimuli that would be harmful. The individual learns a repertoire of avoidance responses that are elicited by fear, and any stimulus that comes to elicit fear will elicit those avoidance responses.

This is an adjustive process, but that does not mean that every emotional response that is learned is adjustive. An example was just given of a deer that learned a negative emotional response to the scent of a lion, so that later such smells would induce running. But this learning may not always produce adaptive behavior. For example, let us say this young deer is standing quietly among some trees and underbrush when it smells a lion that is approaching but that is unaware of the deer. Let us say that since the deer is downwind, if it froze where it stood, the lion would pass by without noting the deer. However, the fear stimuli aroused by the smell may elicit the running response and consequent exposure to the lion and its attack. The evolutionary reason we feel our emotions is because, ordinarily, we learn behaviors to those feelings that enable us to behave in an adjustive manner to our environment. But circumstances can be such that the emotion, or the behavior the emotion elicits, is maladjustive. That may occur in humans, of course, where the learning of emotions or of the behaviors they mediate may be pathological.

In this context it is pertinent to mention that Beck (Beck, 1976; Beck & Emery, 1985) considers anxiety to be a residual of humans' evolutionary history, having protective value long ago, but being primarily maladaptive today. Beck's view arises without considering the present behavioral–evolutionary analysis of the role of emotion. In contrast, PB states that negative emotions are an adaptive part of human behavior, in the present as they have been in the past. Our behavior is guided as much by what we have negative emotional responses to, and thus avoid, escape from, and strive against, as by what we have positive emotional responses to, and hence approach and strive in favor of. Learning is always an adjustment to the particular environment in which it occurs. That environment may vary and make past learning maladjustive, but the emotion mechanism is generally adaptive.

SECONDARY PRINCIPLES OF LEARNING-BEHAVIOR

The two fundamental principles of conditioning have been presented, as well as how the two principles produce three basic functions of stimuli. There are secondary principles that operate in classical and operant conditioning. The commonality of the secondary principles across the two types of conditioning may be noted, with respect to considering whether both principles of conditioning are different types of learning, as treated in Skinner's theory.

Extinction

In addition to the value of knowing the secondary principles of conditioning, these principles help indicate the plasticity of behavior and the great importance that learning plays. The principle of extinction shows this plasticity very clearly.

It is helpful to consider extinction as unlearning something that has been learned, for the process is the opposite of learning. Thus, in learning an emotional response, the conditioned stimulus is paired *with* the unconditioned stimulus that elicits the response. The conditioned stimulus thereby comes to elicit the emotional response; this is the learning. Extinction refers to the process where the conditioned stimulus continues to be presented a number of times, *without* the unconditioned stimulus. Each such occasion is an extinction trial, and on each trial the power of the conditioned stimulus to elicit the response is weakened, not strengthened as in conditioning. The process thus produces the *unlearning* of the response. It is an active process; extinction does not occur simply with the passage of time, and thus is not like the popular concept of forgetting.

The same process pertains to operant conditioning. Each time a motor response is reinforced in the presence of a particular stimulus, that stimulus will come to be a directive stimulus, that is, will more strongly elicit (or control) the response. When the organism has learned to respond to the directive stimulus, extinction can remove that learning. That is, if, for a number of occurrences, the organism makes the motor response in the presence of the stimulus, but the response is *not* followed by reinforcement, the power of the directive stimulus to elicit that response is weakened. If extinction is repeated sufficiently the organism will no longer respond to the stimulus any more than it originally did; the stimulus will have lost its directive value.

We can see that learning and extinction are adaptive for the organism. Organisms that function according to learning principles will acquire new behaviors (adapt) to the stimulus conditions the environment presents. But the environment can change. If the organisms continued to respond as they have learned this will now be maladaptive. In such cases organisms then unlearn their previous learning. The plasticity of their behavior is biologically adaptive, which is why organisms have evolved biologically to have such plastic learning characteristics.

Generalization

In both classical and operant conditioning the organism learns responses to particular stimuli. But how specific is that learning? If it were very specific, it would not be of much value, because stimuli are rarely, if ever, exactly the same each time they occur. Fortunately, organisms are biologically constructed such that when a response is learned to a particular stimulus, *similar* stimuli will elicit the response, to the extent of that similarity. Organisms are so constructed because the characteristic is adaptive. For it is the case that similar stimuli in life usually have the same effect. So it is adaptive that a response learned to one stimulus will generalize to similar stimuli. When a deer has learned to run to the scent of a particular lion, it is adaptive that it will respond to the similar smell of other lions. If the antelope had to learn to respond to the smell of each specific lion that specificity of learning would place the animal in continued jeopardy.

The principle of stimulus generalization applies to both classical and operant conditioning. If a response is conditioned to one stimulus it will occur to similar stimuli. Similarity can vary on multiple dimensions, for example, with a visual stimulus variation can take place on the dimensions of brightness, color, shape, and so on.

Discrimination

The fact is, however, that in some cases, although stimuli are similar their effects may not be the same. I remember a newspaper article about a barroom fight that began when one man entered the bar, then walked over and took a bite out of another's hamburger. It was a case of mistaken identity—the man taking the bite thought the other was a friend. However, the other man only was *similar* in appearance to the friend.

It is thus important that animals' learned behavior is plastic in this respect. Although a learned response to a stimulus will generalize to similar stimuli, experiences that occur with these similar stimuli can modify that generalization. If a laboratory rat, for example, is reinforced for pressing a bar in the presence of a 100-watt light, it will also respond (in decreasing strength) if the light is 95 watts, 90 watts, or 85 watts. This is stimulus generalization. But, if the animal is only reinforced when the light has the 100-watt intensity, and is extinguished at the other intensity levels, the animal will come to respond only to the 100-watt light. This process of unlearning (through extinction) of the response to *similar* stimuli is called stimulus discrimination. Such learning narrows the band of stimuli to which the organism will make the learned response. This principle is involved in learning all kinds of fine sensory discriminations, as in discriminating colors, sounds, smells, and tastes. The same principle applies equally to operant and classically conditioned responses.

Intermittent Conditioning

It also helpful in analyzing human behavior to know that conditioning can be continuous or intermittent in nature. For example, the unconditioned stimulus can be paired with the conditioned stimulus on every trial. Or, the unconditioned stimulus can be presented every other time the conditioned stimulus occurred. That would constitute a case of intermittent conditioning. Conditioning would take place in each case. But the conditioning would not elicit as strong a response in the intermittent case. Although this counters what might be expected, a response learned under intermittent conditioning is *more* resistant to extinction than when continuous conditioning trials have occurred.

Intermittent conditioning, and increased resistance to extinction pertain also to operant conditioning. There are many different ways that the reinforcer can be applied in an intermittent manner. In operant conditioning Skinner names these ways schedules of reinforcement. As examples, a reinforcer can be presented on some proportion of trials (a ratio schedule), or reinforcement can be given on a time basis. Let us say the response of the lab animal will not be reinforced until a certain time period has occurred (this is called an interval schedule). Skinner devoted much of his research career to the study of schedules of reinforcement (see Ferster & Skinner, 1957), as did many radical behaviorists. Different schedules have different effects on the rate of behavior, the characteristic of behavior of interest to Skinner and those who study reinforcement schedules. While the *detailed* work on the many different schedules has not proven significant in the study of human behavior, the *major* principles are important to know. For some types of behavior may involve the principles. Moreover, from a PB standpoint, this work is another demonstration of the fact that the secondary principles of conditioning show plasticity and adaptability. As an example, an animal's behavior that had learned to trace its way to a water hole, that sometimes has water and sometimes not, would learn a resistant response in the face of several occasions when there was no water. The animal with a history of continuous reinforcement would extinguish with fewer trials when the hole contained no water. That behavior becomes more persistent as a function of a variable environment is important in an evolutionary sense. It is also adaptive that animals that are reinforced for a portion of their responses respond more rapidly, because that increases their receipt of reinforcement. Adaptability and plasticity of behavior are shown generally by the various reinforcement schedules.

Time Variables

The time between the conditioned stimulus and the unconditioned stimulus affects the conditioning. When the stimuli are closely paired in time, the strongest conditioning occurs and this decreases as the interval is lengthened. With animals and young children, if the interval exceeds 30 seconds conditioning does not occur. Again, time variables are important to know about when analyzing human behavior. We can also consider time principles in an evolutionary sense. The fact is that, when things occur together closely in time, they are more likely to be related—that is, to occur again together. The longer the time between a ^{C}S and ^{UC}S the less likely in life will the two stimuli have a relationship. It has been suggested that the time principle is different in some animals, at least with respect to some responses. For example, rats that have been presented with a new food (and taste) and then have been made sick at a much later time, will subsequently avoid that food. This finding has been interpreted to suggest that learning principles are not universally general (Garcia & Ervin, 1968) and that this discredits a learning approach. That is a gratuitous interpretation, however. Some animals, especially those that eat foods that may have toxic properties (such as scavengers), can have evolved differently with respect to time principles, for certain unconditioned stimuli. That would be an adaptive development and would not be inconsistent with the present learning approach.

The time variable is also important in operant conditioning—in this case the time between the response and the reinforcer. The greater the time interval the less the strength of conditioning.

Two Types of Conditioning: One Learning

Thus, all of the secondary principles apply equally to classical and operant conditioning. In the PB view this suggests that the two types of principles evolved for the same reasons of biological adaptability. Moreover, this suggests that there are common physiological mechanisms involved. This position contrasts with that of Skinner, who considered that classical (respondent) conditioning took place via the autonomic nervous system and operant conditioning took place via the central nervous system. In the PB view, however, that difference is only relevant with respect to peripheral nerve conduction. The PB position is the learning of emotion takes place in the brain, as does the learning of operant behavior. This organ operates the same for both types of conditioning. Brain damage, for example, can result in the loss of previous emotional conditioning just as it can result in the loss of previous operant conditioning. Thus, in the PB view, Skinner was wrong (and inconsistent—see Skinner, 1950) for considering operant conditioning to be the superior type on the basis of his physiological analysis. The responses have different characteristics, but learning is the same for both and it involves the brain.

MOTIVATION

The study of motivation has been hindered by the fact that some investigators study basic motivation principles on the animal level and others study motivational conditions with humans. Because the two are on different levels of study, different phenomena and different principles are involved. Without recognizing this separation—which is typical (see Keller & Schoenfeld, 1950, pp. 262*ff*)—and without constructing bridging theory by which to bring them together, the two levels of study remain separate.

Those who have studied motivational processes in animals have traditionally considered such study to provide the basic principles by which to explain human motivation. For example, Young (1936, pp. 544–545) took the classic position that the animal and physiological study of motivation provides the basis for understanding motivation for going to a movie, interests, changes of interest with age, attitudes, prestige motivation, sense of inferiority, altruism, and so on. Those are simplistic generalizations.

In contrast, the PB position is that there are multiple levels of theory to be developed between the study of animal motivation and human motivation. Only the basic principles of motivation will be dealt with here. Additional levels of development are necessary before a theory of motivation can be constructed that can deal with motivational phenomena (such as interests, attitudes, and values) relevant to complex human behavior and personality. The basic level of theory aims to be heuristic at the animal level of study, while also providing the fundamental principles of motivation that can serve as the foundation for building to the human level theory.

Emotion and Motivation

The relevance of motivation was recognized early in the context of classical conditioning. It was established that the animal that was not deprived of food did not condition very well. For non-deprived animals pairing the food with the ^{C}S did not result in the stimulus coming to elicit much in the way of salivation. Stated more generally, when the subject has eaten food recently (is satiated), food as a stimulus will only weakly elicit a positive emotional response. When the organism has not eaten for a time, food will more strongly elicit a positive emotional response. Finch (1938) conducted a systematic study and found that his canine subjects salivated increasingly to the food stimulus as well as to the ^{C}S. The strength of the response increased as food deprivation was extended, up to 72 hours. An implication of this principle of motivation is that deprivation increases the extent to which any positive emotion-eliciting stimulus will serve as an unconditioned stimulus in classical conditioning.

The same effect was evident with motor behavior, which was also a subject of study very early. For example, Ligon (1929) ran groups of animals in a maze that were either satiated, or under 6-, 12-, or 21-hour food deprivation. With food as reward, generally deprivation increased the speed of learning. Tolman, Honzik, and Robinson (1930) found that food-deprived rats made fewer errors in learning a maze. Skinner (1938) deprived a rat of food and then ran the rat in an operant chamber and measured the rate of bar-pressing. The only food obtained was the pellets used as reinforcers. Skinner found that over the six days of increasing food deprivation the animals responded more and more rapidly. His conclusion was that food deprivation increased the *strength of the response* that was reinforced by food.

Skinner's theory (1938) is very unclear with respect to defining motivation (drive) in classical conditioning and operant conditioning. His theory stated that conditioning processes strengthened a hypothetical state, the *reflex reserve*, which determined the strength of response (although he gave the concept no further attention). Another condition, deprivation (drive), could also raise the strength of the response. However, Skinner did not consider that drive affected the reserve; drive constituted a variable that affected the display of the behavior, but not its strength, which depended upon conditioning. (Hull, 1943, is basically similar in this respect.) Skinner did not indicate *how* drive affected the display of behavior. Skinner (1938) also mentions emotion to involve variables that affect the strength of behavior, but not the reserve. (Later he states emotions do not affect behavior [Skinner, 1975]). His examples of emotion involve presentation of negative stimuli, not presentation of positive stimuli. The analysis is not clear, but he did not consider motivation and emotion to be the same, and no relationship between them was specified. So, in addition to not relating classical and operant conditioning, Skinner's radical behaviorism has lacked a good basic theory of motivation.

Keller and Schoenfeld (1950) attempted to update and systematize Skinner's theory, including its concept of motivation. They state, *"What is drive?,* we must now answer that drive is the *name* for a fact—the fact that certain operations can be performed on an organism (for example, depriving it of food) that have [a strengthening] effect upon behavior which is different than other operations" (Keller & Schoenfeld, 1950, p. 265). The fact is that this is a generally held conception of motivation; that deprivation just generally *strengthens* behavior (Hebb, 1955; Hull, 1943a; Keller & Schoenfeld, 1950; Skinner, 1938). Hull's theory specified that drive (which is defined by deprivation) multiplies with all of the organism's learned behaviors—thus generally increasing the strength of those behaviors. Keller and Schoenfeld state, "Behaviorally, a drive is marked by *concurrent changes in the strength of many reflexes.* A food-deprived animal not only presses a bar more frequently and eats more vigorously, but many other reflexes change at the same time (e.g., climbing, sniffing, and running about) if the bar is not present" (1950, p. 270).

The PB Conception of Deprivation and Its Motivational Effects

This is not a good theory of motivation, in the present view. For one thing, such a general strengthening would not be adaptive. To illustrate, an organism has many behaviors, many of which have no relevance for getting food. If deprivation of food strengthened all such behaviors—the animal's grooming behavior, sexual behavior, play behavior, and the like—that would be maladaptive. For energy (food) would be consumed in performing such behaviors, even though the food-deprived animal needs to conserve energy. Moreover, those unnecessary behaviors would yield no advantage with respect to securing food. Animals operating according to such a principles would be disadvantaged with respect to survival.

The PB position is that the various findings suggesting that deprivation strengthens behavior actually show something quite different. There is indeed a change in behavior. But the deprivation does not affect the behavior directly. Rather, the changes in behavior are due instead to the fact that food deprivation strengthens *the functions of food stimuli and those stimuli that have been associated with food.* This occurs because food deprivation changes the strength with which food and food-associated stimuli elicit a positive emotional response.

Documentation for this basic effect of deprivation is given by Finch's (1938) experiment. But the behavioral importance of deprivation is given by PB's three-function learning theory. That theory states that anything that increases the extent to which a stimulus will elicit an emotional response will also increase the extent to which the stimulus will function as a reinforcing stimulus. That is why deprived animals learn a maze faster than non-deprived animals. The deprived animals, because they respond emotionally more to the food, are actually receiving larger reinforcers. Size of reinforcement affects learning. In part that is also why Skinner's (1938) rats pressed the bar progressively more rapidly as they were progressively deprived of food. Deprivation was making the food pellets into progressively stronger reinforcers.

But PB states that an emotional stimulus has another function; it serves as a directive stimulus for approach behaviors. The motivation conception states that as deprivation increases, the extent to which a stimulus elicits an emotional response increases. The result is that the extent to which the stimulus serves as a directive stimulus is also increased. *Deprivation of an appetitive stimulus increases its strength as a directive stimulus* (see Staats, 1970a, 1975). This effect can be seen in a number of studies. For example, Seward and Seward (1940) placed a sexually receptive female rat on one side of a barrier and a male animal on the other. They found that the male rat subjects would cross the hurdle to get to the female more quickly if they had been deprived of sex for several days than if they had recently copulated. Such results can be interpreted to show that increased motivation (drive) increases the strength of behavior. In terms of three-function learning principles, however, deprivation of sex made the receptive female rat, as a stimulus, more strongly elicit a positive emotional response in the male rat. The stronger emotional response of the male rats, in turn, more strongly elicited their approach responses—all approach responses—but only to the female rat. The animals would have run, swum, and climbed more rapidly in approaching a receptive female. Those responses were not generally strengthened, with respect to other stimuli. The effect that Keller and Schoenfeld (1950, p. 270) refer to—the general strengthening of "climbing and sniffing and running about"—is not due to a general strengthening of behavior, but due to the increase in the directive stimulus value of specific stimuli.

Of course, increasing the strength of the emotional response elicited by a stimulus also increases the stimulus generalization of that stimulus. For example, the sex-deprived male rat will have a stronger emotional response than usual to the non-receptive female and to male rats. This increase will result in behaving more generally to stimuli than is the case when not deprived. But the effect of generalization should not be confused with the principle that deprivation has the effect of generally raising the activity (behavior) level. Thus, PB's theory of motivation (drive) derives from its three-function learning theory. Let me only add that Hull (1943a) had a concept of the fractional anticipatory goal response that deprivation would increase and that had stimulus properties and would guide behavior. It was developed in the context of particular studies, however, and did not have characteristics for general development, and did not establish a tradition for continued development.

Psychological behaviorism also differs from traditional positions (see Keller & Schoenfeld, 1950; Michael, 1993; Skinner, 1938) in how it considers positive and negative motivation. The traditional concept of motivation does not sufficiently clarify the difference between negative drives and appetitive drives. This traditional view is probably drawn from observations of human behavior. After all, there are things that people strive to avoid (aversions) as well as things they strive to get (incentives). While this is true, there is nothing that corresponds to the deprivation–satiation operation *for aversive stimuli*. The strength with which a negative unconditioned stimulus elicits a negative emotional response depends upon the intensity of the stimulus itself. There are no (or very weak) variables of a deprivation–satiation sort that affect the strength of that elicitation. The same is true of conditioned stimuli. The strength with which a conditioned stimulus elicits a negative emotional response depends on the strength of the classical conditioning that has occurred (for example, number of conditioning trials, the ^{C}S-^{UC}S time interval, and the intensity of the ^{UC}S).

The difference with respect to motivation in the positive and negative case may seem like a strange imbalance, because everything else that pertains to positive emotional stimuli pertains to negative emotional stimuli. But, considered in terms of principles of biological evolution, adaptation and survival, the imbalance is not strange. To illustrate, by increasing the extent to which the positive emotional stimulus elicits the positive emotional response, deprivation increases the reinforcement and directive stimulus value of the emotional stimulus. The result is the increase of the behavior that is likely to obtain the appetitive (positive emotional) stimulus. Gaining appetitive stimuli—like food, water, sex—has biological (species) survival value. When the organism is satiated, however, displaying the same behaviors would be a waste of energy, a drawback for survival. So deprivation effects the changes that are adaptive.

   This is different with respect to aversive (negative emotional) stimuli. These stimuli do the organism biological harm, and avoiding contact is adaptive. Centrally, in this context, the harmful effect pertains *whether or not the organism has just experienced the stimulus.* If organisms were constructed such that experiencing the aversive stimulus resulted in satiation, where the stimulus would not elicit a negative emotional response, this would be biologically disadvantageous. For the reinforcing and directive functions of the stimulus would be lessened, which would lessen the behaviors that would escape and avoid the stimulus. For the sake of the organism's survival, the negative emotionality of harmful stimuli should never be decreased whether or not the organism has recently experienced them. That is why organisms have evolved so that deprivation–satiation operations are not effective for aversive stimuli. Thus, motivation *at the basic level*—that is, deprivation–satiation—concerns only positive emotional stimuli.

Establishing Operations Theory and Motivation and Emotion

More recently, Michael (1993) has presented a motivational theory. Nominally an extension of Skinner's approach, it combines features of Skinner's theory, Keller and Schoenfeld's theory, as well as PB's theory. The principles are presented in a new terminology, and the various combinations of the variables are productively elaborated. In the new terminology Michael refers to deprivation–satiation operations as "establishing operations" (a term used by Keller & Schoenfeld, 1950) along with other operations. Like PB, the theory attempts to interrelate classical conditioning and operant conditioning—although this goal is not made explicit. And his system also includes PB's conception of the functions of stimuli. But Michael's account, like Skinner's, still does not specify the emotional response or its role in the other functions of stimuli. Like Skinner, and Keller and Schoenfeld, Michael also retains the conception of aversive stimuli having a drive-inducing (motivational) property, because such stimuli will bring on certain behaviors. But, as indicated in PB, drive induction pertains only to positive emotional stimuli—the functions of the negative emotional stimulus are not affected by deprivation–satiation. Moreover, Michael's terminological system confounds deprivation–satiation operations with conditioning operations—making everything an EO (establishing operation). This blurs distinctions and makes the system imprecise. And the theory is cumbersome and indirect. Like Hull's (1943a) theory of learning, establishing operations theory (EO) increases complexity unnecessarily. In any event, there is little or no new empirical evidence called for by the theory, or invoked in support of the theory. The field of behavior analysis lacks research in classical conditioning, which leaves the theory which attempts to relate classical and operant conditioning without an empirical foundation.

COGNITIVE PROCESSES AT THE BASIC LEVEL: IMAGES (LEARNING AND FUNCTION)

Let me indicate another schism in the field of learning that has not been resolved by the second-generation behavioristic theories. The schism involves the treatment of cognitive ("mental") concepts. To begin, Watson (1930) rejected concepts that involved inferences concerning the mental processes that traditional psychology considered to be causes of overt behavior. He saw the program of psychology to be that of establishing the relationships between directly observable environmental (stimulus) events and directly observable behaviors. That position alienates many traditional psychologists. People, including psychologists, have their own personal cognitive experiences, as well as experiences of the manner in which these internal "mental" processes influence their overt behavior. It is difficult to convince anyone that those experiences do not occur.

Although this has not been realized, Skinner (1953) has actually taken a very inconsistent position in this area. Seemingly, like Watson, he rejects the consideration of mental processes—processes that are inferred from behavior, and have no other stipulated definition. His methodology, rather, deals with the effects of the manipulation of reinforcement contingencies on the rate of response. Seemingly this is clear. But Skinner provides a loophole by introducing the concept of the "private event" in the consideration of human behavior. The private event, however, is no better defined than other mentalistic concepts. No research is reported to support the inference of such processes. The private event is left unspecified, as well as how it comes about, and how and by what principles it affects the individual's behavior.

An example of another inferred internal process can be seen in his reference to conditioned "seeing." Skinner states that when food is paired with a dinner gong and later the gong is rung, the individual "sees" the food. But Skinner did not provide the empirical specification of this concept—which his methodology demands—even though some specification existed at that time (see Ellson, 1941; Leuba, 1940). As another example, later on, Skinner (1966) introduced the concept of "rule-governed behavior." This concept is that verbal statements that specify reinforcement contingencies for a person will affect the individual's behavior in the same way the reinforcement contingencies would themselves. Again, this suggests that cognitive processes that can affect behavior can be given a behavioral definition. But the concept of the "rule" is very vague and unspecified. Moreover, the concept was never developed by Skinner or given empirical support, so it has been treated differently by different radical behaviorists (see Burns & Staats, 1992). The result is differing interpretations and arguments like that which discredited the mentalistic-introspectionistic work that Watson originally criticized.

Tolman (1932), in contrast to Watson and Skinner, attempted to unify the behavioral and "mental" traditions by his manner of conceptualizing basic animal learning. His plan was to make the cognitive process (intervening event) objective by defining it in terms of preceding stimulus events and resulting behavioral events. His program was to do this on the animal level, such that cognitive concepts like "expectancy" of reinforcement and the "cognitive map" of a maze were basic concepts that could be used in the analysis of human behavior. For example, he rejected the idea that a motor response was conditioned to an external stimulus, because the response was followed by reinforcement. Tolman, rather, saw the animals to be learning stimulus–stimulus associations, which had nothing to do with reinforcement. When animals were put in a maze, without any reinforcement, and they wandered around, they learned a "cognitive map" of the maze. Subsequently, when reinforcement was put at the end of the maze, the animal's then developed an "expectancy" of reinforcement, which activated their "cognitive map" and they ran directly to the reinforcer. Thus, in his view, basic learning involved learning cognitive processes that then determined behavior. He opposed the view of Hull and Skinner that animals simply learned specific responses to specific external stimuli.

In the present view the problem with Tolman's theory was not with its goal of dealing with the cognitive as well as the behavioral, but with the way in which he attempted to accomplish the feat. To say that stimuli are associated with each other in the organism says nothing more than had been said by the 18th-century British Associationists in their philosophical analyses. To simply infer that animals must experience cognitive processes like Tolman's cognitive maps and expectancies of reinforcement, just because we personally have experiences we can label in that manner, is anthropomorphic and empty. And it does nothing to solve the problem, which is to stipulate those cognitive experiences objectively, *behaviorally*. In fact, Tolman's theory is curiously circular, since it derives concepts from personal (human) experience with which to "explain" the behavior of animals, in order to construct a "basic" theory by which to "explain" human behavior. This methodology cannot succeed. Interestingly, although this is not realized, Skinner's (1953) concept of "conditioned seeing" and Tolman's concept of the "cognitive map" are really very similar. The difference arises in that Tolman attempted to establish a methodology for introducing his concepts and Skinner did not. This lack of systematicity acted to Skinner's advantage—introducing his concepts informally and in an unimportant way gave his theory the patina of being able to deal with cognitive matters without presenting a method that would have been rejected if stated formally.

Fortunately, beginning around 1940, experimental findings began to accumulate that provide the basis for the construction of a better founded and better developed theory of such basic cognitive–behavioral concepts (see Staats, 1963a, 1968a; Staats & Lohr, 1979; Staats, Staats, & Heard, 1961). One basic concept, that of the sensory response, is relevant to understanding "stimulus–stimulus associations" as well as "conditioned seeing." In PB theory, it should be noted, stimuli cannot be associated, only stimuli and responses. The basic concept is that any external stimulus to which the organism is sensitive is actually eliciting in the organism a *sensory response.* For example, when the retina is stimulated by light the activity in the visual cortex part of the brain is a *response,* in the sense that it has response characteristics. In addition, however, this response process will also activate sensory nerve fibers, which is to say the response will have stimulus characteristics. What the individual experiences, the sensation, consists of those stimulus characteristics. To recapitulate, a light is shown, the visual apparatus (especially the visual cortex) responds, and the response produces the individual's experience, which is the sight of the light. This may seem a cumbersome description, but placing the process within a stimulus–response framework makes it possible to unify the processes involved within principles that generally apply to behavior.

What is not usually recognized is that sensation is not simply a sensory process; it is a response process that produces a sensory process. What is the purpose of this distinction? Centrally, considering sensations as responses says that they can be learned, that an organism can be conditioned to have a sensory response. As a consequence of such conditioning, a sensory response can be elicited by a stimulus other than the stimulus that ordinarily arouses that sensation. Such a learned sensation, which occurs in the absence of a sensory stimulus, is, in commonsense terms, called an image. (Under some circumstances, an image may be considered to be a hallucination—seeBurns, Heiby, & Tharp, 1983; Staats, 1968a, p. 50). An image is a sensory response that has been *conditioned* to some extraneous stimulus and can be elicited by that stimulus.

This analysis was constructed on the basis of research, from various sources. Because the response and stimulus events involved in the conditioned sensory response are internal and inaccessible to direct observation, the studies involve manipulations that produce conditioning. The evidence of the conditioning is an expected change in the behavior of the subject. In this way, both animal (see Brogden, 1939) and human (see Brogden, 1947; Ellson, 1941; Leuba, 1940; Phillips, 1958; Staats, Staats, & Heard, 1961) studies have shown how images can be conditioned according to classical conditioning principles (see Staats & Lohr, 1979). The present theoretical position is that sensory responses (images) are learned via classical conditioning. The external sensory stimulus is the [UCS]; it elicits the sensory response, which can be conditioned to any other stimulus. A young man, for example, may have an image of a young woman on hearing a song that was played at the time they are dating. The pairing of the auditory sensory stimulus (song) and visual sensory stimulus (the woman) result in their "association." Later the song stimulus, the ^{C}S, elicits the visual image (conditioned sensory response) of the woman. (The sight of the woman would also elicit the image of hearing the song.) The term *association,* then, is defined as the case where presentation of a stimulus elicits a conditioned sensory response (which is the image).

It is important to realize that sensory responses can be learned, but this provides only part of the importance of the theoretical concept. Interestingly, even behaviorists who have employed concepts of images have not systematically addressed the manner in which they affect overt behavior. Let me thus say that the image can elicit the same overt behavior as the real stimulus object itself. That is why we have evolved to experience images, a stimulus to which other behaviors can be conditioned. And therein lies the adjustive value of images. As an example, the individual who has learned an image of where he has left his car keys can be "guided" by the image and go to this place and find them. The image *mediates* the behavior in the same way that actually seeing the keys would. The animal that traces its way through the jungle acquires conditioned sensory responses that will provide it with a "cognitive map" to return to its lair. Studies that are employed in the present theory to define the sensory response/image show that images can serve to elicit other behaviors. For example, Staats, Staats, and Heard (1961), using human subjects, conditioned a sensory response to a nonsense syllable. Later, the subjects' motor responses to the syllable were affected by the conditioned sensory response. Brogden (1939) showed the same effect with animals and later with humans (Brogden, 1947).

There are three parts to this theory. One is to give the cognitive event (the image) a behavioral definition, stating that the cognitive event acts according to known behavior principles. In addition, part of the definition of the image lies in showing how images are determined by conditioning variables. The other part of the definition resides in showing the behavioral principles by which images may mediate other behaviors. The above experiments provide evidence that supports the analysis; that sensory responses can be conditioned, and that conditioned sensory responses have stimulus (image) properties to which other responses can be conditioned.

It is such analyses that lead some behavior analysts (Hayes & Brownstein, 1986) to consider PB to be mechanistic. This position stems from using Skinner's analyses as a model. As has been indicated, Skinner introduces the concept of conditioned seeing, but in an informal manner, without a methodology for doing so, without empirical support, and without an analysis to serve as a basis for gaining that support. However, there should be no advantage to leaving concepts vague, informal, and without empirical definition, as Skinner does. It is time to evaluate critically the differences involved in these positions. The present formulation is that Tolman and others were indeed right in saying that pairing two stimuli together creates an association, but it is not a stimulus–stimulus association, but rather a stimulus–response association. Tolman was also correct in his concern with a cognitive representative of the reinforcing stimulus. But the concept of expectancy is also a concept that lacks the behavioral specification necessary. In PB theory the concept of emotion, and the three-function learning principles that elaborate the concept of emotion, fulfills the role of "expectancy," again within a behavioral framework, and with much specification.

I will only add that if we were analytically accurate we would not say that an operant response was conditioned to an external stimulus. There is no way that the nervous system of the organism reaches out and connects to an external stimulus. The external stimulus elicits a sensory response in the organism, which produces an internal stimulus. The operant response (or what stands for it in brain activity) is connected to that internal stimulus. However, to give this detail to every behavior we wished to analyze would be cumbersome. We can thus simply understand what is involved but simplify our analyses as though external stimuli directly elicit overt responses. Cognitive psychologists should understand this does not slight consideration of the internal processes and when the occasion calls for inclusion in the analysis there are available concepts. For example, we need the image mechanism and conditioning principles in various other cases, such as in analyzing phenomena like hallucinations, which involve sensory responses to stimuli that are not there (see Staats, 1968a, p. 50). The same can be true in projecting research to study the mechanisms involved. We need a rich set of behavior–cognitive principles to deal widely with complex human behavior.

ISSUES IN PB LEARNING THEORY

The foregoing has set forth the PB learning theory, presented in framework form, to serve as the basic level in the multilevel theory to be developed. The principles have not been discussed in detail in the context of the relevant animal literature, and there are various issues that have not been treated. It is the case that the foundation area of behaviorism is involved and some additional comparison to other approaches is important.

Two-Factor Theory and Three-Function Theory

As has been indicated, Skinner took a two-factor approach, stating there were two types of conditioning that are unrelated to each other. A specialized two-factor theory (May, 1948; Miller, 1948; Mowrer, 1947; Osgood,

1953; Rescorla & Solomon, 1967; Solomon & Wynne, 1954) arose, however, associated with Hull's theory. (This was odd since Hull took a one-factor approach.) This two-factor theory, in part, considered the two factors to be related. The theory arose in research with animals in a particular type of experimentation involving a "shuttle box." The animals were first shocked through the floor, learning in response to move from one half of the box to the other half, where the electricity was turned off. This was repeated, after a period, where the new side was electrified and the other side was not. This training was said to condition the animals to make the escape response to the fear the electric shock elicited.

After having learned to escape the shock, the animals were additionally classically conditioned to have a fear response to a buzzer, by pairing the buzzer with electric shock. These animals, then, as a result of the two types of learning, when in the shuttle box would respond to the *buzzer* by running immediately to the other side of the box. The theoretical interpretation was that the buzzer elicited the fear response and the fear, in turn, elicited the escape behavior. The fear conditioned to the buzzer constituted one learning factor, and the conditioned escape response to fear constituted the other learning factor in the two-factor (or two-process) theory.

The customary concept of fear was utilized; that is, a set of peripheral responses controlled by the autonomic nervous system. Thus, to test the two-factor learning theory, a study was run in which animals given the two types of training then had their autonomic nervous systems removed. If fear was involved in the animals performance, it was expected they would no longer make the escape behavior when the buzzer was presented. Unexpectedly, the animals still responded to the buzzer. Rescorla and Solomon (1967) concluded that the experimental effect was not mediated by the fear—that there was no support for two-factor learning theory. These authors raised the possibility that perhaps fear was a central state, but they did so as an afterthought, with no conviction and without further development.

In addition to this disproving evidence, two-factor learning theory suffered other problems. It was developed within a very specific experimental apparatus and was not elaborated as a general theory and applied to various behavioral phenomena. For example, the theory did not tie its behavioral principles in with the physiological/behavioral research showing there are centers in the brain whose stimulation produces emotion *and* reinforcement. As another example, the theory dealt only with fear and was not unified with other relevant experiments involving the positive emotional response (see Brown & Jenkins, 1968; Trapold & Winokur, 1967). Because of these weaknesses two-factor learning theory ceased to be generally used and elaborated.

In contrast, the three-function learning theory is a general theory. It includes a general theory of emotions that is based on physiological as well as behavioral research (Staats, 1975, chaps. 4, 15; Staats & Eifert, 1990). That theory indicated why the Rescorla and Solomon (1967) failure to disrupt the two-process effect was not a crucial experiment. Moreover, the PB theory specifies the concept of stimulus functions, indicates there are three, and stipulates their relationships and how they come about. Because three-function learning theory is a general learning theory it is possible to analyze a wide range of animal *and human* studies using its concepts and principles. For example, PB analyses described the phenomena of autoshaping (Brown & Jenkins, 1968) and transfer of control (Trapold & Winokur, 1967). And PB has added a number of its own studies with humans, both basic studies and those dealing with aspects of complex human behavior. Many basic animal and human learning studies demonstrate the same principles (see Staats, 1963a, chap. 4; 1975, chaps. 3, 4, 5, 7). Because of its construction it is suggested that three-function learning theory provides the foundation for a general theory of animal learning as well as human learning. Very essentially, two-process theory lacked the human perspective, which is necessary to show the very general importance of work on the emotion–behavior relationship. When it is realized that emotion has such general importance in affecting human behavior, there is a basis for a long-term, continuing, and broad program of work to study the principles involved. This will be shown further on.

Skinner's Basic Theory and PB's Basic Theory

Skinner's (1938, 1975) approach—emphasizing that emotional responses (and classical conditioning) are separate from operant responses (and operant conditioning)—became the dominant basic theory in behavioral psychology. Radical behaviorists, social learning theorists, and most applied behaviorists employ his basic theory. However, this conception, its methods, and its empirical work do not provide impetus or direction for focally studying classical conditioning, how it occurs in uniquely human ways, or how emotions affect behavior. For these reasons Skinner's approach does not instruct the applied behaviorist in how emotions can be changed in order to effect changes in behavior.

Psychological behaviorism has pointed to these weaknesses in radical behaviorism's basic theory, and in recent times some radical behaviorists have attempted to remedy the problem—not by accepting PB's theory, but by incorporating aspects of PB into a radical behaviorism framework. As already indicated, examination of the concepts of Michael (1993) reveal reference to the multiple functions of stimuli and to the classical conditioning and operant conditioning interaction. Hayes and associates (see Hayes, Zettle, & Rosenfarb, 1989; Zettle & Hayes, 1982) also introduce concepts like those in the three-function learning theory, although not in clear form. Zettle and Hayes (1982, p. 81) state that words can elicit an emotional response that may alter one's capacity to "find particular events reinforcing or punishing," and that "a good [TV] commercial can literally make your mouth water" (Hayes, Zettle, & Rosenfarb, 1989, pp. 207–208) and affect one's behavior. And Schlinger and Blakely (1987) write even more clearly about the "functions" of stimuli and the role of emotions.

While this is a productive development, these theoretical elaborations more generally reveal weaknesses in the radical behaviorism approach. For one thing there has been a long lag before even beginning to correct the basic learning theory, even though materials by which to do so have been available. For another, radical behaviorists still cannot employ directly the developments in another behaviorism. The developments must be appended to Skinner's theory. That means the new theory statements are set into an inconsistent theory structure, as is the case with Hayes, Zettle, and Rosenfarb (1987), Blakeley and Schlinger (1987), and Michael (1993). Very fundamentally, in addition, radical behaviorism has provided no *research* on the interaction of emotion (classical conditioning) and behavior (operant conditioning), and on the resulting interrelated functions of stimuli. Moreover, with the exclusivity that is part of radical behaviorism, it is not possible to utilize findings, or methods, from other approaches, even other behaviorisms. So the various experiments that have been done on this topic cannot be used in the new radical behaviorism theories. Being cut off from essential avenues of development makes for weak theory formulations.

Theory-Construction in Radical Behaviorism and PB

Differences in basic theory *methodology* constitute a primary reason that many radical behaviorists do not use the PB theory concerning how emotion affects behavior. To illustrate, Hayes (1993) has directly criticized the PB learning theory for being mechanistic—for example, PB analyses indicate that emotional responses (through their stimuli) mediate operant behavior (as in Figure 2.3). This criticism is based on the Hayes and Brownstein (1986) rejection of the use of "behavior–behavior" principles. Behavior–behavior principles (see Staats, 1975, pp. 65–72) are those in which one behavior is seen as the explanation for the occurrence of another behavior. Hayes and Brownstein state that it is better that behavior be explained directly by environmental events, not by the occurrence of a preceding behavior. An explanation that stipulates the environmental causes, so goes their argument, provides knowledge of variables by which to affect the behavior of interest. Hayes and Brownstein state that behavior–behavior explanation of the type used by PB does not provide this possibility.

There is no reason why a chain of events cannot be the cause of a later event. Environmental events may be the explanation of a behavior, and the occurrence of that behavior may be the explanation of another behavior. That is perfectly clear. Moreover, Hayes' position is inconsistent. For Hayes (see Hayes, Zettle, & Rosenfarb, 1986) uses the three-function learning principles in his own theorizing as do others. So Hayes' methodological rejection of behavior–behavior explanation does not agree with the theorizing he accepts in other areas, as shown in Poppen's example of the motorist who reads a set of directions and this behavior then affects his driving behavior. Hayes even says "the driver covertly recites directions he has been given" and this covert behavior controls the overt driving behavior (Poppen, 1989, p. 333). This constitutes just the kind of behavior–behavior explanations that Hayes and Brownstein (1986) criticize in PB. The inconsistency is even more emphatic because PB uses exactly the same example of a driver whose behavior is controlled by his reading and covert verbal behavior (Staats, 1963b, p. 274).

These two accounts are the same. They involve the same methodology. yet the field of behavior analysis, affected by Skinner's methodological statements (see Sidman, 1960) does not recognize that its stated methodology is different from its practices. It will accept analyses if they are considered to be from radical behaviorism and reject the same analyses if they are from another behaviorism. So many things that are inconsistent with radical behaviorism have been incorporated into it that its practitioners do not have a theory framework that provides clear guidelines. Because of this, radical behaviorism cannot develop needed methodology in a systematic way, or use another behaviorism that has already done so.

The PB position is that it was valuable that behaviorism criticize the mentalistic methodology of inferring internal processes as supposed explanations of behavior (see Skinner, 1945, 1953; Spence, 1944; Staats, 1963a, chap. 2; Watson, 1930). It was also valuable that radical behaviorists avoided the type of theorizing of Hull and Tolman that involved "intervening variables." This methodology is frequently just a disguised form of mentalism. PB does not employ mentalistic concepts, or the intervening variable methodology. In PB methodology it is recognized that there are internal behavioral processes in individuals that may not be directly observable, but that nevertheless are causes of behavior. Difficulty in observing internal causal events presents a problem, but it must be faced systematically. Part of PB's methodology involves analysis of the internal processes as response and stimulus processes, and calls for the study of the processes (see, for example, Staats, 1975, pp. 10–11, 46–48; Staats & Fernandez-Ballesteros, 1987). The trick is to conceptualize internal processes—such as thinking, purpose, self-speech (as in planning), reasoning, attitudes, emotion, and so on—in behavioral terms, *to study them empirically,* and to do so within a methodological understanding of what is involved. How PB has done this will be exemplified in various later sections. Radical behaviorism methodological orthodoxies have prevented the approach from developing the systematic work in this area that is necessary.

Empirical Differences in Radical Behaviorism and PB

The conceptual–methodological orthodoxy of radical behaviorism is matched by its experimental orthodoxy. At one time only studies using Skinner's experimental analysis of behavior technology were acceptable in radical behaviorism. To illustrate, I remember well in 1962 an editor of the *Journal of the Experimental Analysis of Behavior* at first rejected a paper of mine because my experimental procedure used "learning trials" rather than "free operant" responding. The paper, when published, laid out an agenda for studying developmental disorders using my token reinforcer system (see O'Leary & Drabman, 1971), but its publication was first questionable because of an orthodoxy. PB's works helped radical behaviorists to broaden that orthodoxy, and to admit various studies of reinforcement using various types of methodology including study in naturalistic circumstances (see Staats, 1963a, 1964).

Methodological orthodoxy still immobilizes radical behaviorism in various areas, restricting the problems that can be studied. The PB approach is that the problem should determine the experimental methodology, not the reverse. Rather than an orthodoxy, the criteria for any experimental method should concern technical attributes—the extent to which the method is public, replicable, reliable, stipulates the events under study, and so on. Data should never be rejected when they provide some knowledge, unless methods are available for obtaining better data.

Today, the radical behaviorism approach, restricted as it has been to operant conditioning methods, studies classical (respondent) conditioning very little. It has not accepted or used at all the methods for studying uniquely human types of classical conditioning, like that which can be produced using words (called language conditioning). When radical behaviorists describe words eliciting emotional responses—as Hayes (Hayes, 1986; Hayes, Zettle, & Rosenfarb, 1989) does—this is done without benefit of evidence, or a means of obtaining it. Radical behaviorism does not accept the verbal learning methodology used in studying word associations, so the corresponding term that has been coined by Skinner (1957), *intraverbals,* has no evidential definition or support. The same rejection is true of the various experimental methodologies of cognitive psychology, the methods of psychological testing, physiological study, psychotherapy, and so on, as will be indicated in later chapters.

In contrast, the PB methodological position is that, in the study of complex human behavior areas, multiple methodologies are apt to be useful. PB's concept of the central emotional response is a case in point. The concept is based on PB studies employing Pavlovian conditioning methods (see Maltzman, Raskin, Gould, & Johnson, 1965; Staats, Staats, & Crawford,

1962; Zanna, Kiesler, & Pilkonis, 1970), PB's human classical conditioning methods (see Cooper, 1959, 1969; Geer, 1968; Staats & Staats, 1957, 1958), PB's combination of classical conditioning and reinforcement methods (see Finley & Staats, 1967; Harms & Staats, 1978; Staats & Burns, 1982; Staats & Hammond, 1971; Staats, Minke, Martin, & Higa, 1972; Staats & Warren, 1974), and also incorporates and draws from other studies using methods of a physiological nature (see Staats, 1975, chaps. 4, 15; Staats & Eifert, 1990). Included in this is the evidence provided by brain stimulation procedures that produce reinforcement (Olds & Milner, 1954) *and* emotional responding (see Kolb & Wishaw, 1984).

Hayes (1993) has labeled PB as mechanistic because it does such things as specify its concept of emotion. That specification is possible, however, because PB draws upon findings that are not considered within radical behaviorism (RB). Without those sources of evidence, RB's concepts of internal events are left vague and unspecified—such as the concept of the "private event" (see Skinner, 1953). RB's methodological orthodoxy has prevented it from gathering evidence by which to support and develop its concepts that refer to inner states. Thus, RB remains mentalistic in this respect.

CONCLUSION

I believe that the work of the first two generations of behaviorists will one day be recognized for having begun one of the great science traditions. The first generation (for example, Pavlov, Thorndike, and Watson) provided the basic conditioning principles. The second generation (especially Skinner and Hull and Tolman) focused on systematizing the basic conditioning principles and made philosophical, methodological, and empirical advancements in doing so. The two generations also contained interest in extending the basic theory to human behavior (especially Skinner but also Neal Miller, John Dollard, O.H. Mowrer, and Charles Osgood). But this interest was undeveloped awaiting the third-generation development. And the first two generations of behaviorists did not provide an understanding of what psychology is as a science and what the task is of making behaviorism into a general approach to psychology. The second-generation behaviorists (like Hull, Skinner, and Tolman) each thought that his theory was a complete foundation for a grand theory. The social learning theorists also have thought that they, too, could use the animal learning theories, along with the addition of the principle of modeling, as the basic theory.

However, in the second generation of behaviorism the basic animal theories were specialized theories directed to the details of the field of animal learning-behavior. They contained much that was superfluous, and did not contain much that was needed. When the theories were employed to deal with human behavior (see Dollard & Miller, 1950; Skinner, 1953) the basic theory was reduced to the bare principle of reinforcement. The PB view has always been that both the specialized animal behavior theories, and the abbreviated versions for human application, are inadequate foundations for generally treating human behavior—the first are too cumbersome and the second too simple.

In the beginning (see Staats, 1963a) PB provided a basic theory that was much richer than were previous behaviorism applications to human behavior and its problems. Later behavior therapy works also use a more complete set of principles than did the second-generation efforts. But those principles are generally still taken from the second-generation behaviorisms, especially Skinner's. The central problem is that none of the basic learning-behavior theories was constructed with the human behavior perspective at hand. In the PB view, the basic learning-behavior theory must be systematically formulated to address the field of animal learning, but also to address the human fields for which the theory is to apply.

That view sets forth a new theory construction task. With these guidelines, for example, it becomes necessary to *distill* the work in the field of animal learning in order to construct a basic theory that includes the heavyweight principles that are significant for human behavior. Moreover, classic behavior theories lack necessary developments. The human perspective is valuable for indicating what theory developments are needed. A central example is the fact that the second-generation theories did not deal successfully with the emotion (classical conditioning) and behavior (operant conditioning) relationship. The human perspective helped indicate the importance of developing this aspect of the basic theory. It should be added, as will be indicated in the last chapter, the PB learning-behavior theory is a *basic* theory, and it has implications for the study of animal learning-behavior as well as the study of human behavior.

As the next chapter will indicate, moreover, the basic theory level does not by any means provide all the basic principles and concepts that are needed to deal with human behavior. Humans learn via the basic principles, as do species lower in the philogenetic scale. But human learning involves much more than the basic principles. Human learning involves principles and concepts that do not apply to lower animals. We can now turn to the consideration of such matters.

CHAPTER 3

The Human Learning/Cognitive Theory

Second-generation behaviorists were wrong in assuming that their principles of animal learning alone could serve as the theory with which to explain all of human behavior. That position created the cognitivism-behaviorism schism. PB's human learning theory resolves the schism by setting the task of explaining cognitive characteristics using basic behavior principles. This requires understanding of the importance of the basic principles, as well as their limitations, in the explanatory task.

To begin, the advantage of laboratory study is simplicity. Because a simple stimulus represents the environment, a simple response represents the behavior, and a simple organism is used whose past environment has been controlled, it is possible to establish elementary principles without interference by uncontrolled conditions. Those principles cannot be seen as distinctly in the complex naturalistic human situation, where the lawful working of the principles is not clear.

But, by the same token, the simple laboratory situation is artificial, distant from the human life situation. Traditional behaviorism did not take adequate account of that large separation, and the need for bridges between the basic laboratory and the complex phenomena of everyday life. The PB position, contrasting with second-generation behaviorism, states that levels of study are necessary to fill the gap. We must move from the study of the elementary principles, in artificially simple situations, to the study of *progressively* more complex human behaviors, in more and more naturalistic situations. It should be understood that when behaviorism's study went to the laboratory a number of levels of study were bypassed. So, in working back from the laboratory to natural human behavior, those levels have to be filled in.

The first level in advancing from the basic learning level is called the human learning level. The principles and concepts of this level derive from the basic level, but they, in turn, are basic to the study of human cognition, child development, and social interaction. These developments, then, will provide the structure of concepts and principles for constructing a theory of personality to use in studying more advanced levels.

COMPLEXITIES AND CONSTELLATIONS OF LEARNING

A first step in advancing the elementary principles of conditioning is simply to generalize them beyond the specific conditions in their establishment. For example, it is necessary to show that classical and operant conditioning apply to various stimuli, various responses, and to various species, including humans. There are many studies that have provided such demonstrations, and the basic principles do apply to humans. Moreover, since the principles have been isolated under the simplest of conditions, it is necessary to advance study to more complex circumstances, which involves additional concepts and principles. Actually, the general field of behaviorism includes beginnings in such studies, even though their role in behaviorism has not been clear; that is, how they can serve in a multilevel theory of human behavior.

Principles of Higher-Order Conditioning

The elementary principle of classical conditioning involves a stimulus, like food, that elicits an emotional response because the organism is biologically structured to respond in that manner. The same is true of the elementary principle of operant conditioning. But we know that humans learn emotions when no biological (unconditioned) stimulus is involved, and the same is true of operant conditioning. We need to understand how this happens.

Higher-Order Classical Conditioning

We repeatedly have the experience of reading something, or having something said to us, that elicits an emotional response—either positive or negative. Words, however, are not biologically determined unconditioned stimuli. This is true of many other emotion-eliciting stimuli. Moreover, frequently those stimuli have not gotten their emotion-eliciting characteristics from having been paired with food or some other unconditioned stimulus. By what principles does this happen? Higher-order classical conditioning is such a principle; it provides a basis for understanding that the significance of classical conditioning extends far beyond the use of biologically based unconditioned stimuli. By this principle we can begin to understand unique human learning processes.

Higher-order classical conditioning, simply defined, is when a ᶜS—a stimulus that has previously acquired emotion-eliciting properties—is used as the ᵁᶜS to produce conditioning to a new stimulus (for animal studies see Davenport, 1966; Kamil, 1969). To illustrate, let us say that the child has been abused by a father who displays a frowning countenance. The father's frown will thereby come to elicit a negative emotional response in the child. Additionally, however, any new stimulus that is paired with his frown will then come to elicit such a negative emotional response. For example, an argument that challenges the father's opinion will be followed by a frown, and thereby will produce negative conditioning. Once this higher-order conditioning has taken place the child will avoid disagreeing with the father. The basic principle is that a stimulus that has become an effective ᶜS for an emotional response can serve to produce later emotional learning. A new stimulus paired with that ᶜS will come also to elicit the emotional response.

Higher-order conditioning—although not studied intensively with animals—provides humans with an extraordinary capacity for learning emotional responses to a huge variety of stimuli. This is a type of vicarious learning, not dependent upon the occurrence of biologically significant stimuli (Staats, 1963a). Vicarious emotional learning—in its variety, ubiquity, and importance—is essentially human, a central differentiation of the species from lower animals.

As has been indicated, classical conditioning of an emotional response imparts all three functions to the new stimulus. This is also the case with higher-order classical conditioning. Thus, vicarious emotional conditioning which, as will be indicated, takes place ubiquitously through language, affects greatly what is rewarding and punishing as well as what acts as positive and negative incentives for the human.

Higher-Order Instrumental Conditioning

Higher-order conditioning traditionally was considered only for classical conditioning. Psychological behaviorism adds that there is a form of higher-order instrumental conditioning as well. The principle is as follows. When a stimulus has become a ᴰS and will elicit a particular motor response, that stimulus will transfer this function to a new stimulus with which it is paired. Let us say that the child has learned to close the door on being told "Close the door," which is to say that the word "close" has become a directive stimulus for the motor response of closing something. Let us also say that the child has never had experience with the word *shut*. If we now tell the child "Shut means close, shut means close," and then later "Shut the door," the child will do so. Pairing the two words will transfer the ᴰS power of the word "close" to the new word "shut." I conducted this very "micro-experiment" with my own child and described the principle (Staats, 1968a). Herry (1984) has since verified the principle in an important experimental study with children. This principle should be studied systematically, on both the basic and human learning levels, since it appears to be necessary for understanding an important way of learning operant behavior.

STIMULUS–RESPONSE MECHANISMS

In the march from the basic laboratory to the study of human behavior an important conception is that organisms, especially humans, learn complex combinations of stimuli and responses via conditioning principles. Moreover, those combinations—which can be called stimulus–response mechanisms—give humans certain characteristics they did not have before that learning has occurred. It is important to have concepts of such mechanisms in understanding and dealing with human behavior and human learning. As one example of a stimulus–response mechanism, humans many times learn more than one response to a stimulus situation. The situation, thus, will tend to call out the several responses. If the responses are compatible they can all occur. If the responses are incompatible only one can be made, which will be the one most strongly learned to the situation. Such a learned mechanism is called a *response hierarchy*. As an example, two children may have been given training in a response to a stimulus, but one may have in addition learned another, stronger, response to the stimulus. The two children will then respond differently to the stimulus because one child has learned the hierarchy. Human behavior involves complex arrays of stimuli and complex hierarchies of responses which, as we will see, produce individual differences in behavior.

There are various types of such mechanisms. Another involves a generally useful concept: that responses typically themselves also *produce stimuli*. So the stimulus produced by one response can serve to elicit another response, and thus be the "cause" of the second response. Such a learned stimulus–response mechanism is called a *response sequence* or *chain*. Long sequences of responses can be learned as in "memorizing" (learning) the sequence that constitutes a poem, the multiplication tables, phone numbers, chemical formulae, algebraic rules, grammatical rules, or driving a car, swinging a golf club, or doing aerobic exercises. Although individual responses may have been learned separately and have functioned in that manner, once they have been learned as a sequence they may function as a unit. Strengthening one response, then, may strengthen them all (see Staats, Staats, & Finley, 1966; Staats, Staats, & Minke, 1966).

Sequences of responses may involve different types of responses, learned via classical or operant conditioning. A stimulus may elicit an image response, whose stimulus elicits an emotional response, whose stimulus, in turn, elicits a verbal response, whose stimulus, in turn, elicits a motor response. Moreover, such sequences may be complex at each point, since the stimulus involved may tend to elicit various responses, rather than just one. Human behavior typically is composed of such complex response sequences and alternatives, and it is thus important to study the stimulus–response mechanisms involved. When we consider complex human behavior—such as reading, concept formation, memory, grammatical speech, problem solving, what constitutes intelligence and other aspects of personality, or the language and thought disturbances of schizophrenia—the concepts of this and other stimulus–response mechanisms are necessary, in addition to the basic conditioning principles.

Without recognizing that it is the operation of response chains that is involved, traditional experimental psychology has studied such phenomena as response mediation, semantic generalization, sensory pre-conditioning, transfer of training, auto-shaping, semantic conditioning, and verbal learning. Radical behaviorism has been slow in undertaking this type of study (see the topic of stimulus equivalence). Because the common principles involved in these various areas of study are not realized, as well as the significance of the study, the studies remain as unrelated works without much general meaning.

In general, behaviorism has not established the need for a general *level of study* of human learning as envisioned in PB. In the PB view the human learning level must study the stimulus–response mechanisms systematically and also study how the principles and concepts involved can be used in the analysis of more complex types of human learning and behavior. An advancing conceptual framework is proposed that moves from the basic conditioning principles to the study of more complex stimulus–response mechanisms. As this complexity is advanced it can be seen that humans learn *repertoires* of behavior. A further advancement involves the conception that the stimulus–response combinations (repertoires) can affect later learning, and study of these repertoires provides concepts of human cognitive characteristics, as will be indicated.

CUMULATIVE-HIERARCHICAL LEARNING, BASIC BEHAVIORAL REPERTOIRES, AND COGNITION

An important characteristic of human learning not evident on the animal level is the tremendous *length* of time involved and, hence, the tremendously complex repertoires that are typically produced. Furthermore, when such long-term learning is analyzed, new principles emerge that animal study does not reveal. One central principle is that complex human learning characteristically is cumulative and hierarchical in nature. The child, for example, learns a language repertoire (Staats, 1968a). This repertoire will then provide the basis for the child learning to count (see Staats, 1971a). And these repertoires will provide the basis for the child learning the number operations of adding, subtracting, multiplying, and dividing. These repertoires (and others), in turn, will be basic to learning algebra, which is requisite to learning more advanced mathematics, which is requisite to learning physics. Decades may be involved in such extended learning. *It is such repertoires that compose cognitive (mental) characteristics.*

Although the basic principles of conditioning are operative throughout, those principles alone are insufficient for understanding or dealing with such complex learning. It is necessary to understand the cumulative-hierarchical learning process. That necessitates isolation of the successive repertoires involved, for preceding repertoires are part of the *explanation* of the acquisition of later repertoires. If there is a problem in the final performance of the individual, understanding and solving the problem requires the knowledge of the cumulative-hierarchical learning process and the *content* of the repertoires involved. This is fundamental, one of the central new characteristics of psychological behaviorism, for it constitutes a new conception of how human nature develops through learning.

There has not been a meticulous, detailed, systematic study of the repertoires that yield human behavioral (cognitive) characteristics or the cumulative-hierarchical learning processes involved in acquisition. Being a reader, being algebraically sophisticated, being a scientist, being a musician, being a mechanic, being a religious person, as well as being intelligent, extroverted, schizophrenic, pedophilic, dyslexic, or depressive, and so on, all involve the cumulative-hierarchical learning of repertoires of behavior. Analysis of cumulative-hierarchical learning and the cognitive characteristics that are thereby formed has been lacking.

THE CONCEPT OF THE BASIC
BEHAVIORAL REPERTOIRE

One of the purposes of this chapter is defining the purview of the human learning level which includes study of the various complex repertoires of behavior that humans acquire in complex cumulative-hierarchical learning. This task must *describe* the basic repertoires, the *principles* by which they are acquired, and the *conditions* of learning in everyday life through which the basic repertoires are acquired. The task also demands the analysis of the principles by which the repertoires work their effects in later behavior and learning. These elements provide a definition of the *basic behavioral repertoire* (BBR) concept that is central in the present multilevel theory.

Psychological behaviorism arrived at this conception progressively, in the process of studying three types of human behavior repertoires. Study of each repertoire yielded a theory, the theory of language (see Staats, 1968a), of emotion (see Staats, 1975, chap. 4; Staats & Eifert, 1990), and of sensory-motor skills (Staats, 1963a, 1975). These three BBRs are very complex. They determine, in part, the individual's ability to learn, to experience, and to behave in the later-life situations that are encountered.

THE PSYCHOLOGICAL BEHAVIORISM THEORY OF LANGUAGE/COGNITION AND THE LANGUAGE/COGNITIVE BASIC BEHAVIORAL REPERTOIRE

Although PB's study of language began in the early 1950s, it nevertheless had new characteristics that preceding behaviorism approaches did not have. As will be indicated, PB was based on a unifying approach that attempted to deal broadly with language. In 1956 and in 1957—the same year Skinner's *Verbal Behavior* was published without any empirical foundation—articles appeared that began PB's systematic series of theoretical and *empirical* analyses of language (see Staats, 1956, 1957a, 1957b; Staats & Staats, 1957, 1958). The PB program of study led to a full theory of language (see also Staats, 1971a; 1972; 1975, chap. 5), based on its own research but also utilizing other behavioral and non-behavioral works.

The concept of the basic behavioral repertoire (BBR) arose in good part in the context of studying language behavior. The theory is that the individual's language is a huge complex BBR, important because it helps determine the individual's experiences, learning, and behavior. Learned via both classical and instrumental conditioning principles, language is not a unitary ability. Different subrepertoires can be distinguished for study, although they are learned and function in an interacting way. The following sections will briefly sketch some of these subrepertoires which together compose the individual's basic language repertoire.

The Verbal-Emotional Repertoire

The ways in which language serves as a stimulus are important, for example, in how some words elicit emotion. We have all had occasions, on reading or hearing a melancholic passage, of experiencing a negative emotional response, sometimes with watery eyes and throat constriction. We have all had the experience, also, of feeling anger or joy at something we have read or heard someone say. How can words—just visual and auditory stimuli—have that emotional function? Words have emotional properties because of classical conditioning. Beginning in infancy humans have innumerable experiences where a word will be paired with some stimulus that elicits an emotional response. Each occasion produces the conditioning of the emotion to the word. I first studied this process with a pet cat by pairing the word "No," with a light punishment (see Staats, 1968a). She came to respond appropriately to the word. I replicated the informal findings in an experiment with human subjects (Staats, Staats, & Crawford, 1962), and other investigators have repeated and extended these findings (see Maltzman, Raskin, Gould, & Johnson, 1965; Zanna, Kiesler, & Pilkonis, 1970). Beginning in infancy humans ordinarily learn a repertoire of positive and negative emotional responses to hundreds of words, the verbal-emotional repertoire.

These words may be nouns (like ice-cream, money, pain, or flu), adjectives (like nice, pretty, bad, or foul), or adverbs (like cheerfully, gracefully, disgustingly, or loudly). This repertoire of words is very important because it affects the individual's experience. That is, humans, with a large repertoire of positive or negative emotional words, can experience extremely varied emotional responses vicariously, through language. For example, we can experience the thrill of an adventure by the skillfully arranged words of a writer or storyteller. Conversely, a person who feels perfectly healthy when told by a doctor that he has terminal cancer will feel the fear and sadness of approaching death, long before that event actually arrives. Part of the unique human character is the ability to experience emotions variably and widely and vicariously, which allows us to be anticipatory, foresightful. Moreover, the emotion can be self-aroused, through self-speech.

The repertoire of emotion-eliciting words also has a great impact on the individual's learning. Because of the verbal-emotional repertoire humans can learn emotional responses to new stimuli easily and rapidly. That is, if an emotion-eliciting word is paired with a neutral stimulus, the latter will be conditioned to elicit the emotion. PB experiments have demonstrated this higher-order conditioning of emotional responses in a number of experiments (see Staats, Minke, Martin, & Higa, 1973; Staats & Staats, 1958, 1959) using its language-conditioning methods. In this method the ^{C}S is paired once each with a number of different ^{UC}S-words—like *vacation, dinner, friend, love, candy, intelligent,* and *rich.* Each of these words, while otherwise different, ordinarily elicits a positive emotional response in the hearer. The ^{C}S comes thereby to also elicit a positive emotional response. This language conditioning has been verified in a very large number of studies (see, for example, Berkowitz & Knurek, 1969; Early, 1968; Hekmat, 1972; Hekmat & Vanian, 1971; Parish, 1974; Sachs & Byrne, 1970; Tryon & Briones, 1985; Weiss & Evans, 1978). In every language there are many emotional words (see Osgood, Suci, & Tannenbaum, 1957). The verbal-emotional repertoire gives humans a unique emotional-learning capacity.

Language conditioning explains various social phenomena. As examples, the child who is told that "sex is dirty and sinful" will thereby learn a negative emotional response to sexual stimuli. Also on the negative side, many people have learned a negative emotional response to the word "abortion" through being told such things as "abortion is murder." The religiously raised child who has heard and read many positive emotional statements about God will be emotionally conditioned to this word (concept), and part of the reality of the concept of God will be given by its emotional impact. Something that is nonexistent may appear to have a reality, because we have a strong emotional response to its name.

Let me add that the language conditioning of emotion can be countermanded. Using the above example, let us say the individual on being told that "abortion is murder," says to herself "I do not believe that abortion is murder, for a new fetus is not a human being." That self-statement will allay any conditioning effect of the first message. While the principles of classical conditioning operate in language, the process is not as simple as the animal laboratory. The human experience is complex, as are its outcomes.

To conclude, the normal human learns a verbal-emotional repertoire that helps determine the individual's emotional experience and the individual's emotional learning, as well as the individual's behavior, the next topic of concern.

The Directive Function of Emotional Words

Psychological behaviorism's basic learning theory states that emotional stimuli tend to elicit approach or avoidance behavior. This holds for the elements of the verbal-emotional repertoire. A word or word combination that elicits a positive emotional response will tend to elicit approach and supportive responses; a word that elicits a negative emotional response will tend to elicit escape, avoidance, and oppositional behaviors. For example, a hungry freeway driver sees a sign up ahead that says RESTAURANT. The word elicits a positive emotional response, and the driver takes the turnoff that constitutes an approach behavior leading to the restaurant. On the negative side a person who has been conditioned to the word *abortion* because it has been paired with the word *murder* will be set up to take negative actions against clinics where abortions occur. The principle has been demonstrated in tight laboratory research (Staats & Warren, 1974).

The Reinforcing Function of Emotional Words

It is also true that any word or word combination that elicits an emotional response can also serve as a reinforcing stimulus. Let us say an individual has been working very hard and an associate says "Working like that will get you a promotion." Delivered contingent on the behavior involved, the words will act as a reinforcer and strengthen the behavior, because the words elicit a positive emotional response.

We use words frequently as reinforcers in an attempt to influence—strengthen or weaken—other individuals' behavior. The parent, for example, says to the child, "See what a mess you made—I really don't like that." If those words elicit a negative emotional response, the child will display the behavior less in the future. The words have to be in the child's verbal-emotional repertoire, however, for the parent's statement to be an effective punisher of the behavior.

It should be noted that PB in analyzing the emotional properties of language deals with cognitive phenomena. My first language-conditioning study (see Staats & Staats, 1957) addressed the cognitive psychology concepts of "word meaning" and "communication." Skinner's *Verbal Behavior* (1957) is quite different. In the present case it does not deal with the emotional functions of language, neglecting even behavioral research (for example, Cofer & Foley, 1942). It is interesting that Blakely and Schlinger (1987) and Hayes, Zettle, and Rosenfarb (1989), radical behaviorists, are now using some of PB's principles of the behavioral functions of the emotion-eliciting properties of words, as though the principles are a part of radical behaviorism. The fact is that Skinner (1975) rejected the principle that emotion and cognition could affect operant behavior.

One further point. The concept of self-reinforcement, as elaborated in the first PB work (Staats, 1963a, pp. 95–97, 315–317), is used widely today in explaining human behavior, but in an indiscriminate way, without indicating what the mechanism is. Self-reinforcement typically involves self-speech where the words elicit an emotional response. The words usually are not said contingent on any behavior—so there is no strengthening of behavior, hence no reinforcement. In such cases the function of the words is that of eliciting an emotional response. In dealing with human behavior, as in behavior therapy, it is important to employ a theory that distinguishes the several functions of emotional words, as well as the other cognitive functions of words to be treated. Only by employing an analytic theory can human behavior be understood.

The Verbal-Image Repertoire

All of us have had the experience of hearing or reading descriptions that make us "picture" or image what is being described. A description such as "jagged, granite, snow-blown peaks" elicit one composite image, and "limpid, green-blue, palm-edged lagoon" another. Why do words have this power to evoke images and thereby produce new experience and learning in us? The fundamental principles of sensory conditioning were presented in the preceding chapter to provide a basis for answering this question. To recapitulate, environmental stimuli elicit sensations, or sensory responses, in us. And these sensory responses are conditionable in the form of images. The important point here is that, for humans, through classical conditioning, images are conditioned to words, a very large number of words. The word *dog* elicits an image in us because the word has been paired with dogs. The same is true of the words *house, book, Dad, spoon, screech, stink,* and many others. (This analysis, again, makes a cognitivism/behaviorism unification.)

Once learned those words are instruments for the arousal of images as various studies have shown indirectly (see Ellson, 1941; Leuba, 1940; Phillips, 1958). For direct evidence Staats, Staats, and Heard (1961) selected words that all elicited the same general image, in one case "roundness," like *globe, hoop, ball,* and *bulb.* In the other case the words denoted "angularity," like *steeple, triangle, zigzag,* and *pyramid.* A nonsense syllable paired one time each with the first class of words was rated as more round than the nonsense syllable when it was paired with the angular words. The results indicated that the similar sensory response (image) elicited by the words was conditioned in each case to the nonsense syllable. This study indicated how new learning takes place on the basis of the verbal-image repertoire. (See also the study by Holzman & Levis, 1991.) The verbal-image repertoire is generally important because it provides the basis for important new learning and also can effect behavior.

For example, through language presentations humans can have sensory (image) experience and learn. To illustrate, most of us never see an aardvark. But we can learn that image in a rough way through reading a dictionary definition that uses words like *short and thick legs, stocky body, powerful claws, large ears like a donkey,* and *heavy tapering tail.* Humans learn a large repertoire of image words and it provides the basis for much vicarious experience. The repertoire is an essential aspect of the "human mind," that is, cognition (Staats, 1968a). Individual differences in the verbal-image repertoire produce observed individual differences in human cognitive characteristics.

In addition to nouns that elicit whole-object images, adjectives and adverbs elicit images involving only parts of objects or events. For example, the word *white* elicits a "whiteness" image because the word has been paired with many different objects that all have one common stimulus characteristic, that of being white. Once learned, the word white can be combined with other words that elicit different image responses and the result will be a combination of images. To the words *white car,* the individual will see the image of a white car, as is the case when the word *white* is combined with most nouns. In such cases the image elicited is the general image of the noun with the specific attribute of the adjective. The same analysis applies to adverbs—such as rapidly, gently, rhythmically.

Communication and joint learning occur through the verbal-image repertoire. As an example, one architect could describe an envisioned building to another in technical terms that elicit images, and the latter could react by suggesting changes, all on a verbal-image level. The same would be true of two choreographers, two artists, and two musicians (where the images are auditory). Such communication depends on specialized verbal-image repertoires shared by the people involved.

It is essential to realize that the images elicited by words can guide the individual's behavior. The soldier who imagines tomorrow's battle scene with himself being mortally wounded has a negative emotional response and goes to battle reluctantly. The individual who reads directions on how to assemble a newly purchased bicycle, with the words eliciting images of the parts in assembly position, is thereby enabled to perform the task. Moreover, the individual can be foresightful and solve problems on the basis of language-induced images—for example, the individual, who, in planning a trip, says to herself, "Let's see, the last time I was in Seattle it was also November." The image the words elicit will get her to pack a raincoat.

The Verbal-Motor Repertoire

One of the functions of language is that words can be used to elicit other people's behavior. One person asks another to go to a movie, to go to lunch, to hand over a book, to close a door, to make love, to be quiet, to go to the store and get several named items, to perform a complex dance, to hold a tennis racket and stroke the ball in a certain manner. And the other person performs the behaviors. The behavior that is verbally elicited may vary in different individuals, and sometimes compliance does not occur. But people direct one another's behavior by their words in a very specific way, rather than in the general approach–avoidance way that applies to emotion-eliciting words.

Again, we must ask, how do words get this extraordinarily important power? This depends upon the individual having acquired another type of language repertoire, the verbal-motor repertoire? The verbal-motor repertoire consists of words that elicit specific motor responses in the individual. How do we learn this repertoire? As an example, I began training my six-month-old daughter to approach me when I said, "Come to Daddy," by holding out to her an attractive object (such as a jangling ring of keys), and then by giving her the object when she approached me (by creeping forward). This fulfilled the requirements for operant conditioning, that is, a situational stimulus (what I said), the approach response, followed by a reinforcer. As other examples, a mother may say to the toddler, "Turn around" while dressing the child, guiding the child to turn. Then the mother tells the child, "Good," or "Thank you." Or, the father, after asking the child to hand him the pliers, guides the child, by pointing, to make the appropriate response, and then also reinforces the child. A child is told many verbs—such as *stand, run, walk, wash, drink, eat, lift,* and *sit*—and is led to make the appropriate response in each case. At least in the beginning, the child is usually reinforced for the action. The child, through this experience, directly learns a specific type of response under the control of a specific type of word stimulus. Each of these is a verbal-motor unit and the child will acquire a beginning repertoire of such units.

This repertoire will be expanded greatly through language. Thus, as an example, the child may be told, "Hop over the lines in the sidewalk," and the child might ask what "hop" means. The answer might be, "Jump up on one foot and come down on it." The child who has previously learned appropriate verbal-motor units to the words "jump up" and "come down on" will perform the new response. We learn a huge number of new verbal-motor units on the basis of verbal-motor units we have already learned. This takes place via the principle of higher-order operant conditioning, which is why the principle was presented in the preceding chapter—because it is so significant in human learning, if not in animal learning.

Part of the complete verbal-motor repertoire involves learning to respond motorically not only to *verbs* but also to *nouns, adjectives,* and *adverbs.* These types of words have special behavioral qualities in addition to the verb in a sentence. The verb determines what response will be made. The adverb determines variations in the response, for example, quickness or slowness. The noun determines to what stimulus the response will be made, and the adjective provides additional specification of the stimulus. The instruction to "Press rapidly the red button" will determine the particular response, the form of the response, and the particular stimulus object to which the response is made. The richer the individual's verbal-motor repertoire, the more finely can her behaviors be directed by language and the more finely she can learn new skills thereby.

Importantly, since the individual can say verbal-motor words to herself, she can thereby direct her own behavior. This analysis makes a central unification with cognitivism, showing how behavior can be *self-directed* cognitively. Self-language can also produce emotions and images via the verbal-emotional and verbal-image repertoires.

An important point in this context is the originality that takes place *through learning,* by means of the verbal-motor repertoire. That is, once the child has learned a large repertoire of verbs, nouns, adverbs, and adjectives, novel *combinations* of motor responses will be elicited when new, original instructions are encountered. Many special work skills—artistic, musical, and so on—that are considered to be creative involve special developments of the verbal-motor repertoire. For example, part of being a trained dancer is having a special verbal-motor repertoire that enables the individual to respond to original instructions of the choreographer with new sequences of responses that constitute an original dance routine. The expert dancer—because of the specially developed verbal-motor repertoire (which involves special sensory-motor development)—can learn new complex dance sequences much more quickly than the lay person. The analysis of original (creative) behavior, introduced early in psychological behaviorism (see Staats, 1956, 1963a, 1968a), involved new combinations of verbal-motor units. Recently Epstein (1991) has used some of the same concepts—for example, the combination of learned responses, richness of repertoires, and so on—in a radical behaviorism terminology, although it is not consistent with Skinner's approach. Psychological behaviorism's verbal-motor repertoire analysis (Staats, 1963a) showed how language can determine behavior in the context of such cognitive activities as problem solving and reasoning. The basic behavioral repertoire (BBR) concepts and principles provide a basis for treating the interests of cognitive psychology in an explanatory way. Many studies are needed that analyze cognitive processes in such terms.

The Speech (Verbal-Labeling) Repertoire and the PB Theory of Speech Acquisition

The several repertoires that have been described thus far refer to the manner in which language *stimuli* elicit responses in the individual. Equally important is explanation of how humans come to speak, a unique ability. Watson (1930) considered speech as conditioned responses, but Skinner (1957) elaborated this beginning analysis significantly by considering speech as an operant, with different classes of speech defined by the controlling stimuli. He called naming things *tacting;* imitative speech was called *echoic* verbal behavior; reading became *texting;* and word associations became *intraverbals.* This second-generation formulation also was incomplete in various ways. For one thing how speech is learned was not addressed. There was no analysis of how the child *learns* to speak or what the parent can do to produce speech in the child. This fundamental weakness stems from disinterest in learning; and Skinner's operant analysis cannot deal with speech acquisition because speech acquisition involves the classical conditioning/operant conditioning interaction, which his theory does not treat.

To elaborate, there are 56 sounds in the English language and the individual must have a repertoire consisting of the vocal responses that produce those sounds. This repertoire is basic in learning new words, that is, new combinations of the responses that produce the sounds. Each of us has the experience of pronouncing a new word. At first novel combinations are difficult, so the first time we pronounce the word we do so haltingly, with errors. With repetitions we learn the new word as a smooth unit.

The PB theory is that the speech repertoire is learned and that both classical conditioning and operant conditioning are involved. The learning is not a simple thing, because speech constitutes a very complex response, which involves various muscular organs such as the diaphragm, intercostal muscles, the larynx, the tongue, jaw muscles, and lips. With simple motor responses, a parent can arrange or guide the response physically—as in helping the child to hold a spoon, walk, or sit on a pottie. But the infant cannot be manipulated to make a speech response—too many organ systems are involved and most of them are unreachable. The complexity and inaccessibility also make unfeasible the use of "shaping" techniques, where the subject is progressively reinforced for making better and better approximations to the desired response.

The parents have an important role at the beginning, but it does not involve reinforcing vocal responses. For the first phase of the child's language development depends upon classical conditioning, not reinforcement (see Staats, 1968a, 1971a). This classical conditioning occurs coincidently as a by-product of caretaking, *when the parent talks to the infant while feeding, cleaning, providing warmth to, giving affection to, and playing with the child.* This coincidence of talking to and caring for the child means the parents' words are being paired with stimuli that elicit a positive emotional response in the child. Through classical conditioning the parent's words thereby become positive emotion-eliciting stimuli. When the parents' words come to elicit a positive emotional response, that makes the parents' words positive reinforcers. This is the source of reinforcement that trains the child to make vocal responses that produce sounds like the parents.

The process is that at the beginning the infant will utter a variety of vocal sounds of a "random" nature. Some of those sounds will be like those that occur in the language and many of them are not. Some of the sounds the child makes will be *similar to the sounds the parent makes in speaking.* These particular sounds that the child makes, however, will be reinforcing, because the parents' words through the classical conditioning now elicit a positive emotional response in the child. As a result, when the child happens to make a vocal response that produces a sound like that of the parent, the sound itself will be reinforcing and will strengthen that vocal response. The child is actually learning speech because the sounds produced are reinforcing stimuli. Through this self-reinforced learning the child will gradually begin to make sounds like those in the parents' language.

This process takes the child into the babbling stage (approximately six months of age). As the process is carried forward the child begins to make utterances that noticeably resemble words, and it is at this time that the parents recognize and begin reinforcing vocal responses that the child makes. What the child says is cute, and the parents are delighted with the child's progress. When the child says something like "ma-ma-ma" or "da-da, da-da" or whatever, even though the response is not perfect—or even made to the correct stimulus—the parent will respond with enthusiastic attention, an effective reinforcer. This reinforcement, from self and parent, will strengthen the child's vocalization.

The parents will also refine the sounds by repeating back a better pronunciation, rewarding the child with affection when an improved response is made. The parent will also commence to reinforce the child for saying the word in the presence of the appropriate stimulus, and through this the child will learn to say words under progressively finer stimulus control. Children first learn single words in this manner. The child is reinforced for saying approximations to such words as "milk," "cookie," "Mama," "Dada," "pottie," "bottle," "water," "no," "bye-bye," "look," "come," "all-gone," and "eat" in the presence of the appropriate stimuli. The child thus begins to learn its verbal-labeling repertoire, which consists of stimulus-controlled vocal word responses. The various stimuli, in the presence of which the appropriate word-responses are reinforced, are familiar objects or events.

The child begins in this way to acquire a verbal-labeling repertoire. Some stimuli are internal rather than external, for example, when the parent gets the child to say "pottie" (when its bowel is distended), then reinforcing the child. As a consequence of repetitions of this training the internal stimuli will come to elicit the speech response "pottie." The child will learn to label various types of internal stimuli. This will include the stimuli produced by internal emotional responses, which the child learns to label in terms of the intensity of the emotional response and whether it is positive or negative. To illustrate, when the parent consoles the child who has bumped herself, saying, "Hurt, oh, that hurts," the parent is training the child to label those negative emotional feelings with the word "hurt." When the child is eating chocolate pudding and the parent says "Good, m-m-m, good," the child learns to label that positive emotional response as "good."

The Verbal-Imitation Repertoire

The first words of the child take a long time to learn, because of the complexity of the response and the several types of learning involved. Since the child lacks imitation skills, there is thus no way to get the child to make a particular speech response. But, as the child learns to make speech responses, the child also receives experience that begins to produce a verbal-imitation repertoire. This learning occurs because the parent many times utters a sound just before the child makes a vocal response that produces the same general sound. The parent will hear the child saying "da-da-da-da-da," for example, and say, "Da-da, yes, da-da." and the child who has been making the response will say "da-da-da-da-da" again. When this occurs the parent will be pleased, express that, and this will constitute a reinforcement of an imitational response. I will not go into the extensive learning that is involved, but simply say that, through such experiences, the child will progressively acquire the repertoire—that is, will be able to repeat on command all of the sounds in the language as well as combinations of sounds in imitating new words and phrases. After the child has learned to imitate words that the parent says, speech learning can progress much more rapidly, because the parent does not have to wait for a particular verbal response to emerge in the child.

There is an acceleration in word learning when the child is about a year-and-a-half or two years of age, and PB theory attributes this to the child's acquisition of the verbal-imitation repertoire. For now the parent simply needs to say the word, while the child is attending to the object (or event) the word labels. The child repeats the word, the parent reinforces the vocal response, and the response is conditioned to the object or event. Intermittent reinforcement soon comes to suffice. The imitation behavior comes to be maintained by its function. That is, learning new words becomes reinforcing, because those new words enable the child to get desired (positive emotional) things and avoid negative things. Speaking, in general, is maintained by the reinforcement that language makes possible.

Progressively the parent can present more complex (multiword) verbal stimuli for the child to imitate and learn to the appropriate stimuli. More difficult words can be introduced, such as adjectives and adverbs that label only a part of the object (for example, the color of or number of objects). And other grammatical word classes (such as articles and prepositions) will be learned similarly and by hearing them used by parents and others. There is now abundant evidence (see Rondal, 1985) supporting the psychological behaviorism analysis that there is a progressively increasing complexity in the experience and training provided to the child by the parents (see Staats, 1971a).

As the speaking repertoire is acquired the child becomes able to interact verbally with others, children and adults, and will learn through these experiences. Most of the learning trials that occur will be informal, that is, there will be no attempt to train the child. When a father says, "Hand me the pliers, please," pointing to the tool, and the child says "pliers," while giving them to the father, the child has received training in saying a new word without any educational intent on anyone's part. In the present view, after the child's basic language repertoires are learned, it is not even necessary that the child repeat the word at time that it is heard. Simply having heard a new word in association with an object can establish the learning.

The functions of the speech repertoire are quite evident. We interact with others on the basis of speech. We make our "wants" and "feelings" evident through speech. Moreover, this repertoire in the form of self-speech is the basis for planning, reasoning, decision-making, and so on; that is, this repertoire is the basis for various cognitive abilities of the individual. The individual's self-speech may elicit emotional responses in her, or image responses. Self-speech may also elicit motor responses. More will be said of these topics. It should be understood that spoken language is essential to behaving as a normal human being. Few activities do not require that the individual have an adequate speech repertoire (or some replacement, such as sign language). When speech is absent, or distorted, the individual will suffer grave social difficulty. Moreover, individual differences in the goodness and richness of this repertoire are at the root of individual differences in human behavior and human achievement (and cognition), from normal to abnormal, as will be indicated later.

The Verbal-Association Repertoire

So far I have described the learning of speech in terms of individual word responses. Language is much more complex than that, of course. Individuals emit long sequences of individual word responses, as in conversation, giving a lecture, or in writing a book or an article. Although more is involved here than word associations, they are important. It has long been known that humans *learn* associations of words, that people differ in the associations that they have, and that associations are involved in cognitive activities. The study of word associations became a central area of study in psychology, beginning with Hermann Ebbinghaus in the 19th century (see Boring, 1950), who considered associations to be contents of the mind. Many hundreds of experiments of word association learning were conducted in early cognitive psychology. That is what happens when an experimental technique is produced, as in the case of the many studies of reinforcement schedules. Word association (verbal learning) study, in any event, produced a host of disconnected experiments (see Bindra, 1984; Deese, 1969; Gergen, 1984; Grauman & Sommer, 1984; Staats, 1983b) that now have only archival interest. What was not realized is that word associations are important, not because we can do an infinity of experiments on them, but because word associations are involved importantly in human behavior. And that is what still needs to be studied.

A guiding framework is needed for this study. It is thus suggested that word associations should be studied as they are actually learned and as they *function* in real human behavior and cognition. With respect to learning, the child first learns single-word responses. But the child will hear word combinations that will produce word association learning. And the child will also be prompted to learn associations. For example, let us say the child can say "cookie," in making a request. The parent may respond, "Cookie please," and give the cookie when the child has made the two-word utterance. This will produce the word association under control of such stimulus circumstances. As the child receives more language experience she will hear and read a huge number of sequences of words. Such experiences lead us to emit a huge number of word sequences ourselves. Through these things we learn words as associated strings.

These word associations will be functional in such things as grammatical speech, mathematics repertoires, reading, communication, problem solving, thinking, knowledge, beliefs, opinions, humor, and so on (see Staats, 1963a). Using grammar as an example, many times the child hears such statements as "The boys are playing," when more than one boy is involved, and "The boy is playing," when only one boy is involved. As a consequence the child learns a word association between the "s" at the end of the "boy" (or whatever) and the "are" (plural) form of the verb. The absence of the "s" has an association to "is" (singular) form of the verb. This is the learning basis for the child speaking grammatically with respect to such things, as well as for responding appropriately on grammar tests. "The boys are playing" comes to sound better than "The boys is playing." Whether the child speaks in a correct or an incorrect manner, we know the child's learning opportunities have produced the word associations responsible for that form.

Word associations affect content as well as form. The historian learns the word associations "The Battle of Hastings was fought in 1066." The engineer learns the word associations "r equals *i* divided by *e.*" Problems can be solved by such associations, and the problem-solving ability of the individual depends, in part, on the kinds of associations that have been learned. Psychological behaviorism (Staats, 1963a) interpreted an experiment (see Judson, Cofer, & Gelfand, 1956) to illustrate the manner in which the content of associations affects individuals' thinking and problem solving. One group of subjects learned a sequence of word associations that included "rope–pendulum–swing" and another group learned the same words, but separated by one or more nonsense syllables, in a different sequence. Then both groups were presented with a problem that demanded taking a rope, constructing a pendulum, and swinging it. The group that had learned the rope–pendulum–swing word association sequence solved the problem better than the group that had not. This word association can be said to have *mediated* the overt problem-solving behavior, and there are a number of experiments showing such mediation by implicit verbal associations (see Russell & Storms, 1956, for another example.) This work provides a model for understanding important parts of human cognitive activity. Skinner's (1966b) later concept of rule-governed behavior is an attempt to address problem-solving also, but it is vague and lacks an empirical foundation.

Repertoire Interaction in Functional Language

It is valuable to analyze language into the several repertoires. By so doing the learning of and the function of each repertoire can be seen more clearly.

But, it should be understood, the individual does not separately learn different repertoires that function independently. Rather, the learning takes place in overlapping ways, the individual's repertoires are learned in combinations, and the repertoires also function in interacting ways. To illustrate, when the child is given training in saying "dog" in the presence of a dog, the child learns an element in the verbal-labeling repertoire. At the same time, however, the word dog is also being paired with the actual dog. Since the dog elicits a sensory response in the child, the sensory response will be conditioned to the word and henceforth constitute an element in the child's verbal-image repertoire. Also if the dog elicits an emotional response in the child that emotional response will be conditioned to the word, and the child will have a new element in her verbal-emotional repertoire. The child will have learned three aspects of language in the one experience.

Moreover, language performs multiple functions. Let us say the individual has said, "Andy says this movie has exciting horse-racing scenes and is funny, and that I have to go and see it." This statement includes or will arouse elements from the verbal-labeling, verbal-association, verbal-image, verbal-emotional, and verbal-motor repertoires. The verbal repertoires can also be involved in very complex combinations that may function as units themselves; for example, a complex statement like "government of the people, by the people, and for the people." The combination of words has become a unit for many of us, and it elicits a stronger emotional stimulus than the words do singly. This unitization principle holds for all the language repertoires.

The Verbal-Emotional and Verbal-Motor Repertoires

Interaction may be illustrated further with two repertoires—the verbal-emotional and verbal-motor—to make several general points. As has been indicated, words in the verbal-emotional repertoire have strong controlling properties for approach behavior. But this control is not specific. The verbal-motor repertoire, on the other hand, is made up of words with specific controlling properties. The two language repertoires work together in eliciting the behavior of the individual. Take the following statement: "There is a valuable prize for the contest; two tickets to the Super Bowl, all expenses paid. To sign up call the athletic office, or put your name and address on a card and drop it in this box." The first sentence includes elements from the verbal-emotional repertoire; that is, words that elicit the emotional response that will activate approach behavior, but the words give no direction. The verbal-motor elements in the second sentence will elicit specific behaviors, but the control is weak. Putting the two together is necessary to produce an effective language stimulus that has strong *and* specific control.

This example has also been given because it defines what is commonly called "intention." Most people discard behavioristic explanations of human behavior because they make people into automatons. Present the stimulus and the person responds. That seems to belie our common experience, which is that we do things because of our intentions, which are experienced before we do something. That experience suggests our feelings determine our behavior. The PB analysis provides an explanation of "intentions." That is, if the individual has a strong positive emotional response to the words "Super Bowl ticket," then she has the experience of "wanting" the ticket. And that emotional response will mediate behaviors to get the ticket. In a sense the subject determines her behavior by how she feels, but that feeling itself depends upon past learning. This account behaviorizes the mentalistic concept of intention and also makes the approach cognitive.

Veridicality (Reality) and Language

Individuals' language repertoires perform many functions, in widely varying degrees of "goodness." Let us use as an example the business columnist who analyzes economic data and then writes, "World markets are glutted with manufactured goods, factory production is going to decrease, unemployment will increase, further lowering demand, stocks will fall, a depression will occur, real estate prices will decline, so this is the time to sell one's properties." The statement will elicit selling behaviors in some readers. The point here is that the reasoning sequences are not the same thing as the actual economic events the sequences describe. The reasoning sequences may or may not parallel (be isomorphic with) the actual events. And that is central. Reasoning sequences are valuable for mediating behavior appropriate to the world when they *parallel* the actual events of the world. In that case, when they occur prior to those actual events, the events are predicted. If the reasoning is awry (not parallel) then predictions will be awry. And faulty predictions can elicit behaviors that are not adjustive, that is, are not appropriate for the actual events that occur.

Human language repertoires have a central role in individual and group reasoning, communication, and perception and consequent effects on behavior. But the adjustive value of that role depends on the veridicality (truth or reality) of the language. This is true for the various language repertoires. For example, emotional words in the individual's verbal-emotional repertoire should elicit the same emotions as the actual events the words label, otherwise they are not veridical. The same is true of the verbal-image repertoire. "Words that elicit conditioned sensory responses [images] may be combined in ways that yield a composite [image] that has no real counterpart in experience. . . . [N]o one has ever experienced referents for GOD, DEVILS, FLYING SAUCERS . . ., [y]et for many people these words elicit vivid sensory responses" (Staats, 1968a, p. 50). In addition, sequences of words must parallel the events they supposedly describe, or the sequences are not veridical. Language, although correct in form, cannot serve its functions unless it is veridical. There are great differences in the veridicality of language as it is employed by different individuals and groups, and as it varies over historical, ethnic, cultural, and other variables. These differences are important in understanding individual differences in behavior, including abnormal behavior. This is also a cognitive unification.

Psycholinguistics and the PB Theory of Language

Watson (1930) considered language to be composed of learned responses. Other second-generation behaviorists made analyses or studied phenomena in the area of language. Some studies dealt with generalization that occurs between words and between words and objects (see Cofer & Foley, 1942; Russell & Storms, 1955). Dollard and Miller (1950) used such studies to consider more naturalistic forms of behavior relevant to clinical psychology. Mowrer (1952, 1954, 1960) and Osgood (1953), also working within a Hullian learning theory, attempted to deal with traditional topics of experimental psychology such as word meaning, communication, and how language includes symbolic functions such as concepts (see Hull, 1920, 1930). While these accounts employed learning principles, they were concerned more with traditional topics than with the phenomena of natural language. And they did not project the study of conditioning principles in that context. Skinner's (1957) account interpreted certain types of verbal behavior as operant behaviors. There were also those who followed the word association tradition and studied the effects of many experimental variations on learning and retaining verbal chains (see Postman, 1971; Underwood & Schulz, 1960).

Early in the 1950s linguists and psychologists of a learning orientation began an interdisciplinary effort (see Osgood & Sebeok, 1954) called *psycholinguistics*. A "Group for the Study of Verbal Behavior" was formed whose members were of various traditions, including those indicated above (with the exception of Skinner) as well as linguists, developmental psychologists interested in language, as well as the present author. The research programs of some of the group members were supported by the Office of Naval Research, as was a 1961 conference on verbal behavior (Cofer & Musgrave, 1963). This interdisciplinary phase began to break down when Chomsky (1959), a linguist, criticized and rejected Skinner's (1957) *Verbal Behavior* as though the learning-behavioral tradition was generally discredited. Skinner never answered that rejection, and neither did the other leading learning-behavior theorists of that generation. This had the effect of shutting down the incipient study of language within the learning-behavior framework. Chomsky's (1959) article was one foundation of the resurgence of cognitivism, in its opposition to behaviorism, and various psychologists whose work had been in the learning tradition became cognitivists.

As has been indicated, the PB program of research in language began in the early 1950s with interests wide enough to encompass what had been done, regardless of theory orientation. The PB view was that each approach dealt with interesting matters, but that each was incomplete and each approach contained errors as well as unusable parts. For example, in PB word associations were considered important, but not the endless studies that dealt with trivial experimental variations. The same was true with respect to mediation studies. Likewise, linguists observed important language phenomena, but left out others, and the theory was deficient. To illustrate, Chomsky's theory of language acquisition considered that the child had a human brain that was made to produce language and all the child had to do was "break the code," like a linguist would do. So language acquisition involved a rational act, not learning. Similarly, Skinner (1957) described some interesting categories of verbal behavior and said they were operant in nature, which implied that reinforcement principles played a role in their existence. But he did not analyze or study the development of verbal behavior through learning, he did not address the phenomena others had studied, and his theory was very incomplete and undeveloped. None of the approaches dealt with how language (as cognition) affects human behavior.

In the PB view, while there were individually important elements in each type of study, they were isolated from each other and competitive. A theory framework had to be constructed that could incorporate these elements so they would interrelate with each other and with the other principles and concepts of the theory. Let me give some examples. Following Chomsky's lead, psycholinguists undertook the general task of rejecting learning approaches to language. For example, Slobin (1971) described a number of phenomena in language development that were said to be unexplainable by learning. One phenomenon involved the child saying things like "Allgone shoe." The analysis stated that parents do not say such things, so children could not *learn* them. The PB view was that this assumption was made because linguists study adults speaking to each other, not parents to children. Parents do indeed say such things as "Allgone shoe"—but they say them *only to children.* The PB analysis urged linguists and psycholinguists to observe parent–child speech interactions, because adults speak differently to children than to adults, in accord with the age and competence of the child (Staats, 1971b).

Although the psycholinguists rejected the PB learning analysis of language, PB's suggestion to study the learning produced in parent–child interactions was actually followed (Ervin-Tripp, 1971). Psychological behaviorism's prediction that parents talk differently to their children than they do to adults was tested and substantiated, and the new learning/linguistic unification opened a large research field in psycholinguistics. Some years later Rondal's (1985) book acknowledged the PB role in initiating the new field of research. But, while the PB initiative in joining linguistic problems with behavioral analysis was productive, the general potential of the approach has not been used.

As another example, Slobin (1971) said that learning could not explain the fact that children first correctly say the past tense of the irregular verbs—like ran, drank, and sat—but later on begin to err by saying "ranned," "dranked," and "satted." They start adding the regular verb endings to the irregular verb forms. According to Slobin (1971), this proved that the child did not *learn* her grammar, because his view was that the learning process only progresses from incorrect responding to correct responding, not in the reverse.

The problem, of course, arises from a simplistic definition of learning. The PB analysis, in contrast, was that in the historical development of our language the irregular verb forms have been shortened, because those verbs are so commonly used. Because they are the most used verbs their irregular past tense forms are the first learned to the past-tense stimulus situation. Later, when a number of regular verbs are introduced, the child has accumulating experience with them. Their ending, *-ed*, is always the same, and the repetitions make the *-ed* response strongly elicited by the past-tense situation. Later, when a situation elicits the past-tense irregular verb, it also elicits the *-ed* verbal response. So both responses occur together, producing the incorrect combination of irregular verb with regular ending. It takes further training before the child learns not to add the regular ending. What this illustrates—and this has implications for the study of all cognitive processes—is that to understand the child's language development one must be prepared to make a detailed analysis of the complex behavior and learning involved. The importance of learning for cognition cannot be seen via oversimplified analyses using commonsense concepts. The PB analysis of this particular phenomenon of learning past-tense verbs has also been supported recently by David Rummelhart in the context of neural network computer models (see Peterson, 1993, p. 141; Tryon, 1995). Again, however, the potential of the PB theory of language for analyzing cognition is being overlooked.

A third example of the value of PB's behaviorizing of cognitive (linguistic) phenomena is the psycholinguistic study of the child's ability to pluralize nouns. This was originally described as a cognitive development that takes place with age, yielding a mental "grammatical rule" (Brown & Fraser, 1961). As an example in English, words that end in an unvoiced consonant are made plural by adding the unvoiced sibilant sound (the hissing *s* sound), as in pronouncing *picks, pats,* and *mops.* In contrast, when a noun ends in a voiced consonant it is pluralized by adding the voiced consonant (the *z* sound) as in *pigs, pads,* and *mobs.* The PB analysis (see Staats, 1963a, pp. 177–178) stated rather than biological maturation of the mind, the child's "grammatical rule" consisted of learned word associations—those between the voiced consonant and the voiced sibilant responses and the unvoiced consonant and the unvoiced sibilant responses. Although Skinner did not analyze such topics, this PB theory of the grammatical pluralization "rule" was substantiated in a series of studies conducted by behavior analysts (Guess, 1969; Guess, Sailor, Ruthersford, & Baer, 1968; Sailor, 1971; Sailor & Tamar, 1972). (Since these researchers were radical behaviorists they also did not utilize PB's general position, that linguistic-cognitive knowledge should be generally subjected to PB behavioral analysis.)

Grammatical speech generally involves hordes of complex and subtle word associations. Such associations guarantee that the individual's speech follows the patterns established by the language community. An individual who has not learned those associations, or who has different associations than are customary, will speak differently (ungrammatically). It is in the context of such important aspects of language, as these examples treat, that word associations should be systematically studied.

With this as background, it is possible to characterize further the PB approach to language. The position is that there are various groups who study language and cognitive phenomena. This generally takes place with each group interested in its own phenomena, and theories and methods, and not in others. In fact, the formulations of the different groups are in competition. The end result is a divided field, chaotic pieces of unrelated knowledge, and a plethora of antagonistic endeavors. No general theory of language centrally has unified the cognitive and behavioral positions.

Psychological behaviorism's position is that this makes for ineffective science. Use of an overarching theory would yield great productivity. PB was constructed to be a comprehensive framework theory of language. Its program in this area was to incorporate relevant findings from various approaches within its principles. Examination of the PB theory of language indicates that this has been done, such that the diverse and conflicting principles, concepts, phenomena, and methods of the various approaches are represented, by employing an overarching theory that makes these elements complementary and unified. The general suggestion is that the PB theory is capable of generally integrating cognitive study within its framework, in a manner that is heuristic, theoretically and empirically. The potential of such unification suggests a general program of research.

Cognition and Intrapersonal (Self-) Speech

Let us now turn more generally to personal language (or intrapersonal or self-language). We all have had the experience of talking to ourselves. And we all know that what we say to ourselves is part of what we call processing, thinking, reasoning, planning, deciding, judging, and perceiving—and that these activities affect what we feel and what we do. The tradition of cognitive psychology is the study of the processing and the contents of that processing. The cognitivism/behaviorism schism began with Watson's rejection of cognitive concepts and cognitive study. Skinner followed that tradition, but strangely enough introduced the same type of concept, that of "private events," seemingly to suggest there was a behavioral explanation to be found in his theory of mental events. But Skinner never specified what private events are, never studied them, or indicated how they could be studied. And he did not consider them to be determinants of behavior. The concept of private events, thus, is useful for debate, but not for science.

The same type of prejudice exists on the cognitive side. Anything that is labeled behavioristic is rejected out of hand by many cognitive psychologists. Cognitive psychologists have not been interested in analyses of mental processes as response and stimulus processes. In the present view this stance contributes also to the separation of behaviorism and cognitivism. Psychological behaviorism offers a program for constructing a bridge between these opposing traditions.

There are various ways to study objectively behavioral processes that occur within the person. A primary way is to train some subjects to particular responses or repertoires that the other subjects do not have. Differences in overt behavior between the two groups then can specify the action of the responses or repertoires. The present theoretical position is that all of the cognitive characteristics that humans have—and that are studied by cognitive psychologists—are composed of the types of basic behavioral repertoires being described. The "characteristics of the mind" that cognitive psychologists study are not givens—genetic gifts of humanness—they are learned. The human is an organism who can profit from that learning experience, but does not have human cognitive characteristics without that human learning experience. We need a great deal of study in the analysis of human cognitive behavior repertoires—applied as well as laboratory samples. However, the concepts of the language repertoires that have been described have, and can be, used to analyze "the working of the human mind." The schism between cognitivism and behaviorism can and should be resolved, not by treaty but by additional research and theory. When this is done psychology will make a huge step forward as a coherent, unified science.

Rule-Governed Behavior

Skinner (1957) does not indicate how verbal behavior *functions* in affecting the individual's behavior. For example, Skinner (1957) presents the concept of *intraverbals* (more usually called word associations), but he does not indicate how single words or intraverbals can mediate overt behavior. Without using the concept of how one behavior can elicit another, his position lacks the means by which to understand the concepts of cognitive psychology. A very central aspect of his theory is that his categories of verbal behavior are never considered in terms of (1) individual differences or (2) as causes of other behaviors of the individual.

In contrast, the PB theory of language indicates, for each of its language repertoires, how the repertoire can determine overt behavior—a characteristic that makes it suitable for unification with cognitive psychology. For example, in the PB treatment of purpose the individual's verbal-labeling and verbal-association repertoires constitute the "purpose" mechanism, as they mediate other behaviors (see Staats, 1963b). Skinner (1957) at first did not deal with such phenomena, and when he did (Skinner, 1966b) he attempted to channel the analysis into his reinforcement framework, in proposing his concept of rule-governed behavior. A rule is a contingency-specifying verbal statement, such as "If you do this, you will get that," indicating a behavior and a reinforcement contingency. The idea is that the individual behaves to the rule as she would if her behavior were directly reinforced.

It is revealing that there is disagreement among various behavior analysts (Blakely & Schlinger, 1987; Brownstein & Shull, 1985; Catania, 1989; Glenn, 1987, 1989; Hayes, 1986; Hayes & Hayes, 1989; Parrott, 1987; Schlinger, 1990; Schlinger & Blakely, 1987; Vargas, 1988; Vaughan, 1987, 1989) concerning just what rule-governing entails (see Burns & Staats, 1991). The problem arises because the concept of rule-governed behavior is vague and deficient. Why a rule affects behavior is not stipulated. So, we must ask, why should a *statement* of contingency have the same effect as the contingency? It could be said that the reason the rule is effective is because the individual in the past has been reinforced for behaving the same to the rule statement as to the actual contingency. But this definition makes the "rule" the same as any discriminative stimulus; so no new term is needed. Moreover, such a definition would not indicate why the individual would respond appropriately the *first time* a rule statement is presented. Centrally, however, there is no evidence showing rules are discriminative stimuli. (The weakest part of Skinner's theory of language is that twenty-seven years after its publication radical behaviorists admitted that it had produced no research. See MacPherson, Bonem, Green, & Osborne, 1984).

The PB position is that words do not affect behavior because they state a "rule" of environmental reinforcement for some behavior. Words affect the individual's behavior if the individual has previously learned the necessary language repertoires. An example was given above of instructions for signing up to win tickets to the Super Bowl. It was said that whether this statement elicited the behavior depended on the nature of the individual's verbal-emotional and verbal-motor repertoires. This is generally the case. It is after having learned the various language repertoires, that the individual is prepared to respond widely to language. Then, words can be put together in new combinations and elicit new combinations of behavior. The individual can experience emotions and images and word associations on the basis of language, and these, in turn, can affect overt behavior. Moreover, the PB concepts and principles are not vague; they are backed up by empirical demonstration, and they suggest new types of empirical investigation. Behavior analysts should abandon the very weak conception of rule-governed behavior and avail themselves of a detailed theory of language that addresses specifically the effects of language on behavior.

The PB Theory of Language and Unified Theory

As has been indicated, the PB theory of language is a unified theory in the sense that it incorporates concepts, principles, and findings from diverse works. It is also unified in another sense. As will be developed further, the theory of language is the basis for consideration of other aspects of human behavior, in child development, social interaction, personality, personality measurement, abnormal behavior, and clinical treatment. There is no other theory of language that is developed from the basic to human learning level of study and on to the consideration of advanced levels of study.

ADDITIONS TO THE PB THEORY OF HUMAN EMOTION-MOTIVATION: THE EMOTIONAL-MOTIVATIONAL REPERTOIRE

The PB theory of emotion-motivation has multiple levels (Staats, 1975, chaps. 4, 15; Staats & Eifert, 1990). So far, the biological and basic conditioning levels of study have been outlined. (Lang's [1995] theory of emotion contains concepts and principles on these levels that are much the same.) In addition, however, those principles must be elaborated at the human learning level of study, the next topic. And, as later chapters will indicate, these several basic levels will provide the foundations for personality, personality measurement, abnormal psychology, and clinical psychology developments in the theory of emotion-motivation.

Theory and Human Research on Basic Principles

Actually the concept of motivation differs at the human and animal levels. Deprivation, for example, is central at the animal level. But the principle is left out in theories of human motivation or is changed. As an example of the latter, Maslow (1954) proposed that humans have a hierarchy of "needs," where the most basic need must be satisfied before the next is activated. Another approach is to list the areas of human need with vague explanations for their existence (Murray, 1938, pp. 127–128). A number of other terms, such as values, have been introduced as motivation concepts (see, for example, Cuber, 1955). Generally there is little linking of the animal and human levels of study. The term "motivated" is not defined clearly, seeming to involve cataloging what the individual likes or dislikes, or what the individual will strive for or try to avoid.

Psychological behaviorism takes the position that animal behavior principles are basic and that these principles must be elaborated in additional levels of study, beginning with the human learning level. This level was the beginning focus of the PB theory. Its basic study of emotion-motivation used a "human preparation," that is, a type of emotional stimulus sensitive to deprivation–satiation manipulations in humans. This was based on the PB analysis of language, which revealed that humans' ordinary language experience produces classes of emotional stimuli. For example, our experience repeatedly involves the pairing of food with food words. This should result in the "human preparation," where food words become conditioned stimuli that elicit a positive emotional response.

On the animal level Finch (1938) showed that for dogs deprived of food, both the ^{UC}S and ^{C}S more strongly elicited the salivary (and general emotional) response. If food words are stimuli that reliably elicit an emotional response then food words can be used to test the principles of motivation with human subjects. For example, if food words elicit a positive emotional response, then subjects who are deprived of food should have a stronger emotional response to food words than non-deprived subjects. A first study was conducted to validate the "human preparation." One group of subjects did not eat for 15 hours prior to the experiment, while the other group ate within an hour of the experiment. Food words mixed with non-food words were presented one at a time to the subjects, and the extent of their salivary response was measured in each case to .001 gram accuracy (Staats & Hammond, 1972). The results showed with human subjects that deprivation increased salivation to food words, a ^{C}S.

In three-function learning theory, a ^{C}S should also be a reinforcing stimulus. Thus, food words should function as stronger reinforcing stimuli for food-deprived versus non-deprived subjects. Harms and Staats (1978) showed this to be the case where a food word was presented to subjects contingent on making a motor response and a non-food word was contingent on making another motor response. Subjects deprived of food learned the food-word-reinforced response more than did non-deprived subjects.

Finally, another study tested the effect of deprivation–satiation on the third function that positive emotional stimuli have, that of serving as a

directive stimulus for approach behavior. It was expected that food deprivation would make food words stronger directive stimuli for approach
responding. Either food words or non-food words were presented to subjects who had to learn to make an approach response to one and an avoidance response to the other. The rapidity of responding was timed to the
thousandth of a second. Food-deprived subjects learned the approach
response to the food words more rapidly than the non-deprived subjects.
Subjects, on the other hand, who had to learn an avoidance response to the
food words did so more slowly if they had been deprived of food than subjects
who had not. Both results showed that deprivation increased the strength with
which food words elicited approach behavior (Staats & Warren, 1974).

Thus, PB's basic principles of motivation were formulated in the context of laboratory experiments with human subjects. Deprivation of food
does increase the emotion-eliciting, reinforcing, and directive value of a
class of stimuli that has been paired with foods. It should be noted that
animal study, when dealing with deprivation–satiation, employs primary
stimuli—such as food, water, and sex. Animal study does not deal very well
with how deprivation–satiation operations affect the strength of learned
reinforcers or directive stimuli. These principles, thus, have not been available for extension to human behavior. Psychological behaviorism provides
the basic principles and supporting evidence that animal learning study
has lacked.

Classes of Human Emotional-Motivational Stimuli

Those basic principles should be studied in a programmatic manner on the
animal level. But additional development at the human level of study is
needed also for a general theory of human emotion-motivation. For example,
food words are uniquely human stimuli and it is important to demonstrate
that deprivation of a primary stimulus (food) affects them. (For example, how
would anorexics respond?) The study, however, raises the question of whether
other primary deprivations would affect other classes of word stimuli. For
example, if a person was deprived of sexual contact, would sexual words
become stronger emotion-eliciting stimuli, stronger reinforcers, and stronger
directive stimuli for approach behavior? That expectation of PB theory
raises other implications (and studies), as will be indicated.

Humans Unique in Number of Motivational Stimuli

More generally, we need to consider *what classes of stimuli can be involved in
human motivation.* The fact is that humans are unique in the great quantity
of stimuli that for them have emotional (and hence reinforcing and directive) power. This is such an important part of being human, no other animal comes close with respect to sheer number of emotion-eliciting stimuli.

Moreover, there are such huge differences in people, both individuals and groups, in *what* stimuli are motivational, positive or negative, and what stimuli are not; that is, what will elicit an emotional response, what will have rewarding or punishing effects on behavior, and what will be positive or negative incentives (that is, will attract or repel behavior)?

There are differences in the particular stimuli that are involved, and there are differences in the number of such stimuli. There are differences in the intensity of the emotional response. And there are differences in *relative* intensity also. For example, two individuals could have positive emotional responses of equal intensities to movies, but one of the individuals could have an even stronger positive emotional response to symphonies and operas. This *relative* difference in strength will produce differences in the behavior of the two individuals, the former going to the movies more than the latter, who will divide time between movies and classical music events.

In this theory of emotion-motivation, normal humans learn a vast quantity of emotional stimuli, which can be called affective-reinforcing-directive (ARD) stimuli, or emotional-motivational stimuli. Part of the task of understanding human behavior involves understanding the emotional-motivational stimuli that are operative, for these stimuli, in an important way will determine that behavior. To illustrate, the individual who has a very positive emotional response to movies will, other things being equal, spend time watching movies and expend money in that pursuit, for such behavior will be reinforced. The person who has very positive emotional responses to symphony music stimuli, on the other hand, will have the same behavior controlled by that class of stimuli. A determinant of the human's behavior thus is the positive emotional response that has been learned. We thus need a systematic study of the major types of affective-reinforcing-directive stimuli that function for humans. Some of the types of ARD stimuli may be indicated briefly here.

Biologically Based Emotional-Motivational Stimuli

Contemporary belief is that individuals' preferences are largely biologically determined, certainly for stimuli like food and sex whose biological significance is clear. We can see this orientation in contemporary beliefs about homosexuality, that the individual's sexual attractions are explained by some biological mechanism, as yet unfound, but sought in many research efforts. The inevitability of biologically determined homosexuality can be seen in the common view expressed by a popular columnist. "You did not choose to be gay any more than I chose to be straight . . . and whether you act on your feelings or not, you are a homosexual" (Van Buren, 1980, p. B3).

The PB theory of motivation takes a different position, which can be described, using food as an example. The infant has biological structures in the sensory organs of taste and smell, whose stimulation will elicit a positive or negative emotional response. Most everyone starts out approximately equal in terms of biological response to food stimuli. But learning will later produce very large differences in food preference. Some tastes and smells will come to be positive for some ethnic groups, but not for others. Other stimuli—visual (like color, shape, and size) and tactile (like crispness, softness, firmness)—will come also to elicit a positive emotional response (including salivation). The differences in what food stimuli elicit positive and negative emotional responses will dictate "food behavior," what foods are purchased, what foods are prepared, what restaurants are patronized, and what TV food programs are watched. Learned food motivations are long-lasting, resistant to change.

Is sexual choice any different? There is not good evidence to the contrary. Although differences could be expected in terms of the intensity of sexual emotional responding as well as cultural views of sexual preference, the fact is humans learn the things to which they respond emotionally—even in the cases where a primary (biological) stimulus is involved. Although the basic stimulation that will elicit sexual emotional responses on a purely biological basis is limited, the stimuli that through learning can come to elicit such emotional responding appears to be tremendously variable. Visual, auditory, tactile, gustatory, and olfactory stimuli can become sex emotion arousers, virtually anything for different people. Even stimuli that basically are antagonistic to sexual arousal—such as painful stimulation—can come through complex learning conditions to have sexual emotional properties. Since a large class of emotional stimuli are of a sexual nature, and these stimuli have a heavy influence on behavior, understanding how the stimuli *come* to be that way and how they *work* is important. Let me add here that sexual words also have motivational characteristics. To illustrate, pornography can elicit easily measured physiological sexual responses, serve a reinforcing function (in maintaining reading), as well as elicit overt sexual behavior (as in practicing what has been read).

Let me only add here that the categories that have been described—food and sexual stimuli—include much more than might be commonly considered as such. For example, the names of foods, pictures of food, descriptions of food, and so on, would be included in that category. This has been shown very clearly in the series of studies involving food words that has already been described. What this means is that there are a very large number of learned stimuli in the food category, and the same applies to the sexual category.

Language Classes of Emotional-Motivational Stimuli

A principle of the present theory is that when any stimulus has positive or negative emotional value, the word denoting that stimulus will also elicit a similar (but less strong) conditioned emotional response. For this reason in every language there are hundreds of words that have positive or negative emotional value (see work on word meaning, Snider & Osgood, 1969). There are various *classes* of actual stimuli, and words denoting those stimuli, that have important motivational functions. For example, there is a class of religious stimuli, which for the religious person are very large in number. There are material objects, such as buildings and the many parts of buildings (such as stained-glass windows), the garb and accoutrement of religious personnel, religious symbols, icons, jewelry, art works, and other paraphernalia, as well as real and conceptualized religious figures. In addition, there are rituals, music, customs, and holidays. And, most of all, there are religious language stimuli in the form of stories, preachings, conceptual positions, and so on, of great complexity and range. Through a complex learning history that extends over many years an individual can acquire positive (or negative, in some cases) emotional responses to this huge complex of stimuli, in various levels of intensity. This aspect of the individual's emotional-motivational system can have a heavy influence on the behavior the individual displays. Those with strong positive emotional response to religious stimuli are reinforced by such stimuli and have strong approach behaviors to such stimuli. The result is much religious behavior. The behavior, in turn, results in having additional religious experiences and consequent learning of various kinds.

It is important to indicate that there is no specific primary (biological) stimuli involved for religious words, as there is in the case of food words or sex words. So no biological deprivation can be involved. That raises interesting basic questions. For example, would the person with positive emotional responses to religious stimuli be affected motivationally by deprivation of those religious stimuli? Would deprivation increase the extent to which religious stimuli would become stronger emotion-elicitors, stronger reinforcers, and stronger directive stimuli? PB research (Staats & Burns, 1982) shows that religious words have incentive functions, and Staats, Gross, Guay, and Carlson (1973) have shown the three functions with words relevant to work preferences. There are many classes of non-biologically based emotional stimuli and they affect behavior in many ways. But there have been no studies of possible deprivation effects, although this is fundamental in constructing a theory of human motivation.

Additional Classes of Emotional-Motivational Stimuli

Recreations provide another class of numerous and variable ARD stimuli. Reading, for example, provides an endless fund of positive emotional-motivational stimuli for some, and many spend thousands of hours in that behavior. Athletic participation can provide an abundant source also of positive ARD stimuli. Movies, plays, art exhibitions, concerts, parties, television, viewing athletic contests, lectures, gardening, and on and on, constitute recreational stimuli that elicit positive emotional responses in some people. It is important to realize that in each case there are many stimuli that are involved. Individuals who surf have a positive emotional response to many stimuli that are associated with the sport; to the ocean, states of the ocean, the weather, the view of land from the sea, the crisp clean sensations, the feeling of robustness and well-being, as well as the variable thrills from the rides. All of the equipment involved, people who participate and compete in the sport, stories, movies, and television about the sport, knowledge about the sport, and on and on, will have positive emotional-motivational value. The same is true of the person who is a gardener, tennis player, music buff, or movie fan.

Another important class of ARD stimuli is constituted by people. As is well recognized, the emotional "investment" in our loved ones plays a central role in human behavior, mothers, fathers, husbands, wives, children, siblings, grandparents, cousins, nieces and nephews, friends, business associates, acquaintances, community, national, and international leaders, movie stars, and so on. In addition to particular individuals we learn emotional responses to aspects of people, that is, their physical and behavioral characteristics. To illustrate, a child may learn a positive emotional response to beards, or to a deep and hearty voice, or to quick movements through having a father with those characteristics who is many times paired with positive emotional experiences. That emotional conditioning will generalize; other men with a beard or a hearty voice or quick movements will thereby elicit a positive emotional response in that child that will remain in adult life. People have many different physical and behavioral characteristics and we learn emotional responses to many of them. Individuals can differ greatly in the breadth and depth of the emotional responses they have for people and for the different behavioral characteristics that people have.

Another class of ARD stimuli may be called economic. Money is perhaps the most general of these stimuli, serving as a good example because we can easily see how a suitable amount of money elicits a positive emotional response, attracts behaviors that approach (gain) the money, and strengthens behaviors that are followed by the receipt of money (such as working). Money has these ARD functions in such strength, however, because it can be exchanged for (is paired with) all kinds of different material goods and services. There are vast numbers of such goods and services, and they can all be positive emotional-motivational stimuli for some individuals. Some of the principles of economics very much coincide with this analysis, as I have indicated previously (Staats, 1963a, 1975). For example, the basic law of diminishing utility (supply and demand) states that the more one has of some commodity the less satisfaction an additional unit of that commodity will bring. This is actually a paraphrase of the principles relating deprivation–satiation to the ARD functions of a stimulus (see Staats, 1963b, p. 309; 1975, p. 497). In our terms the economic principle would be that the more one has of something (the more one is satiated on something) the weaker become the ARD functions of that something.

Cognition and Motivation

Having described language stimuli that have motivational functions, this provides a basis for considering cognition and motivation. And this brings us to the final category, those aspects of the individual's emotional-motivational system that are "cognitive" in nature. I have said that words as units can be emotion-eliciting stimuli. But we know that the individual's "cognitive" nature consists of more than a compendium of the positive or negative emotional words the individual has learned. The individual learns complexes of organized language that refer to complex objects (such as institutions, countries, corporations), people, behaviors, actions (such as wars and legislative decisions), and events (such as AIDS and earthquakes). These complexes of words with respect to such things may be called values, beliefs, opinions, ideas, knowledge, worldviews, themes, or schemas. In the present terms they constitute statements that elicit emotional responses and hence serve as incentives and reinforcers. For humans such "systems of thought" will cover many occurrences in life and help determine the individual's emotional response to those occurrences. As examples, different individuals will have different emotional responses to the welfare system, abortions, school lunches, the right to possess firearms, protecting whales, progressive taxation, legalizing drugs, disarmament, war in general, the economic blockade of Cuba, particular wars, labor strikes, street people, mandatory AIDS testing, gay marriage, economic protectionism against foreign imports, men doing housework, prayer in the schools, women's rights, evolution, themselves, and many others. People have different ideas (complexes of verbal statements) with respect to such occurrences.

The emotional response elicited by the language is part of how the individual experiences the things denoted by the language and how the individual thus responds to those things. An individual who has extensive language experience concerning the evils of war will respond emotionally to the outbreak of a war in a different manner than a person whose language experience has been of a patriotic nature concentrating on the nobility and heroism of war. And their overt behavior will be affected by this motivational difference.

It is important to recognize that the emotionality of the individual's cognitive constellation will determine what the individual approaches and avoids. The "liberal" subscribes to and reads different things than the "conservative" (see Staats, Gross, Guay, & Carlson, 1973), because each has an extensive language-emotional complex with respect to the positions espoused by liberal and conservative media. And, as will be indicated further, the differences in such choices will, in turn, affect the individual, for each will learn language-cognitive things as well as emotional-motivational things from the reading. The "cognitive-emotional nature" of the individual is thus a most important determinant of the individual's behavior.

Environmental Conditions That Affect Emotional-Motivational Differences

Emotional-motivational differences have been called various things—values, attitudes, interests, needs, satisfactions, preferences, fetishes, goals, desires, and so on, as well as fears, phobias, anxieties, stresses, pressures, and the like. We recognize there are wide individual differences with respect to such things. The suggestion that they are learned raises the question of the environments involved. This should become a topic of systematic concern. Here it is relevant to indicate that human experience can differ along a variety of different lines. There are huge cultural differences, ranging from peoples living in the limitations of a stone-age culture (in some places in New Guinea, the Amazon, and the Philippines) to peoples who have access to the cultural achievements of humans from the stone-age to the present. There are many different cultures and being raised in one imparts certain emotional learning to the child. There are different national groups, religious groups, social class groups, occupational groups, socioeconomic groups, peer groups, neighborhood groups, political groups, recreational groups, gender groups, familial groups, and the like. And each passes many emotional-conditioning experiences to its members. Within a particular industrialized society there are many institutions, educational, judicial, artistic and cultural, welfare, penal, and journalistic, each with variations, and each of which provides experiences to those who in some way contact the particular institution. A large society potentially provides an unlimited number of different experiences, and each individual experiences only a small subset. The individual's emotional-motivational repertoire is formed through exposure to the particular subset of experiences encountered.

The Learning of Emotional-Motivational Stimuli

The principles involved in learning new emotional-motivational stimuli are always the same, that is, the principles of classical conditioning. In the laboratory the procedures are simple. But for humans emotional conditioning circumstances are much more complex, subtle, and evanescent. A fleeting smile or a surprised or puzzled look may elicit a positive or negative emotional response, which will be conditioned to other stimuli in the situation.

The sight of someone in pain can elicit a negative emotional response that will be conditioned to associated stimuli (Berger, 1962). An emotional response can be conditioned to someone or their actions by a subtle statement with implications that elicit an emotional response (see Berkowitz & Knurek, 1969; Early, 1968). A preacher's sermon, a propagandist's statement, a parent's lecture, an editorial writer's article, a government spokesman's release, a friend's opinions, may involve complex and subtle emotion-eliciting stimuli that effectively condition the listener to new stimuli. Such conditioning occurs each day in many ways, and we are unconscious in many cases of what has happened (Staats, 1969). Later, the conditioning may persist although we no longer remember the specific words and particular occasion when the conditioning took place. As an example, an individual raised in an Afrikaner community in South Africa could not remember the many times she had experienced the word *kafir* paired with a word that elicits a negative emotional response (such as *stupid, promiscuous, lazy, untrustworthy,* or *dangerous*), but the negative emotional response that has been learned will be strong and long-lasting, even more resistant to change because there is no way of remembering (and then countering) the conditioning circumstances that produced the emotion.

Psychological behaviorism's central inclusion of the classical conditioning of emotional responses in the explanation of human behavior creates a very different behaviorism from Skinner's radical behaviorism. This difference is enhanced because PB indicates *there are various ways by which classical conditioning can occur, including that which occurs through language.* We cannot understand human behavior well until we understand the ways that new emotions can be formed vicariously, through language-cognitive conditioning. The verbal-emotional repertoire, with its many emotional words, provides a mechanism by which new emotional-motivational stimuli can be learned ubiquitously and easily. The individual's language-cognition constitutes an important part of the emotional-motivational repertoire as well as a mechanism for additional learning.

Concept of the Emotional-Motivational BBR

Let me introduce the concept that each human—primarily through learning—acquires a very large "system" of stimuli that will elicit an emotional response, and will also serve as reinforcing and directive stimuli. This system is called a basic behavioral repertoire (BBR), for it affects the individual's experience, learning, and behavior in the life situations that are encountered. Since the emotional-motivational repertoire explains so much of human behavior, it is essential that a theory of personality formulate the principles involved. This must be done explicitly, in an empirically stipulated manner. Human motivation theories have lacked those qualities.

Additional analyses will further develop the theory of emotion-motivation and its relevance for personality.

BASIC THEORY OF BEHAVIOR AND
THE SENSORY-MOTOR REPERTOIRE

In life, we do not experience another person's thoughts, ideas, or emotions. Those occur inside, inaccessible to ordinary observation. We may infer cognitive and emotional states, make judgments of character and personality, but it is behavior that we observe or contact, what the individual does and says. When we see a person cry, that is what we observe—we only infer that the individual is sad. When we say a person is aggressive, dependent, athletic, gifted musically, artistic, mechanically inclined, a passionate lover, a protective mother, brutal, timid, or whatever, we are referring to the behavior displayed. That realization guides us to examine how people differ behaviorally and how those differences are learned. So far, theories of the language-cognitive and emotional-motivational BBRs have been presented. It now remains to present the PB approach to behavior, that is, the sensory-motor basic behavioral repertoires of which behavior is composed.

Just as with the language-cognitive and emotional-motivational repertoires, humans also have sensory-motor repertoires of different types. Let me take a straightforward example, vocational occupation—which involves wide differences in sensory-motor skills. We can see that easily in plumbers, electricians, lifeguards, professional athletes, doctors, engineers, chemists, dentists, musicians, artists, dancers, and actors. With respect to physicians, skills ranging from drawing blood to diagnosing slides of pathological tissue constitute sensory-motor skills. Long-term, complex training is necessary to produce the sensory-motor skills that are involved in a vocation.

There are sensory-motor skills of a recreational nature. Individuals, to differing degrees, can do such things as knit, play tennis, hike, bowl, scuba dive, dance, garden, cook, hunt kangaroo, skin crocodiles, spear fish, and repair and rebuild cars. It is interesting that there are anthropologists who consider tool use, and the anatomy of the hand for this purpose, to be central factors in human evolution (see Aiello, 1994). The sensory-motor skills involved in recreations may also require extensive cumulative-hierarchical learning. Such developments ordinarily have various by-products that affect the individual generally. The person who has high-level skill in tennis, for example, will be sought after by friends to play, will be in better physical shape than if sedentary, will receive social approval of various types, will have a "self-concept" that is influenced by such experiences, and will acquire generally an emotional-motivational system that includes positive emotional response to many stimuli in the world that non-players do not have.

There are also sensory-motor skills involved in the mechanics of living. Men usually acquire a repertoire of skills involving repairing things. Women usually acquire a repertoire of household- and baby-care skills. (These differences have been changing.) People also learn sensory-motor skills concerned with self-care, grooming and cleaning, with transportation (by car, bus, etc.). There are sensory-motor skills involved in such things as operating televisions and VCRs, household appliances, computers, and bicycles. We take these for granted, but people without that learning will lack the skills. Prejudiced people sometimes complain about public housing, on the grounds that poor socioeconomic classes of people do not know what to do with modern conveniences and will quickly turn a modern apartment into the hovels to which they are accustomed. The point here is that living in a modern society demands many sensory-motor skills that are learned informally. Even though not every individual in our society will receive the necessary experience, anyone without them will be perceived as disabled. In the present view what is involved is simply a matter of learning (although that learning may not be so simple)—a society that desires certain sensory-motor skills in its members has to provide the opportunity for learning those skills.

The above examples include sensory-motor skills on which there are sex differences. This point may be given emphasis here by indicating that there are differences in the sensory-motor skills that groups acquire, including the groups that are formed by gender. Such differences may change over different cultures and over time, but there typically are differences. In our society, men have different ways of speaking, of gesturing, of moving, sitting, and so on, than do women. We sensitively detect when a man displays the sensory-motor skills that are common to women, and vice versa. There are also sensory-motor skills involved in love-making for men and women which are of some moment. Some of the skills of being a good lover are of a sensory-motor nature. There are differences here within each group and between the groups. There are sensory-motor skills involved in responding to other people of various kinds. For example, there are the skills of caring for a baby, being affectionate, playing with children of different ages, expressing camaraderie. And there are important sensory-motor skills that are unique to the person, the types of gestures made, the facial expressions taken, the individualistic way the individual walks and moves, and the other distinctive ways of doing things.

Finally, let me add one other type of repertoire—that of imitation. Humans learn a great deal from others by way of imitation, as has been well recognized for a long time. In recent times (see Bandura & Walters, 1963; Bandura, 1969) imitation or modeling has been considered as a basic principle, innately given, on par with the principles of conditioning. The present approach is that imitation or modeling is not a basic principle; it is a secondary principle, like higher-order conditioning. The ability to imitate consists of learned repertoires of skills, some of them of a sensory-motor nature (Staats, 1963a, 1968a, 1975; Staats, Brewer, & Gross, 1970; Staats & Burns, 1981). (Bandura [1971] modified his original view in a manner that is in the direction of the psychological behaviorism position.)

The imitation repertoires involve specific imitation skills and general imitation skills. As an example of the former, one might be able to imitate the specific sensory-motor mannerisms of someone else, like the walk of Charlie Chaplin. We all acquire a repertoire of such specific sensory-motor skills—our own sensory-motor mannerisms have been formed to some extent in this way, for example, in the gender-specific gestures that are, in good part, learned through imitation.

General imitation skills, on the other hand, are more properly to be designated as constituents of a basic behavioral repertoire, because they provide a basis for additional learning through imitation. An example of a general imitation skill is that of *comparing* for similarities and differences the stimuli produced by someone else's behavior and the corresponding stimuli produced by oneself. To illustrate, the person, even after learning a foreign language, frequently will not discriminate a difference in what is spoken from that which a native speaker says. When that occurs the person will have a "foreign accent." For example, a Greek person who has learned English as a second language will typically use a shorter "ee" sound than Americans—sounding like "Grik" instead of the long vowel sound in the American "Greek." This is funny when a word like *sheet* is said. The person with that accent does not discriminate the difference in the two sounds and hence does not imitate perfectly. Of course, there is an American accent in foreign languages—for example, in Spanish when the final *a* at the end of a word is said as "uh," as in saying "cameruh" instead of the Spanish "camerah."

Thus, there are general "perceptual" (discrimination) skills that are involved in imitation. There are also response skills. It would be possible, for example, to discriminate the difference between the response made by a model and the response that one has made without being able to make the correct response. Using the example of language again, I know someone who discriminates the difference in the way she pronounces the Spanish *rr* from the correct way, but she cannot make the vocal response that produces the correct sound.

The person who is a good imitator has acquired both stimulus discrimination skills and sensory-motor skills that produce a stimulus that matches the model. Some people learn the imitation repertoire in an extraordinary manner, as impersonators do. If basic parts of the repertoire are missing, the individual will not imitate, or will do so poorly, in which case the learning ability of the individual will be correspondingly poor in various situations.

One further point should be made regarding imitation or modeling. That is, Bandura (1969, 1977) has used the concept of modeling as an explanation of all kinds of human interactions that produce learning— instruction, communication, and reading—as examples, without specifying differences in what is involved. Calling something modeling does not constitute an explanation. PB takes a different approach. The same principles of conditioning are involved in instruction, communication, and reading. But complex repertoires are involved, as well as various stimulus circumstances. Each of these types of human learning, and others, must be analyzed for what they are, not simply labeled with a generic term. For that blurs what is involved, producing a vague and undifferentiated theory. PB requires specification and analysis of complex human behavior and human learning.

Approach and Avoidance Sensory-Motor Skills

It has been said that a stimulus that elicits a positive emotional response will further elicit a class of approach behaviors and a negative emotional stimulus will elicit a class of avoidance behaviors. But whether a behavior is an avoidance or approach behavior is not determined by the behavior itself. Running, walking, reaching toward, jumping, whatever, may be made under the control of a stimulus that elicits a positive emotional response, in which case an approach behavior is involved. Or the same behavior may be made under the control of a stimulus that elicits a negative emotional response and the result is to avoid the stimulus.

Whether a behavior is an escape behavior or an approach behavior depends upon whether the behavior brings the stimulus "closer" or takes it further "away." (And a stimulus may be made closer or further away in different ways.) The conception is that the individual's sensory-motor behaviors are *available* for responding to the stimuli of the world, whether the stimuli elicit positive emotional responses or negative emotional responses and thus whether the responses have the effect of increasing or decreasing "contact" with the stimuli.

The Sensory-Motor Basic Behavioral Repertoire

There are many sensory-motor skills that almost all humans learn—for example, walking, talking, running, jumping, hitting, swinging something, and so on. However, even in these cases the behaviors can be learned in a greatly different manner. Moreover, there are many sensory-motor skills that humans display, too many for any one individual to learn. So each human only learns a subset of those sensory-motor skills that can be learned, constituting her sensory-motor basic behavioral repertoire.

It has been said that the learning of the language-cognitive and emotional-motivational BBRs varies greatly, depending on the individual's learning experience, which can vary widely. The same is true of the sensory-motor repertoire. For example, the child may be introduced to playing tennis at the age of four, by someone who is a very good teacher and who is very skilled in the sport. This experience may continue until the individual is a world-class tennis player. The relevant sensory-motor skills acquired will be enormously different than those acquired by a person who has only casual experience in playing tennis. Huge individual differences occur in the very complex sensory-motor repertoire, such that the repertoires of individuals are unique.

Nature and Nurture in Sensory-Motor Skill

It is generally thought that language-cognitive characteristics and emotional-motivational characteristics are, in good part, inherited genetically. The same is true with respect to sensory-motor skills—from playing the piano to playing baseball. It is said that there are "born athletes," for example. The nature–nurture question will be considered additionally in developing the present approach to personality. It is only relevant here to indicate that there is little evidence of the heritability of skill in any of the areas of the sensory-motor repertoire.

It is certainly clear that, in the sport of basketball, someone who is seven feet tall has an advantage over someone who is five feet-eight inches tall, other things being equal. A small-boned, slightly muscled, short male is unlikely to develop much skill in sumo wrestling, where size and weight are so important. Champion male gymnasts are not usually tall, large, and big-boned; rather they tend to be compactly built. This is to say that certain builds are favored in the development of certain types of sensory-motor repertoires. Individuals with inappropriate builds are not likely to develop skills in certain sports. There also appear to be biologically based differences in the muscular strength and explosive force that are important in certain sport performances.

But the PB position is that sensory-motor *skills*, whatever they are, are learned. No unusual complex sensory-motor repertoire comes about through heredity. Such a repertoire can only come about through an unusual set of learning opportunities. There are no "born athletes," no "God-given talents." More will be said concerning the role of biological variables in developing the PB theory of personality.

CONCLUSION

With respect to the various human learning principles, it is necessary to investigate responses and stimuli that are uniquely important in human behavior and, especially, how complex combinations of stimuli and responses are learned and how they can function. There are basic human learning principles that do not emerge from the study of animal conditioning. It is also necessary to state principles and make experimental demonstrations of how some of the individual's behavior (or behavioral repertoires) can affect other behaviors of the individual, as well as the individual's learning. An essential concept in understanding human behavior is how behavior that has itself been acquired plays a causative role in the learning of other behaviors and behavioral repertoires. Our study must deal with progressively more complex repertoires that affect broad realms of the individual's experience, learning, and behavior of the type that is considered to involve cognition and, as will be shown in later chapters, personality itself.

A central drawback of the behaviorism revolution of Watson, presently carried on by radical behaviorism, is rejection of consideration of human cognitive characteristics that are determinants of behavior. But cognitive psychology has produced many studies of important characteristics that explain human behavior. It is true that cognitive psychology does not study what those characteristics are in behavioral terms. Moreover, cognitive psychology does not study how those characteristics are learned. And cognitive psychology errs in assuming that those characteristics are given by the nature of the human mind (presumably through biological inheritance).

But those needed developments and corrections can be made within a behavioral approach designed for that purpose. It is the psychological behaviorism position that the cognitive characteristics that have been isolated in cognitive psychology involve learned basic behavioral repertoires. PB has already shown that to be the case with various cognitive phenomena. This position provides a foundation for the productive unification of cognitivism and behaviorism. And that position calls for many theoretical and empirical studies by which to constitute that unification.

Achieving a cognitivism/behaviorism unification requires specific analysis that makes connections and theory that projects research. Only in this way can a program of development be established. Cognitive-behavioral approaches, in clinical psychology, by using that name suggest unification. But it is in name only; for they are eclectic combinations, without behavioral analyses of basic cognitive phenomena, and they lack a program for making them.

CHAPTER 4

The Child Development and
Social Interaction Theories

In the PB multilevel theory approach there are two additional levels of development needed in the conceptual foundation with which to consider personality and personality measurement. One involves a conception of social interaction, as focally studied in the field of social psychology, and the other a conception of child development. Although these constitute separate fields in psychology, in abbreviated form they will be included in this chapter.

THE PB SOCIAL INTERACTION THEORY

The human learning/cognitive level of study is necessary to extend the conditioning principles past the simplicity of the basic animal laboratory. However, both the basic animal learning and human learning levels deal with the behavior of individual subjects. But most human behavior and learning is social, involving individuals in interaction. It is thus necessary to extend the basic conditioning principles to constitute a conception of what social interaction is and the principles by which it takes place.

Three-Function Learning and Social Interaction

In extending behaviorism to the consideration of social interaction, the three-function learning principles play a basic role. The secondary principles and the human learning principles also apply, but elaborating all the principles in the context of social action would demand a longer account than can be presented here. So the analysis will be largely restricted to the basic principles, although various human learning mechanisms are also involved.

118

The PB conception of social interaction is that each person serves as a "stimulus" for the other. A person, of course, is a very complex stimulus—visual, auditory, tactile, even olfactory and gustatory at times. As physical stimuli people differ infinitely, and their behavior can vary infinitely also. Thus, people not only have voices with different physical qualities but, behaviorally, they also say different things. The sensory-motor behaviors of individuals also differ widely, providing differing stimuli. Sensory-motor and speech behaviors constitute different stimuli for the other person, visual, auditory, and sometimes tactile.

In addition, the person may also be a stimulus by virtue of associated things. For example, people dress in a variety of ways, have different titles, have different friends, possessions, bank accounts, jobs, political parties, and such. Whatever the ways that people vary as stimuli, those stimulus properties follow the basic three-function principles advanced in Chapter 3 (see Leduc, 1980a,b; Staats, 1975, chap. 7).

The Person as an Emotion-Eliciting Stimulus

In social interaction the emotional responses that individuals have for one another are central. This is recognized in social psychology with various concepts, such as *attitude*. Many studies examine the nature of attitudes and the manner in which attitudes affect social interaction. PB theory defines attitudes as a classically conditioned emotional response—positive or negative—to a social stimulus. An early study showed that an attitude could be conditioned via language, by pairing a visually presented national name like *Dutch* or *Swedish,* as the ^{C}S, with either positive or negative emotional words serving as the ^{UC}S (see Staats & Staats, 1958). This method of language conditioning of emotional responses has been used widely in social psychology. For example, Byrne and Clore (1970) and Sachs and Byrne (1970) showed that an attitude can be conditioned to the pictures of people as PB hypothesized (Staats, 1964, p. 335). Bugelski and Hersen (1966) and Carriero (1967) used the language conditioning method to produce attitudes toward opinion items. Coleman (1967) did the same for concepts.

Attitudes can also be established through other conditioning procedures, as Lott and Lott (1960) showed with children who received a primary "reward" (really a positive emotion-eliciting ^{UC}S) in each other's company. Staats and Higa (1970) employed individuals' verbal-emotional repertoires in another way to create attitudes. Forty photographs of women were shown to three groups; in one the pictures were labeled with a positive emotional title, such as *social worker,* in the second neutral titles were used, such as *cocktail waitress,* and in the third the title elicited a negative emotional response, such as *alcoholic.* The results showed the subjects' attitudes toward the photographs were determined by the emotional value of the labels employed.

The evidence that attitude formation can occur through language conditioning indicates the *social* as well as cognitive character of the individual's BBRs. In the above studies the individual has to have learned emotional responses to the ^{UC}S words used in language conditioning for the attitude formation to occur. Understanding attitude formation necessitates the concepts and principles of the human learning/cognitive level of study.

The Person as a Directive Stimulus

The three-function learning theory states that an emotion-eliciting stimulus will also function as a directive stimulus. This should apply to people, considered as stimuli. There are a number of studies demonstrating this principle. As one example here, Early (1968) employed the present author's language conditioning methods to establish a positive attitude in school children to the *names* of two socially isolated classmates. The result was that the isolate children were approached and interacted with more than before. Other studies to be illustrated have also shown the negative directive effect of attitudes.

The Person as a Reinforcing Stimulus

There are times in everyday life when a person as a stimulus is contingent on the behavior of another, and serves a reinforcing function. As one example, many men have had the experience of glancing at an attractive woman walking by, only to immediately look back. The first glance (eye-movement response) has been reinforced, strengthened, by the sight of the woman. So the response occurs again. This type of behavior, called the "double take," has been lampooned in movies. We could easily demonstrate the principle by presenting the male subject on each trial with a picture of a pretty woman if a button is pressed with the right hand, and some neutral picture if a button is pressed with the left hand. The heterosexual subject would be conditioned to make the right-hand response.

Psychological behaviorism set forth these principles and suggested that people or their names or their pictures will have reinforcement value, if these stimuli elicit an emotional response (Staats, 1964). In one study people's names were used as reinforcing stimuli. Positive emotional names like Bill Cosby, Albert Einstein, and Ernest Hemingway were employed along with a group of neutral names, like Paul Tillich, Pancho Villa, and Richard Daley. On each trial, when subjects made one response a positive emotional name was presented, the alternative response was followed by one of the neutral names. The positive emotional words acted as reinforcers and strengthened the response (Staats, Higa, & Reid, 1970). Lott and Lott (1969) also demonstrated the principle employing photographs of classmates who were liked, neutral, or disliked. The liked classmate pictures served as positive reinforcers, and the disliked peer pictures reduced responding below the neutral conditioning.

In addition to the person herself, the behavior of the person can act as a reinforcing stimulus for another individual. For example, the person may behave affectionately, may make compliments, may give approval of some action, and so on. Affection (a stimulus) from someone we love is more reinforcing than affection from someone for whom we have a neutral emotional response. Affection from someone to whom we respond with a negative emotional response will act as a negative reinforcer—that is, it will weaken the behavior upon which that affection has been contingent. An experiment conducted by Insko and Butzine (1967) can be interpreted in this way. In the study the experimenter had a negative interaction with the subjects. PB theory states this would be expected to condition a negative emotional response in the subjects toward the experimenter. The experimenter, hence, should not be able to reinforce the subjects by saying something positive (socially reinforcing) to the subjects. This was confirmed.

These several principles have not been studied in the systematic way needed. As examples, it is important to know the ways that individuals reinforce each other, as well as the manner in which that reinforcement is affected by the extent to which the individuals elicit an emotional response in each other.

Types of Social Interactions

The field of social psychology, as part of the disunified science, has isolated various types of social interaction as independent topics of study. Phenomena such as attraction, prejudice, leadership, communication, persuasion, impression formation, and love have been investigated. The result is a host of unrelated studies, with little study of deeper, unifying, explanatory principles. The PB approach is that the three-function learning theory as developed in the context of social interaction can be used to analyze various phenomena of social psychology in a unified manner (see Staats, 1975, chap. 7).

Attraction, Group Cohesion, and Love: Positive Social Interactions

"We endlessly wonder what makes our affections flourish and fade and how we can win the affections of others" (Myers, 1986, p. 576). In pursuing this interest social psychology has studied a number of phenomena. For example, Walster, Aronson, Abrahams, and Rottman (1966) arranged a dance for which participants had been assessed for physical beauty. Pairs were formed who spent two hours together. It was found that physical beauty affected liking and desired contact of each member of a couple for the other. Byrne, Ervin, and Lamberth (1970) had male and female subjects in pairs talk to each other for a half hour. Physical beauty influenced how close the couples stood to each other, memory of each other's name, the extent to which they talked after the experiment, expressed desire to date each other, and evaluation as a prospective spouse. Landy and Sigal (1974) showed that essays supposedly written by pretty girls (as identified by picture) were evaluated more highly than essays supposedly written by not-so-pretty girls. Landy (1973) also found that a male with an attractive partner is evaluated positively by others, and a male with an unattractive partner is evaluated negatively. These studies and many more are unified by the PB analysis; that when the person elicits a positive attitude (emotional response) in another individual, the person will function as a directive stimulus and elicit a large repertoire of approach behaviors in the individual.

Another phenomenon, group cohesion, in the PB view involves the members of a group having a positive emotional response to one another that affects their behavior. As an example, Lott and Lott (1960) conducted a study in which groups of three children played a game in which "reinforcements" (actually positive emotional ^{UC}S's) could be presented individually. When the child's playmates had been paired with positive emotional stimuli the playmates were chosen more on a sociometric test than was the case when positive emotional stimuli were not presented.

Research on love is currently a "hot" topic, tending to be studied as a new topic. However, the basic principles are the same with love phenomena as they are with liking, attraction, and attitudes. The underlying mechanism in the several phenomena is the emotional response that one individual has for another person, except that with love the emotional response tends to be more intense. Romantic love, for example, involves sexual emotional responding, which is notably strong. Rather than being studied in isolation, love phenomena should be studied within the same set of principles and concepts as those in attraction, attitudes, and group cohesion. In each case, however, there are differences, along with the commonality that results from an emotional response being involved.

Other Types of Positive Social Interaction

A PB framework theory of social psychology cannot be presented here (see Staats, 1975, chap. 7). But two other social interaction phenomena can be mentioned.

Leadership. The PB position is that in a free situation the emotional response of others to the person is a determinant of the person's leadership potential. For that will determine the extent to which that person can reinforce others and can have directive power over their behavior. For example, Raven and French (1958) studied elected versus assigned supervisors. (The act of election indicates there is a positive emotional response, at least relative to the other options.) They found the elected supervisors evoked better work output than did appointed supervisors. Fiedler (1967) found that leaders who were more permissive and considerate (positive emotion-eliciting behavioral characteristics) were more effective leaders.

Imitation as a Type of Social Interaction. Another behavioral phenomenon is that of imitation. There are differences in the extent to which the actions of one person (the model) will be imitated by another. In the PB view "imitation power" is simply another measure of the directive power of the person, which depends upon the extent to which the person elicits a positive emotional response. This principle receives support from various studies (conducted under other theoretical perspectives). For example, Lefkowitz, Blake, and Mouton (1955) dressed the model either in high-status (positive emotion-eliciting) or low-status (negative emotion-eliciting) clothes and found that the model was imitated more in the first condition. Models with high ethnic status (Epstein, 1966) and with high competence (Gelfand, 1962; Mausner, 1954a,b) have also shown stronger imitation evocation than models with less positive emotion-eliciting characteristics. Bandura, Ross, and Ross (1963) have replicated these results with children. Thus, imitation is another type of social interaction that can be analyzed in three-function learning principles.

Prejudice and Discrimination: Negative Social Interactions

An example of a contemporary definition of prejudice is that it is "a learned attitude toward a target object, involving negative affect (dislike or fear), negative beliefs (stereotypes) that justify the attitude, and a behavioral intention to avoid, control, dominate, or eliminate those in the target group" (Zimbardo, 1992, p. 599). Although not formulated within the context of a general theory of behavior, this definition is coincident in essential ways with the PB definition (Staats, 1968b; 1975). In PB terms individuals and groups can elicit negative emotional responses in others. When that is the case, those others will behave in a negative (avoidance) manner to those individuals and groups—in their verbal behavior as well as in their overt actions.

Additionally developing the principles, there are two types of stimuli that affect the group with the prejudice. First, the prejudiced group members have a positive emotional response to the members of their own group, and they have a negative emotional response to the members of the "outgroup." Traditionally, the study of prejudice has been concerned only with the negative emotional response, how the prejudiced group members treat the outgroup members. However, the difference in the emotional response to the two groups is important. Because of this difference the members of the two groups are treated differently. Sometimes it is only the *difference* that defines *discrimination*. As an example on the positive side, a white high-school student is more likely to approach and sit at a cafeteria table with other white students, rather than at a table with black students. Other things being equal, the individual will display more helping behavior for, will work harder for, will vote more for, will make better business recommendations for, and so on, for the members of the ingroup than for those not in the ingroup. Various studies can be seen through this analysis to involve these principles (see, for example, Byrne, Bond, & Diamond, 1969; Griffitt & Jackson, 1970; Pandey & Griffitt, 1974).

The opposite treatment is given those who are in the outgroup, the group toward which the individual has a prejudice (negative emotional response). A study by Berkowitz and Knurek (1969) can be used to support this analysis of prejudice. Their study was based in the principles of PB theory and employed PB's language conditioning method with which to establish the negative emotional response of a subject toward a *name*. Then, in another setting, the subject participated in a discussion with two confederates of the experimenter, one of whom had this name. Each confederate, unaware of the experimental condition, then rated how friendly or hostile the subject had been toward him. It was found that the subjects exhibited more hostile reactions toward the confederate who had the disliked name. The negative emotional response elicited by the name generalized to the confederate with that name (Berkowitz, 1970, p. 107). The ratings of "hostility" were based on different types of behavior of the subjects, so the results showed that the negative attitude evoked a *class* of negative behaviors. Another type of prejudiced behavior was shown in a study by Geen and Berkowitz (1967). They conditioned subjects to have a negative emotional response to a confederate by having the confederate insult the subject. Then how much electric shock the subject would deliver to the confederate was measured. Again, the negative attitude evoked stronger "punishment" behaviors.

What particular behavior will occur will be determined by the other stimuli in the situation. For example, LaPiere (1934) showed that individuals with negative attitudes toward Chinese, who indicated they would not admit them to a restaurant, would nevertheless admit a Chinese person who was well dressed and accompanied by a Caucasian. Whether or not a negative attitude will result in discriminatory behavior depends also on the nature of supporting stimulus circumstances. This effect can be seen in a study by Berkowitz and LePage (1967). Subjects with a negative attitude displayed more punishing behavior toward another person when a gun was present in the room than when there was no gun.

Since the PB theory of prejudice centers on the negative emotional response to outgroup members it is important to study the existence of such responses in people who are prejudiced. Rankin and Campbell (1955) and Porier and Lott (1967) have shown that persons with stronger negative attitudes toward black people, as indicated on an attitude scale, responded with a more intense physiological emotional response when touched by a black person. Westie and DeFleur (1959) also showed that prejudiced subjects showed an increased galvanic skin response to photographs of black people. PB studies also link attitude ratings and emotional responses (see Staats, Minke, Martin, & Higa, 1973; Staats & Staats, 1958; Staats, Staats, & Crawford, 1962; Staats & Hammond, 1972).

To summarize in specific terms, the absolute intensity of the negative emotional response will help determine the extent of negativity of the behavior that is made to the social stimulus. Second, discrimination can be defined as the difference in behavior made to a member of the ingroup compared with a member of the outgroup. Third, the greater the difference in emotional response to the two groups, the greater the difference in overt behavior to be expected. Thus, the behaviors of attraction, group cohesion, following a leader, imitation, and conformity occur to ingroup members and discrimination behaviors to outgroup members. This unified theory needs a specific program of research. One implication is that social organizations (such as religious and political groups) that form a strong positive emotional response in their members for the ingroup, in doing so create unequal emotional responses to other groups, thus fostering discriminatory practices. Discrimination involves positive and negative conditioning.

Theory of Attitudes and Disunity

As already indicated, psychology is a disunified science and this pertains to social psychology (see Staats, 1968b, 1984). In commenting on the early PB theory of attitudes, Greenwald (1968) presented a number of prominent definitions of attitude. His discussion indicated that the various definitions boiled down to PB's two principles—that attitudes are emotional responses, and that they act as directive stimuli that control approach or avoidance behaviors—even though the definitions are considered to be different. (No definition referred to the reinforcement function of attitudes.) For unification to occur the underlying principles must be formulated.

Negative Emotion and Social Interaction

Let me suggest, as another example of the fractionated state of social psychology, that the social effects of negative emotions (attitudes) are mostly not connected to the effects of positive emotions. While it is recognized that there are positive attitudes and negative attitudes, the concepts are not clear and thus do not lead to explicit unification. Thus, prejudice and discrimination phenomena are not related well to attraction, liking, and love phenomena.

The PB analysis, in contrast, clearly indicates that with emotion where there is a positive case there is a negative case. As examples, conformity phenomena deal with the positive case, but there should also be a case of non-conformity involving negative attitudes. Imitation or modeling deals with the positive case also, but what about the case where the *modeler* does the opposite of the model rather than the same thing as the model? This constitutes *negative imitation,* a new social concept proposed in PB (Staats, 1975). (Bandura [1986] has since added the negative case to his theory.) The same is true of leadership. There can be *negative leadership,* where the leader is opposed. Also a communication message may be followed, which is a case of persuasion. Or a communication can result in behavior the opposite of that which the sender intended, which would be a case if *dissuasion.*

Generally negative cases of social interaction phenomena have not been conceptualized and have not been studied. The PB view is that understanding why people have a negative impact on others is as important as understanding why they have a positive impact.

Need for Unification of Social Phenomena

Social psychology needs theory by which to understand its phenomena in a related way, which means the establishment of common, underlying, explanatory principles. The PB analysis provides such a theory. We can see the relationship among attraction, group cohesion, love, leadership, and such. And we can see the relationship, also, of these phenomena to the negative social phenomena. The chaos of diverse principles, concepts, theories, and findings in social psychology calls for the type of unification PB can provide.

BBRs in Social Interaction

The three-function behavioral principles by themselves, it should be added, are not sufficient with which to account for the various interests of social psychology. For one thing, social psychology is interested in individual differences in social interaction. As an example, there are individual differences in "leadership," as was illustrated in some of the examples. The same is true in imitation phenomena, conformity, love, persuasion, prejudice, and so on.

Important questions involve explaining such differences. Some involve person variables, which are a subject of interest in social psychology. One example is the study already referred to where leaders who were considerate and permissive had better results (Fiedler, 1967). Some types of individual difference effects have been studied under the concept of role. "[R]ole is the set of expectations held by perceivers for the behavior of a person who fulfills a particular social function. So the roles of "friend," "student," and "child" are actually in the eye of the beholder, not specific to you as an individual" (Shaver, 1987, p. 238). Translated to PB concepts, classes of people are discriminated within a culture as social stimuli, distinguished by common features—for example, old people, children, pregnant women, pretty women, handsome men, policemen, nurses, men, women, girls, boys, fat people, people with southern accents, oriental people, and so on.

Our cultural experience trains us to respond to classes of social stimuli in certain ways that are different. As one example, PB stated, in analyzing language development, that adults speak to children differently than they do to other adults. Many studies verify this hypothesis (see Rondal, 1985). The general principle is that we ordinarily learn a repertoire of responses with respect to the classes of social stimuli, such as a repertoire of baby talk, speaking in a high tone, making faces at the infant, holding the infant, and playing with the infant in various ways. As another example, we learn a repertoire of behaviors that will tend to be evoked by pregnant ladies, bosses, fathers, mothers, waitresses, and so on. Such repertoires would be describable for a culture, and cultures could be compared on that basis. It is said that the Chinese culture reveres old people more than Western cultures. In PB terms this means that Chinese people generally learn different BBRs with respect to old people than do Americans.

The social psychology definition of roles given above also suggested that there is a "set of expectations held by perceivers for the behavior of a person who fulfills a particular social" role (Shaver, 1987, p. 238). In the present terms it may be said that pregnant women have characteristic movements; it would be unusual to see a late-stage pregnant lady moving lithely like an athlete. Toddlers toddle. Priests do not swear like sailors. And men move and gesture like men, women move and gesture like women. Deviations in behavior from that which is usual by the members of a social role will be seen as deviant. For example, the man who moves and gestures like a woman will be an unusual social stimulus, and will be responded to as such. As will be indicated, there are learned repertoires involved in these differences.

This is not to say that there is homogeneity of behavior to the classes of social stimuli. There are individual differences in learning even though there are intercultural differences. For example, some people learn a fear response to policemen and avoid them, while others do not. As another example, we may see some people responding very easily and naturally with a priest, but not a rabbi, for these people have not learned a repertoire to the latter.

As this discussion indicates, certain social phenomena are like personality phenomena and are treated with "personality-type" concepts. Thus, role is used as an explanatory concept in social psychology in the same way that personality is in the general field of psychology. This discussion suggests that such concepts can be analyzed in PB's principles and concepts, helping lay a foundation for later treatments of personality.

Types, Settings, and Durations of Social Interactions

There are various kinds of social interactions. There are interaction types which have varying degrees of generality, such as parent–child (and other familial combinations), boss–employee, priest–parishioner, doctor–nurse, major–lieutenant, and boyfriend–girlfriend. While there are many variations in each type, there may also be certain characteristics that have a good deal of commonality. For example, the contemporary concern with sexual harassment in the workplace brings to focus the fact that there are super-ordinate–subordinate relations involved that extend farther than occupational responsibilities. The individual in the superordinate position has high emotion-eliciting value or can manipulate positive and negative conditions (emotional stimuli) that are important for the subordinate. In the language of political science (see Staats, 1975, pp. 503–507) that means the superordinate person has power over the subordinate. That power, furthermore, can be abused, as in requesting sexual favors. Psychological behaviorism calls for the study of the various important types of social interactions, for the purpose of abstracting principles that have generality for understanding the nature of the interactions.

Environmental Effects on Social Interaction

Psychological behaviorism also calls for the study of the setting of the interaction. A priest drinking with a parishioner in a bar, or attending a football game, will be responded to differently than is the case when in an official situation. The husband and wife alone in their bedroom have a different interaction than when in the presence of their children. The sexual-harassing supervisor behaves differently to his secretary when they are alone or accompanied by another employee, his wife, or the boss. Strangers interact differently at a cocktail party than if seated together at a movie or on a bus. As the study by LaPiere (1934) showed, people with negative attitudes toward Chinese people behaved differently, depending upon the social situations. The ways that environmental conditions have general effects need empirical stipulation.

Large Group Characteristics and Interactions

Some of the foregoing discussions have involved groups as stimuli, not just individuals, as in considering social roles. We need further study of how groups can be involved in social interactions. For example, in Bosnia (in former Yugoslavia) there are currently three warring groups, the Serbs, the Croats, and the Muslims. The groups are contesting the territory that will be under the jurisdiction of each group, and in the contest members of each group have perpetrated cruelties upon the members of the other groups. In such a case, the perpetrators of cruelties will be identified as the members of a particular group. As stimuli they will come to elicit a negative attitude in the victim group.

That negative attitude will be elicited by all members of the perpetrator group, whether or not they participated in the cruelties. The 1961 Sharpesville Massacre in South Africa, where many in a group of unarmed demonstrating blacks were killed and wounded by government soldiers, can be used as an example. "Such experience and the resulting learning can be transmitted through the group on the basis of the simple language description of the happening" (Staats, 1975, p. 529). Through language the experiences of a small percentage of the group can condition the general membership of the group to the same emotions learned by those who actually experience an event. So group experience can be carried far and wide. It can be conveyed over generations. So the PB principles are intended to apply to large as well as small group interactions.

Intensity of Social Interaction

The interactions studied in social psychology are generally of short duration. This does not allow for the formation of intense emotional responses of individuals to each other. However, many social interactions are characterized in important part by the frequency of contact and the length of time involved. The group–group examples given above are of such duration. For example, the Serbian, Croatian, and Muslim populations in the Balkans have been interacting with each other for hundreds of years, during which time negative emotion has been learned by each group for the others. The same is true of the black and white groups in South Africa as well as in the United States. While the events of the past are gone, and need play no role at the present time, the attitudes that have been conditioned through the ages are transmitted, via language conditioning, to the present. And they constitute a strong determinant of present-day behavior of the members of the groups involved. Intergroup behavior cannot be understood without taking into account such past conditioning, and the human learning mechanisms that have conveyed the learning through the generations.

Many individual interactions are also of long duration and much frequency. The husband–wife relationship is of this type. That provides the opportunity for intense conditioning with respect to emotional-motivational, language-cognitive, and sensory-motor learning. Social psychology should consider social interactions in terms of frequency and duration, and analyze interactions that produce important social repertoires. As will be indicated, the longitudinal study of social interaction is very important.

CHILD DEVELOPMENT THEORIES

The traditional field of child development has assiduously studied many ways in which the child changes as a function of age. Children from birth on have been observed systematically, over extended periods. This has been done with single children, in what is called *longitudinal study*. A variation (the cross-sectional method) studies groups of children of increasing ages. As a consequence, much is known about behavior development: the child holds its head erect and steady at three months of age, sits with support at about four months, sits alone at about six months, stands with support at about six months, walks holding on to furniture at about nine months, walks alone at about a year. Studies to establish general norms of development were conducted very early (see Gesell & Thompson, 1929, 1938). But finer-grained studies continue today. For example, one study compares reaction times of two- and three-month-old infants in response to repeated presentations of a picture, showing the older infants to be faster (Wentworth & Haith, 1992). Ruff, Saltarelli, Capozzoli, and Dubiner (1992), in studying infants' exploratory behavior, found there to be a decreasing use of mouthing as an exploratory contact in infants between 5 and 11 months. Such developmental works stipulate important sensory-motor skill developments.

The development of language also has been a focus of study; for example, that the child babbles at about six months and says her first words at about a year of age, that additional words are slowly acquired during the first year-and-a-half or two, and then there is an acceleration in the rate of acquisition. Some of the behaviors have been broken out for finer-grain studies, as in the case of babbling (Blake & Boysson-Bardies, 1992; Levitt & Utman, 1992). And many aspects of the developing grammars of children have been investigated.

There are many studies also of social and emotional development processes in children. As an example, there are studies concerned with the effects of mothers' messages on emotional and instrumental response to novel stimuli in their children (see Rosen, Adamson, & Bakeman, 1992). Personality and emotion are topics of interest as well. For example, Casey (1993) set up a situation in which a peer would give subjects (mean age seven to 12) mild positive or negative "feedback" concerning the subject's performance on a video game. "Feedback valence influenced emotion expression, self-report, and the subjects' understanding of emotion" (Casey, 1993, p. 119).

These are but examples of the multitude of studies done of a myriad of topics in the field of child development. *Developmental Psychology*, one of the major journals in the field, now publishes studies in various topic areas such as early development, social cognition, personality and emotions, gender, behavior problems and adjustment, social development processes, language development, cognitive processes, social perception, and behavior genetics.

There are also various theories of child development involving different types of psychological or behavioral phenomena. One of the early theories was that of Sigmund Freud. His psychoanalytic theory posited that the child's personality is formed on the basis of the child's developing psychosexual needs in four periods or stages, and the manner in which the parents handle the child during those stages. Freud formulated this theory on the basis of what his patients told him concerning their early experiences. Piaget (1932), on the other hand, studied children's responses to certain types of problems and constructed a theory of cognitive development involving four stages of development. Piaget, like Freud, considered his theory to be very general, not only to the field of child development, but also to psychology in general (Piaget & Kamii, 1978). Kohlberg (1981) studied the child's "moral development," suggesting that there are six invariable stages involved.

There are many theories in the traditional field of child development. But there is a general belief that the child develops, in good part, as a function of biological maturation. Moreover, while it is behavior development that is actually studied, generally that development is considered to be an index of underlying psychological development.

The Behaviorism Conception of Child Development

As indicated earlier, John Watson rejected traditional psychology *en masse*, its philosophy, its methods, and its knowledge products. Interestingly, Watson (1930) presented a very traditional position with respect to inheritance of traits, employing the conception of a geneticist. Watson thus states that "There are combinations of [genes] giving every intermediate type, some yielding slightly imperfect individuals, lazy, stupid or silly; and there are combinations that produce genius" (Watson, 1930, p. 51). This hereditarian position seems inconsistent, because Watson's most widely known position was his "environmentalism" with respect to child development. "Give me a dozen healthy infants, well-formed, and my own specified world to bring them up in and I'll guarantee to take any one at random and train him to become any type of specialist I might select—doctor, lawyer, artist, merchant-chief, and, yes, even beggar-man and thief, regardless of his talents, penchants, tendencies, abilities, vocations, and race of his ancestors" (Watson, 1930, p. 104). Moreover, Watson eschewed traditional developmental research—rejecting a study by Gesell (1929), of identical twin infants with striking similarity in behavior patterns, because the study lacked controls.

Watson also made naturalistic interpretations of how children could learn different behaviors. But he did little study of child learning and did not establish a research tradition for that purpose. The second generation behaviorisms (Hull, 1943; Skinner, 1938; Tolman, 1932) focused on the animal laboratory, not child development through learning. Skinner, in taking Watson's place as the leading radical behaviorist, has been generally thought to take the Watsonian environmentalist position and to have led a tradition of studying how children develop through learning. This view is quite erroneous. There is very little in any of Skinner's writings on the *learning* of behavior. His most detailed analysis of a type of human behavior did not analyze how verbal behavior is learned (Skinner, 1957). In support of the popular belief that Skinner dealt with child learning there is common reference to Skinner's "baby box." But the baby box was really a way of controlling temperature, humidity, and sanitation. It did not involve analyzing or producing learned behavior in the child. There is no evidence that Skinner studied the learning of any children or how to produce such learning or that he made theoretical analyses regarding such matters. Mentions of child learning are few—examples occur in *Walden Two* (Skinner, 1948), of children being reinforced for participating in learning activities, and in Holland and Skinner, of how children who are reinforced for crying will be conditioned to cry and that this behavior can be extinguished (Holland & Skinner, 1961, p. 47). Skinner did not deal with the field of child development or attempt to resolve the issue of nature or nurture.

Generally, the various studies that were done with children in the pure Skinner tradition were of several types. Several involved the demonstration that the basic principles of reinforcement applied to children (see Bijou, 1957; Gewirtz & Baer, 1958). Another studied analogues of behavior such as cooperation (Azrin & Lindsley, 1956). The programmed instruction studies (Holland, 1960) were concerned with developing technology by which to improve academic learning, not with the nature of the child's development through learning. Only after applications of reinforcement principles to functional human behaviors had begun (see Eysenck, 1960a; Staats, 1957a) were radical behaviorism studies of this type conducted with children (see Williams, 1959).

Skinner's experimental work and theory dealt with behavior principles, not learning. His experimental analysis of behavior technology was not for studying the *learning* of the simple responses employed, but for stipulating how reinforcement variables affect the rate of the response. Skinner's concept of successive approximation is a principle of learning, as is the programmed instruction principle that the items in the program should advance in small steps. But these principles were not part of a systematic effort and deal very little with the study of child learning. These characteristics are reflected in the radical behaviorism book *Child Development* (Bijou & Baer, 1961), which was devoted largely to presentation of an abstract summary of the principles of operant conditioning and a general statement that child development involves a progressive interaction between the child's responses and environmental contingencies. Analyses of or work on the child's learning of functional behaviors were not included.

   In the past 40 years there have been many works in the field of behavior therapy that deal with child learning that are couched in radical behaviorism terminology (see, for example, Dupaul, Guevremont, & Barkeley, 1994; Kazdin, 1994; Schreibman, 1994; Walker, Greenwood, & Terry, 1994; and Wells, 1994). As will be indicated in Chapter 9, this work actually derives from a combination of the behaviorisms, especially PB and radical behaviorism. The focus of this work is on the treatment of various types of behavior problems in children *after* they have arisen. Child behavior therapy/behavior analysis, thus, has not centered on the study of the child's development through learning, on dealing with the traditional field of child development, and on construction of a theory of child development. These are important gaps.

The Traditional-Versus-Behaviorism Schism

The traditional approach was constructed to study the facts of child development, not to study either learning or biological causes. Behaviorism, too, despite its study of conditioning principles, has not created a conception of child development through learning, a methodology for studying how this learning occurs, or a research program for carrying out that study. Rather, behaviorism has rejected or ignored the work of the traditional field, just as the traditional field has rejected behaviorism. Following Watson's environmentalism traditional psychology expended much effort in showing that behavior development is not learned but comes about through biological maturation (see Carmichael, 1926; Gesell & Thompson, 1929). On the other side there has been effort to bolster a general environmentalist position, for example, with studies showing that enriched environments raise intelligence (see Dawe, 1942; McCandless, 1940; Peters & McElwee, 1944). Neither orientation provides a way of incorporating two productive traditions of study. Theoretical, methodological, and empirical advancements are needed by which to affect such a unification.

THE PSYCHOLOGICAL BEHAVIORISM THEORY OF CHILD DEVELOPMENT

One of the characteristics that makes PB a third-generation behaviorism is its approach to child development. Unlike radical behaviorism, PB accepts the child development domain of phenomena. And the PB position—a primary example of its behaviorizing approach—is that there is much that is valuable in the traditional studies of these phenomena. In contrast with radical behaviorism, the PB conception is that the detailed study of learning can explain developmental phenomena, cognitive, emotinal, and behavioral.

A major problem has been that both the traditional field of child development and behaviorism have only applied learning principles to simple behaviors in short-term studies. To see the huge differences that learning can produce in human behavior, we need to deal with complex behaviors that require long-term learning. And we need to deal with the case where the individual must learn a set (repertoire) of complex behaviors that is necessary for learning another set, which, in turn, is necessary for learning another set. This type of learning has not been generally studied, which is why the importance of learning in child development is not understood.

Another new characteristic of psychological behaviorism is its focus on studying *functional* human behaviors and how they are learned. Accomplishing these goals in child development called for new methods, which the author began to formulate when still a graduate student studying language learning in a pet cat, as has been described. A single subject was employed, the training was stipulated, as was the resulting behavior. The control consisted of comparison to usual, untrained cats (subjects). Called the *experimental-longitudinal method of study,* this type of research extended over a period of time and involved multiple training trials. The birth of the author's children (in 1960 and 1963) and the detailed study of their development through learning provided a basis for elaborating the methodology. The research was experimental. Development was produced that was valuable for the child. Moreover, like the traditional field, this study was done in a longitudinal way, involving complex behaviors and long periods of time. These were the first children systematically and comprehensively raised within a third-generation behaviorism.

This experimental-longitudinal research with two subjects was as important in the development of the PB theory of child development as were PB's formal studies, and yielded findings that could not be obtained otherwise. The sensory-motor, language-cognitive, and emotional-motivational BBRs were described in the preceding chapter. The following sections will summarize some of the experimental-longitudinal procedures for producing and studying learning in these three basic repertoires.

Sensory-Motor Development

Traditional norms of development heavily involve sensory-motor skills, generally thought to develop as a function of biological maturation. The following sections will summarize some classic sensory-motor developments as they are learned, employing experimental-longitudinal research methods.

Walking Development: Maturation or Learning?

When my daughter and son were only a couple of months old I would hold either under the arms while standing on my lap. The child would support some weight for a brief period and then withdraw her or his feet. When this is done, a child will progressively support more of its weight, for longer periods. Furthermore, the child will learn skills, for example, like flattening the feet when standing. (Infants at first curl their toes and feet under.)

When the child was three to four months old I would let the child support her or his weight on a carpet and move the child forward, as shown in Figure 4.1. By tilting the child, first on one side and then on the other, it was possible to get an alternating leg movement. Further practice in this yielded increased skill in those alternating, walking-like leg movements. The child was also trained to hold on to my thumbs while being pulled up to a standing position. Then the child was given experience in holding on to the railings of the crib while standing, and later in pulling into a standing position. Both children did these things earlier than usual as a consequence, as shown in Figure 4.2 when my son was four-and-a-half months old.

By four-and-a-half months, when holding in each hand one of the author's fingers the child could haltingly take a few steps forward, when my support was moved in that direction. The child put a good deal of weight on the hands. With additional learning trials the child's skill increased and more weight was supported on the feet. By five-and-a-half months the child could take halting steps while holding on to the basket on the back of a stroller, as the stroller was moved forward. Figure 4.3 shows my daughter doing this at seven-and-a-half months, at which time she had developed considerable skill and confidence and needed little if any support. Figure 4.4 shows the same child walking freely at the age of nine months, and Figure 4.5 shows my son at a similar age.

Infants on the average begin walking at 12 months. The experimental-longitudinal research shows that time is not fixed by biological maturation. Thus, the same learning opportunity with the two children yielded the same 33%–50% savings in the developmental time required for walking. Let me suggest that learning to walk involves a complex skill, of various muscular groups that have to be coordinated. Walking also involves learning "balance," that is, learning to make balancing movements under the control of visual stimuli as well as stimuli that arise in the semicircular canals of the inner ear (Staats, 1963a, pp. 369–373). The PB position is that the developmental norms for walking are in good part determined by the learning opportunities the culture provides its infants. Even systematic but brief training can markedly advance the development of this sensory-motor skill. Let me add that these results have been supported by Zelaso, Zelaso, and Kolb (1972), whose training of parents resulted in a similar type of training for infants and yielded walking at the age of ten months.

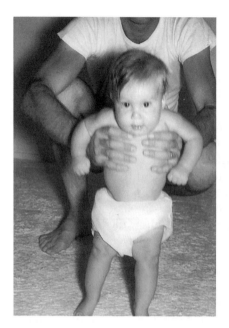

FIGURE 4.1 The author providing training to his daughter Jennifer in making alternating "walking" leg movements.

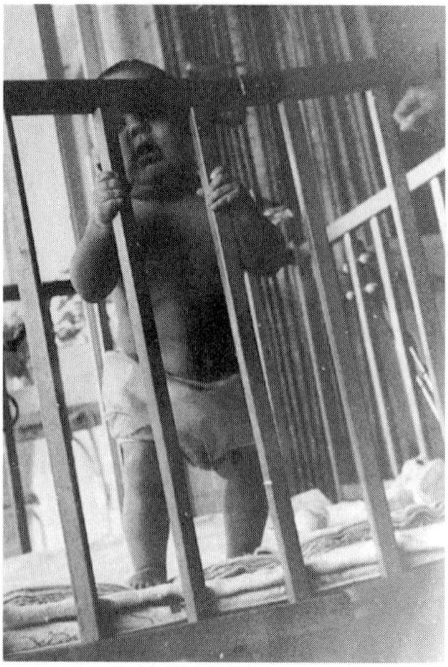

FIGURE 4.2 The author's son Peter standing at four-and-a-half months of age.

Handedness

Handedness is considered by many to be biologically determined and to have important significance with respect to the individual's brain function and personality characteristics. There is a division of function between the left and right hemispheres of the brain, and those functions tend to be switched in left-handed people. This has led to the idea that in infants one side or other of the brain is dominant and this determines handedness. A popular view, also, is that changing handedness disrupts the expression of the biological characteristics of the individual, with deleterious results.

The author's observations, however, revealed that the infant at the beginning is equally unskilled with both hands, in grasping, banging an object on a table, in carrying things to the mouth, and such. With my children, for example, when learning to eat with a spoon I placed it in the right hand, and ensured that this was the hand used. When done very early, when the hands are equal in skill, which hand is selected makes no difference. But systematic treatment results in the child having more experience with the selected hand and thus becoming progressively more skillful with this hand. That difference in skill will then determine the child's "preference" for this hand, for using the more skilled hand results in quicker, less effortful

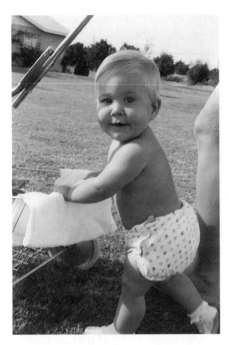

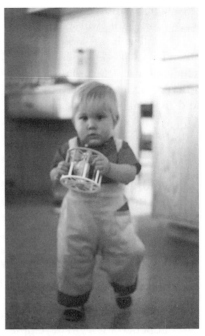

FIGURE 4.3 Jennifer walking behind a stroller at seven-and-a-half months of age.

FIGURE 4.4 Jennifer walking freely at nine months of age.

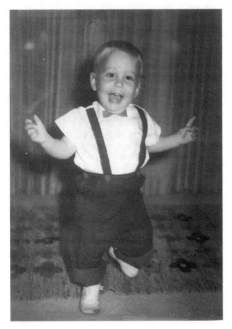

FIGURE 4.5 Peter walking freely at nine-and-a-half months of age.

(stronger) reinforcement. Soon the skill difference will become appreciable, and the child will systematically pick up the spoon more with this hand.

The skill with the spoon with the right hand, moreover, will generalize to other uses. These experiences will further develop the skill of the right hand, and its preferred use. For example, when introduced to using crayons for coloring, chances are the child will hold the crayon in the right hand. And that will set the stage for the child learning to write with her right hand. (I did not leave this to chance, however, but followed the type of procedure I used with the spoon.)

The same pertains to throwing a ball and many other skills. The child who picks up things with the right hand is likely to throw more with the right hand, and thereby develop the skill more with that hand. (Again, I saw to it that the right hand became the throwing hand.) The non-preferred hand, however, never falls into complete disuse, being employed in many tasks, such as reaching for something which is on that side, and skills will develop. It is interesting that this can involve complex skills, like typing, or playing a piano, where the non-preferred hand may be as skilled as the preferred. The PB position is that what handedness involves is the development of special skills on a number of tasks, eating, writing, tool using, and so on. The reason why some people are right-handed but left-footed is because they happened to begin developing skill with that hand and that foot.

There is a strong belief in the biological determination of handedness but, again, the role of learning has not been systematically explored. When the learning of the child is studied, as in the experimental-longitudinal study described, a different view emerges. *The long-standing PB conception is that learning with respect to the preferred hand affects brain development, not the reverse.* When this position is taken different conclusions ensue. I suggest that the learning study of (and production of) handedness can be conducted without problem, when done in infancy, from the beginning, in accord with the PB learning analysis. It would be possible to show that handedness learning produces brain hemisphere dominance. The outcome will be different if the parent waits until the child has developed a skilled and preferred hand, and then tries to change the preference. Done correctly, handedness can be arranged for the child, to the advantage of the child.

Toilet Skill Development

In Freud's theory toilet training assumes a particularly important role because it defines the second stage of psychosexual development. In this stage the child's eliminatory needs, and how the child is treated in this respect, are focal. The view held by most child psychologists and psychiatrists is that biological maturation determines toilet skills, not learning. Traditional advice to the parent is to be patient, not force the issue, and wait until the child's maturation kicks in.

The author made a PB analysis of toilet skills and trained his children accordingly, both with respect to diurnal (see Staats, 1963a, pp. 377–380) and nocturnal toilet skills (Staats, 1975, pp. 348–349). My analysis is that elimination consists of certain sensory-motor responses that are controlled by certain stimuli. The stimuli in defecation include those arising from the distension of the lower bowel as well as environmental stimuli. The young child has already learned the defecation responses in the presence of the diaper; such that the diaper is an eliciting stimulus (for sphincter relaxation and such). In toilet training, the eliminatory responses must be learned to other stimuli, for example, being undressed below the waist, being seated on the pottie, as well as the stimuli arising from the distended colon. The learning is straightforward.

With my children, I first established the time at which defecation usually occurred. The next step is to place the child on the pottie shortly before this time, explaining that she is going to learn how to go to the bathroom (like mommy and daddy or an older child). The child should be entertained, as the reinforcement for the response of sitting on the pottie. The parent can read to the child, tell a story, have the child color a coloring book on her lap, or whatever. The first time should involve a very brief period on the pottie, followed by praise, which reinforces the behavior and conditions a positive emotional response to the pottie chair. No forcing or restraint should be employed. When done successfully, the sessions can be gradually lengthened. The experience should always be positive and the child should choose to participate because of being reinforced for the behavior. If this is continued, sooner or later the child will score a "hit," which should be reinforced by the parent's delight and praise. The hits will then increase in frequency. The comparative natural reinforcement for defecating into the pottie versus into a diaper strongly favor the former. After a sufficient number of successful pottie trials the child will become toilet-trained. The child should also be trained to say when she needs to go pottie. This is an essential part of the toilet skills. Some years after this behavior analysis was published, a radical behavioral method of toilet training also based on reinforcement principles was set forth (see Azrin & Foxx, 1974).

Nocturnal Toilet Training. Many interpretations of bed wetting have been made. Again, the PB analysis is that the skills that must be acquired are simple, consisting of *waking* up under the control of the stimuli produced by distension of the bladder, and then *walking* into the bathroom and urinating. My experience is that the child can be trained to these skills when the child is a couple of years of age. The training is very simple when it is conducted before the child has developed a problem. The child should urinate before going to bed. Presumably this will be several hours before the parent retires. Then, when ready to retire, the parent should *awaken* the child and guide the child to walk into the bathroom and urinate and then walk back to bed. At the beginning the child will not awaken easily, and thus will not walk on her own to the bathroom. But that is exactly what must be learned, to wake up, to get out of bed, and to walk to the bathroom, and so on. So some persistence is necessary in waking the child and getting her started on the walk, supporting her while walking, but not carrying her. After this has been done a sufficient number of times the child's distended bladder and temporal cues will awaken her, and she will go to the bathroom. If the parent does not really awaken the child, however, but simply carries the child into the bathroom, the child will stay asleep through the whole episode and the necessary learning will not occur. This is one of those cases where it is important to adhere closely to the specifics of the training.

As with pottie training, after the child is nocturnally toilet-trained if there are any accidents the training can be resumed to strengthen the desired behavior in its competition with the undesired behavior. Toilet training of both varieties can be conducted earlier than is traditionally thought. Again, the PB view is that it is not biological maturation that is involved, but learning.

Attention Span

A traditional rule of thumb in developmental psychology and education was that a four-year-old child only has an attention span of five minutes. This reasoning suggests the child cannot be given training that calls for longer periods of attention. PB research (Staats, Staats, Schutz, & Wolf, 1962), however, showed that four-year-old children can work diligently for 40-minute periods *when they are reinforced for the behaviors of attending to the stimuli and participating in the task.* Moreover, when reinforcement ceased their attention and work deteriorated and became typical for children that age.

Limitations on attention do not appear to be biologically based. The PB view is that the length of time a child will remain at a task without reinforcement, and the goodness of attention during that time, depend upon the child's previous learning. The PB position is that the child learns to work by being reinforced for doing so, for increasing lengths of time. This was shown in a formal experimental-longitudinal study by Staats, Brewer, and Gross (1970) with four-year-old children reinforced for participating in learning to read the letters of the alphabet. Over the 60 training sessions (12 weeks) it was found that the children made a progressively greater number of responses per unit of time. Staats and Butterfield (1965) found the same effect during four-and-a-half months of reinforced reading learning with an adolescent child with developmental reading disorder, and this result has been replicated with various other children (see Staats, Minke, & Butts, 1970).

It may be concluded that attentional and perceptual skills (see Collette-Harris & Minke, 1978) are learned and are under the control of behavioral variables, rather than being determined by biological development. Such skills advance with age because with advancing age—on the average—children have a greater opportunity for the necessary learning to occur.

Swimming

Psychological behaviorism training was extended to other sensory-motor development with my children in experimental-longitudinal research. For example, I had a multi-step program for training a young child to swim, which my children did before the age of three (see Staats, 1971a, pp. 241–242). Briefly, the training began with accustoming her or him to playing in water and having it bathe the child's face. Later, at about the age of 10 months my daughter, for example, was taught to put her face underwater, in a little play pool. At that time another experience was that of being supported in a large pool, as shown in Figure 4.6, in positions that became more and more like swimming, including having her face in the water. Still later, in that same pool she was taught to hold me around the neck while I swam underwater, and also to push herself off from the side of the pool toward me, with her head underwater. She then learned to do so over a farther distance while kicking. The next step was kicking and paddling at the

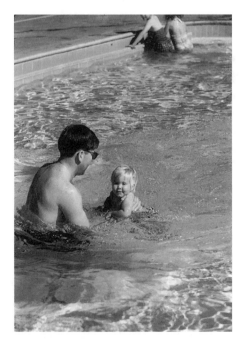

FIGURE 4.6 Jennifer entering the water for pre-swimming training.

same time, then doing so and coming up for air. All of the training, as in the other examples, involved positive emotional experience for the child; and the outcome is the joy and confidence that are displayed by my daughter at the age of three years and five months (see Figure 4.7A), and my son and I in Figures 4.7B and 4.7C.

Visual-Motor Skills

Many sports involve visual-motor skills. For example, catching a ball is a visual-motor skill that a child of two years will ordinarily not have. This can easily be ascertained by telling the child to catch the ball and throwing it to her. The child will not visually track the ball in the air and will make no motor movements to catch it. Such skills do not come from maturation, but they can easily be developed in a young child. When my son was two years old, for example, I used a balloon full of air as the ball. I stood a few feet away, asked him if he could catch the balloon, pretended to loft it to him, but actually guided it into his arms, and gave him social reinforcement. With instructions about watching the balloon and grabbing it, over successive trials where the balloon was thrown the child began to develop those skills. With the game quality as the reinforcement, as well as attention and praise for participation and for catching the object, and with guidance, the child will become progressively more skillful. When the child can watch a lofted balloon and move to catch it, it is then possible to advance to a smaller,

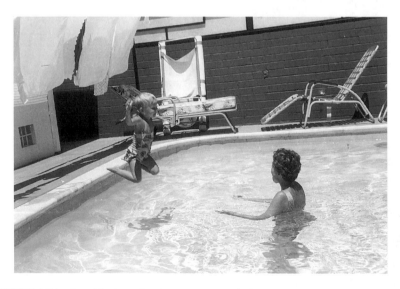

FIGURE 4.7A Jennifer jumping into water to splash.

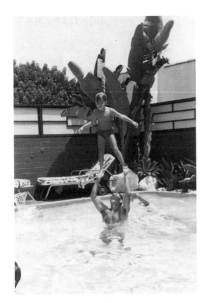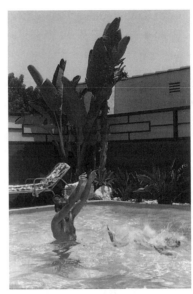

FIGURES 4.7B, C   Peter preparing for and diving into a pool. These are follow-up examples indicating the children's confidence in and love of swimming.

somewhat heavier, faster moving, large rubber ball. When this can be watched and caught, the parent can advance to smaller and smaller balls. With corresponding tuition in throwing, it is possible to train the child to catching and throwing skills at a very young age (Staats, 1971a, p. 57).

Let me conclude by saying that although the training I extended was not rigorous or arduous, it was done systematically and it began a cumulative-hierarchical process of sensory-motor development that culminated in both Peter and Jennifer becoming excellent athletes—Peter in tennis, basketball, tae kwon do, and surfing, and Jennifer in tennis (where she was a state woman's champion at age 17). It is suggested that rigorous, systematic, and continuing training that commences early can produce professional-class skill with any child whose body characteristics are suited to the sport. When children are studied in this experimental-longitudinal manner it is clear that childrens' sensory-motor development occurs through specific learning, not unspecified "maturation."

Language-Cognitive Development

Traditional child development norms have concerned language development, a study that has become a large field. This field, however, does not generally study how learning produces language development. Some of PB's experimental-longitudinal research, derived from its theory, whose target was language development, can be briefly exemplified. The findings call for a change in conception.

Speech

I began studying, and producing, language development in my children from the beginning, systematically talking to the infant during feeding or while engaged in anything that would elicit a positive emotional response. This was done in order to make the sound of my voice a positive emotional stimulus, and hence a positive reinforcer. For these developments would ensure that any vocal response the infant made that sounded like my speech would be positive self-reinforcers and thus strengthen the vocal response.

Very early I also provided the infant with additional experience that would make the sound of my voice a conditioned stimulus for a positive emotional response. For example, when my infant daughter had been asleep in her crib, and I heard her waking and stirring, I would station myself out of her view and then say "Daddy," "Daddy," and then I would enter her field of vision, pick her up, and have an affectionate interaction. The effect was apparent. Soon when I said "Daddy" under such circumstances she would stop her activity, orient toward the sound, and smile and coo, ready for the affectionate play. In this way my voice became a salient directive stimulus, as well as an emotional stimulus.

Later, when I fed the baby with a spoon, I would say "Eat" before "delivering" a spoonful. Many repetitions occurred in one sitting. I would also name anything the child looked at, and I would verbalize our activities. In addition, I would reinforce (by my social response) the child's vocalizations. Many times I would imitate the sound the infant had made, as part of this reinforcement. We would engage in sequences where she made a sound, then I made the sound, and then she made the sound again, repeated a number of times. The result of these systematic procedures was the early appearance of syllable vocalizations (babbling) in the child. And I responded to these vocalizations with special reinforcement (attention, affection, and play). Her vocalizations that had no English counterparts were not so reinforced.

When the child began saying things sounding like the name of some object, I began special training with respect to the vocalization in the presence of that object. An early vocalization was "dah, dah, dah, dah." Whenever she said that I would say "Da-da, yes, da-da, da-da," and give her delighted attention. She was reinforced for the vocal response. And the two syllables were paired with my attention, which elicited a positive emotional response in her. I also would play a game with her when she had been by herself for a period. I would say "Da-da, da-da," and then when she paused and looked around I would suddenly appear, repeat the word a couple of times, and begin playing with her, to her delight. (This was an extension of what I had done when she awakened from a nap.) If she said "Da-da" when I was within earshot I would immediately go to her and repeat the word and play with her. Finally, she began saying "Da-da" appropriately, when she looked at me, or wanted me, or approached me.

Another early word was "eeh." That arose from my saying "eat" prior to giving her a spoon of food. This experience was expected to make the sound a positive emotional stimulus, thus providing a source of reinforcement when she made the sound. She began saying "eeh" during feeding, and I began waiting for her to say it before giving her the food, or prompting her to say it by saying it myself. She was thus reinforced strongly for this vocal response, and she began saying it frequently and appropriately, as a request for another spoonful of food. This was a game enjoyed by us both.

Strengthening these word responses made it easier to train additional words. By the time she was nine months old she had 12 words in her repertoire that were under the control of the appropriate stimulus object—*Mama, Dada, wahwah* (for water), *moo* (for moon), *doh* (for a toy dog), *dah* (for doll), *eeh, spooh* (for spoon), *mil* (for milk), *cah* (for a toy car), *bah* (for a ball), and *key* (for a ring of keys). The usual time for the first word of the child is 12 months. Again, systematically arranged learning opportunities—even though brief—can significantly accelerate the traditional developmental time. Since this is a most central area of development, this topic deserves systematic study. There are children who begin to speak several months before 12, and there are children who do not begin to speak until two years of age and later. The PB position is that these differences do not arise in different rates of biological maturation, but in different learning opportunities. Moreover, the development of speech is very important in the child's learning of other cognitive skills so understanding what is involved and being able to produce it is valuable.

Verbal-Motor Learning

Saying "Daddy" outside the child's room, waiting for the child to attend to and orient toward the sound, and then reinforcing the child by appearing, actually trained the infant to her first verbal-motor response. That is, the word "Daddy" thereby became a directive stimulus that controlled the attentional and orienting behavior. When the infant was five months old I said, "Come to Daddy," and when she crept toward me I reinforced her (in a variety of ways). With repetitions, the words came to be a directive stimulus for her approach behavior. In addition, as she sat in her high chair looking around during feeding, when I said "Eat" and she looked at me and opened her mouth I gave her a spoonful of food. That training made the word a directive stimulus for those responses. Also, when I said "Look," and then directed her attention toward some object or event that had reinforcing properties (such as a favored doll), that brought her attentional behavior under the control of the word as a directive stimulus. This was the beginning of the training that resulted in the learning of a large verbal-motor repertoire. Moreover, for the child so trained, words (language) begin to become an important type of stimulus. Without that training the child will attend less to language stimuli, be considered to be unresponsive, and hence receive fewer training trials. Patricia Kuhl recently (see Boodman, 1995, p. 166) has shown that eight-month-old children can orient to objects that are named. PB research has shown how this development is learned and how it can be accelerated by systematic training.

Verbal-Imitation

In verbal imitation the child must learn to make a particular vocal response to the sound produced by someone else who has made the same vocal response. The child produces this type of learning herself when repeating syllables. The parent can also produce this type of learning by repeating sounds that the infant says, for sometimes the child will then make the same vocal response again. For example, when my child had learned to say "Eeh" during feeding, I would sometimes repeat the word, and wait for her to say it again, before providing the next spoonful. Later, when first sitting down to begin feeding I would ask her "Eat?" and when she had repeated "Eeh" the feeding would begin. (Let me say when these types of interaction are done appropriately, there is no laboriousness about it—rather it is a gamelike communication for both parties. There was no pressure. If the child did not make the vocal response the feeding commenced anyway.)

Such training provided learning experiences that help create the early verbal-imitation repertoire. This repertoire may also be improved in quality through training. For example, one of the first words my infant daughter learned was "wah-wah," under the control of water. She would say it when she saw water, as in a bath tub (and later when she wanted to drink water). At this point I began to improve the vocal response. When she asked for "Wah-wah" I would said "Wah-dah, say wah-dah." Whatever she said in reply I would then provide the water. After some repetitions of this experience she began saying "Wah-dah," which I reinforced immediately (while still asking her to say "Wah-dah" if she said "Wah-wah"). When she began saying "Wah-dah" the next step was to introduce "wah-tah." She later learned the standard pronunciation through her informal experience. The point is that the child's pronunciation can be progressively improved by training, and this also involves imitation training. Normally such learning occurs through the child's informal experience, but knowledge of the process can allow systematicity and provide additional opportunities for positive parent–child interactions.

Let me add that the child may learn incorrect pronunciations (speech defects) that persist. The methods I have described may then be used effectively to treat speech pathologies such as lisping (see Staats, 1971a, pp. 146–148) before they become a problem.

Reading Development

The standard view is that a child is not biologically ready to begin to learn to read until at least the age of five or so. I began training my daughter to read at the age of two in 1962. The first step was to place small pictures of objects, which she could name, individually on three-by-five cards. Then I typed the letter **A** on several different cards, using a primary typewriter. I mixed the letter cards into the picture cards. Then I presented the cards to the child one at a time, beginning with several picture cards. I asked her to tell me the name of the object, which she did. When the letter **A** appeared I told her what it was and asked her to name it (for the actual instructions see Staats, 1968a, pp. 280*ff*). Soon she would say the letter when it appeared. Each response to a card was reinforced (see Staats, 1968a, pp. 270–273, for a description of the reinforcer system employed).

Training sessions were very brief. When she could say "A" to the letter, she was told she had learned the first letter in learning to read, and now she was going to be shown the second letter which was **B**. She was shown the card and asked to say its name, as she did. Again letter trials were mixed with picture-card presentations. After this training she was told the letter **A** comes first—it was shown and she was prompted to say its name—and the letter **B** comes next—and this was shown and she was prompted to say its name. Then, mixed with the pictures, she was shown a card with **A** on the left and **B** on the right, and under guidance asked to name them successively and point to them. Later the letters were presented separately in order, then separately in any order, always with guidance to ensure that mistakes did not occur (which is important). When she could read the two letters presented by themselves, intermixed with picture cards, the next letter was introduced in the same manner. With this training—involving voluntary participation, reinforced responding, and brief sessions—the child learned to read 16 letters of the alphabet.

At this point words were introduced into the training. When she could read a group of words they were combined into sentences that were read. After additional words had been learned little stories consisting of several sentences were introduced. As the words increased in number the stories became longer. At the age of two years and ten months of age she could read the 16 letters of the alphabet, ten single words, and various sentences and stories composed of these words, with understanding and appreciation. At this time my daughter began learning additional upper-case letters and the lower-case letters. Later, phonetic training was begun where she learned to read single letters, like the **s** at the end of a word, as in *boy* or *boys*. At the age of four years and three months she had "a reading vocabulary of 121 words . . . , 52 letters (upper- and lower-case) and six phonetic responses (Staats, 1968a, pp. 292–293). One of the stories she read at that time contained 173 words. The training program continued for several years, even after the child had entered school. The child's participation in training was always voluntary and she progressively became an avid pleasure reader.

Writing Development

By the time my daughter was three I had tentatively experimented with training on writing the letters of the alphabet, but not in a continuing program. The training, employing reinforcement, involved copying the letters and writing them independently when given the letter's name. Samples of her writing are presented in Staats (1968a, p. 296–297).

Number Concept Development

I first began training my daughter Jennifer in number concept skills when she was 18 months old. Since she liked raisins, I held one raisin in the palm of one hand and two raisins in the palm of the other. I asked, "Which do you want, *two* raisins (displaying that hand), or *one* raisin (displaying the other hand)?" When she said "One" I started to give her the one, but she indicated she wanted the two. So I said, "You want *two* raisins?," showing them. She said yes. So I said, "Say two raisins," which she did, and I gave her the two. This occasionally conducted training was also done with different objects. Sometimes the reinforcement was simply praise, as when I asked her the number of fingers I held up. In this manner she learned to name one and two objects. Then three objects were introduced. She had to say whether she wanted two or three objects, for example. She was also given training in saying the number of objects held (one, two, or three) without comparison to another amount.

When the number of objects increases past a certain point, it is not easy to discriminate how many are involved. That is when counting is necessary. In the present case, when the child could unerringly name the number of objects up to three, she was introduced to counting. Many times parents attempt to teach a child to count just by naming the numbers in sequence. That is not good training; it does not produce the number concept or counting skill. The words are non-functional. The child will thereby only learn to say the numbers, usually too rapidly, and this interferes with learning a real number repertoire.

The child must learn three things in counting—(1) naming numbers of objects up to three or four; (2) number responses learned as a verbal chain; (3) responding one at a time to each object in a group; and (4) the coordination of these two sequences of responses, so that each time a number is said the child takes one object out of a pile for each number said. When the child has learned to count objects up to some small number, it is then possible to extend the repertoire solely by verbal training, by adding additional numbers to the sequence (see Staats, Brewer, & Gross, 1970). This should be done one number at a time, maintaining strong learning throughout. My daughter had learned to count up to 13 unarranged objects by the time she was two years and ten months of age (although Piaget says that this develops only when the child is six). When the child has a counting repertoire number reading can be introduced. My daughter learned additional aspects of the number repertoire and was trained to read the numbers when she was three-and-a-half and then addition skills were added (see Staats, 1968a, 398–301).

These skills constitute a basic behavioral repertoire, the "concept of number." Having learned such a repertoire, the child will react finely to quantity, and the child is prepared to learn additional repertoires on the basis of this BBR. This changes the child cognitively. For example, her grandmother could quickly teach her the card game "War," because she had the number repertoire and could read numbers.

Supporting and Follow-Up Evidence

The results of this training have been presented elsewhere (see Staats, 1968a, chap. 13), and the following illustrates what a child can learn through five-minute training interactions enjoyed by both parent and child.

> To summarize . . . at the age of 4 years and 10 months she had learned to follow directions, to attend and work in a concentrated manner, to make close discriminations of various kinds. In addition, she had an increased picture naming repertoire, a rudimentary writing repertoire, a rudimentary number concept repertoire; she could copy abstract symbols, she could read all the letters and numbers, and she could read words and sentences, and paragraphs made up of those words, and she had a small phonetic reading repertoire as well as some of the skills in sounding out words. (Staats, 1968a, pp. 301–302)

In entering the second grade my daughter's standardized reading test scores (inadvertently revealed) were at the 99th percentile. Having said that my daughter and son were the first to be reared—systematically, comprehensively, and in a detailed manner—within a learning theory conception, with learning procedures, it is relevant to indicate more generally that both children entered a school that had highly competitive requirements. In both cases the transition to the classroom was smooth. Both enjoyed school, had good school adjustments, did well academically all the way through, and are now doctoral-level professionals.

But the results might be specific to these children and not depend upon learning. To make the findings general, other children had to be given the same training, by other "trainers" (see Staats, 1968a, pp. 306–320). At Arizona State University I standardized the training methods, apparatus, and recording methods. A graduate student, with no special experience in teaching children, trained three additional children—one three-year-old and two five-year-olds—in part of the material, with similar results (see Staats, 1968a, pp. 306–320). And three years after beginning the reading training with my daughter I employed three additional graduate students in a full research project with a group of four-year-old culturally deprived children, selected because their siblings had already had problems learning in school. A traditional preschool program (that employed behavioral techniques for behavior control—several of the children having behavior problems of varying severity) was provided. During the day the children at different times received five-minute training periods each in reading, writing, and number skills. Like my own children, the culturally deprived children learned complex repertoires (see Staats, 1968a, pp. 321–346) in the three areas. The effects of the training were measurable via standardized tests. That is, during the period of training, which lasted seven-and-a-half months, the children advanced in IQ by a mean of 12 points, advanced in readiness scores from the second to the 23rd percentile (see Staats, 1968a, pp. 321–346), and learned BBRs that would be important to them on entering school. This study was done while I was at the University of Wisconsin. A year later I repeated the study with Headstart children at the University of Hawaii, obtaining the same results (see Staats, Brewer, & Gross, 1970). Later, this work was extended in three studies by Staats and Burns (1981).

These findings indicate that children within a wide range of measured ability can be taught, in standard form, to read, to write, and to have number skills using the experimental-longitudinal methods, as adapted for use in schools. Sub-professionals who are not teachers can provide the important training and gather the behavioral data. PB's findings suggest a new type of educational organization for the beginning years (Staats, 1970b). The closest use of such methods, and others done in PB with older children (see Ryback & Staats, 1970; Staats & Butterfield, 1965; Staats, Minke, Goodwin, & Landeen, 1967; Staats, Minke, & Butts, 1970), however, has been by a private company (the Sylvan Learning Centers) that is concerned with remedial teaching. In addition, similar language training procedures have been used for work with autistic children (see Lovaas, 1977).

Emotional-Motivational Development

Emotional-motivational development has not been as explicitly studied as motor and language development. However, there are basic studies that support the PB view that the emotional-motivational BBR begins to be learned in infancy. For example, there are various early studies that show that classical conditioning occurs in infancy (Brackbill & Koltsova, 1967; Jones, 1930; Kaye, 1967; Krasnogorski, 1907; Lipsitt & Kaye, 1964; Watson & Raynor, 1920), possibly *in utero* (Spelt, 1948).

Classical Conditioning, Bonding, and Attachment Theory

In addition, there are studies like that of Mills and Melhuish (1974), which shows that the mother's voice is a reinforcer for three-week-old newborns. Such results are generally interpreted as evidence that the child is biologically prewired to bond to the mother. We can see that learning is the explanation when realizing that it is previous classical conditioning that has made the mother's voice a reinforcing stimulus. The mother's voice has come to be a reinforcer by being paired with feeding and such and thereby coming to elicit a positive emotional response in the infant. Even by three weeks the infant will ordinarily have many such conditioning trials. The PB analysis makes *learning* the important process, not biological prewiring.

Knowing the principle of classical conditioning, and with the objective of conditioning the child's "love," I systematically talked to my own children when I fed them. And the results were observable. When the infant heard my voice after a period of absence she would show evident signs of positive emotionality (in vocalizations, in facial expression, and in orienting). The topic of emotional conditioning calls for systematic study with neonates.

Supported by the evidence, the PB position is that emotional conditioning begins at birth. For example, it is important that the child learn a strong positive emotional response to the parents, so the parents can be strong sources of reinforcement in the training of the child. The parents also must serve as primary directive stimuli for the child in many training interactions. Both of these stimulus functions depend upon the extent to which the parent has come to elicit a positive emotional response in the child. The parent who does not pair abundantly her or his stimulus properties (appearance, touch, voice, behavior) with positive emotion-eliciting stimuli loses important opportunities to condition the child to a strong positive emotional response. That parent will be a less effective reinforcing or directive stimulus, and thus less effective in the child's learning.

Attachment Theory. One of the prominent theoretical approaches in the field of child development is called "attachment theory." Theorists of this persuasion are interested in the attachments the infant makes with a few central figures, primarily the mother. It is said that the relationship to this person (or persons) is then the model for other later relationships. Typically, it is thought that there is a special propensity for a mother–child bonding that is biologically built into the two, so bonding occurs very quickly and does not rely on the incremental process of learning. This is also the general opinion in our society. A study by Tronick, Morelli, and Ivey (1992) suggests otherwise. The study reports that the Efe (commonly called pygmies) in Africa do not follow the usual Western manner of child-raising. Infants and toddlers spend half their time with other children and adults, and only eight percent of the time with their fathers. By the age of three the child spends seventy percent of the time with non-parents. This arrangement is inconsistent with the attachment theory view of a mother–child biological bond. However, in the present view bonding is not a biologically based process; the emotions the child comes to have for the parent depend on the conditioning experiences that occur, which are widely different.

Shyness and Differential Parental Conditioning

Kagan (Kagan & Snidman, 1991), working with human infants, and Suomi (1990), working with monkey infants, have suggested that shyness (the avoidance of strangers) is an inherited trait. From the PB position, however, the view that shyness is genetic has not involved analysis or study of the infant's emotional-motivational and social skill learning. We must analyze this learning from the beginning to understand the nature of emotional-motivational development, especially the emotional response to people. There are very large differences in emotional conditioning that children can receive from the very beginning. To illustrate, there are parents who spend much time in playful, affectionate, and vocal interactions with the infant. These are primary ways for conditioning positive emotions in the child. Such parents may observe what the child can do, such as attentional and perceptual responses in looking and listening, reaching for things, or rolling over. They can find out how to get the infant's attention and make her laugh. On the basis of knowledge of the infant's behavior, they may then invent little games to play. For example, a parent may say a long, drawn-out "A-a-a-a-a-h" and then terminate the sound by saying an explosive "Boo," and rub the baby's tummy, or some such game. The infant who has been introduced to the game will attend to the parent when the "Ah" sound begins, become more focused as it continues, and then laugh when the "Boo" and tummy rub occur. The child, importantly, through such "games" will learn attentiveness, responsiveness (including laughter) to the funny things adults do and say, and will look to the parent for stimulation. The infant in so doing will herself become "attractive," eliciting "funny" behaviors from adults. Such a child is learning, early, responsive play skills that will generalize to other adults.

To continue, let us take the case of parents who also enjoy having others interact with their infant and who, from the start, pass the infant to others and ensure the child's pleasure when that occurs by helping in the interaction. Let us say they are skilled in facilitating such situations, first remaining close and supportive and making the interaction fun. They are not fearful with respect to the child, how the child may behave, or the effects the others may have on the child (such as the child crying). If this is the case the child will learn a positive emotional to various other adults, and play skills as well.

The course of events, however, from the beginning, may be quite different. The parent may love the child just as much, and take care of the child's needs just as well as the above-described parent—but not be playful and warm, a close observer of the child's behavior, sensitive to the development of "game" interactions, and not articulate. Let us also say that this parent is shy and not comfortable with others—even in-laws and some family members. Let us say that this parent is also fearful concerning how others may hold the child, and the possibility that their interaction with the child will not go well and the child will cry. Such parents will keep the child close to themselves. And when someone else does take the child, the parent will be uneasy and hover anxiously, ready to grab the child as soon as the child shows signs of feeling a strange presence. The parent will make others uncomfortable. The learning is likely to be negative for all. The child will not develop a positive emotional response to other adults or play skills. Rather than presenting a picture of playful expectancy, this child will appear sensitive, withdrawn, and hesitant. Adults will be edgy with the child and will not initiate playful interactions. Those who do will meet rebuff by the child's withdrawal and if they persist the child will cry.

In both examples (as is generally the case) this type of beginning sets the stage for continuing learning. The jolly, playful, responsive, expectant infant is responded to in a different way from the infant without these behaviors, or the infant who is wary, unresponsive, and on the brink of crying. This constitutes a beginning in differences in shyness. This analysis suggests that traditional research on shyness has not begun to study how the child's complex learning can be the determinant.

Punishment and Negative Emotional Conditioning

Punishment in child-raising is a central topic that needs study. Let me begin with the extreme case of child abuse. Frequently the parent lacks training (and sometimes child-care skills). The child consequently cries and the parent has learned to treat undesirable behavior with punishment. The problem is that punishing an infant elicits crying, the crying elicits further punishment—the result can be a mutually aversive interaction to the point of criminal parental behavior. Punishment should not be employed at all with infants.

The use of punishment later, in the best of circumstances, is a tricky business because, while it can decrease behaviors in the child that are dangerous or undesirable, the child also learns a negative emotional response to the parent through classical conditioning. The stronger and more frequent the punishment, the more the parent will become a negative emotional stimulus. The author presented an analysis of punishment in child training (see Staats, 1971a, pp. 232–241) which included benign uses, one of which was the "time out" procedure which he used regularly with his children in the 1960s. "It will act as punishment to the child to be removed from the presence of the family members by being restricted to his room" (Staats, 1971a, p. 236). Properly used time-out procedures constitute a mild negative reinforcer that is effective but that does not involve corporal punishment. It elicits a negative emotion, but this occurs mostly when the parent is not there, so the negative emotional *conditioning* to the parent is less than with punishment administered by the parent.

The Negative Verbal-Emotional Repertoire

A central aspect of the PB approach to punishment for controlling behavior, however, is the creation of the language repertoires. With children it is possible to terminate or prevent behavior simply through words if they have learned an appropriate part of the negative verbal-emotional repertoire. That is, it is important that the child learn a negative emotional response to words like "No," "Don't do that," "Stop that," and the like. That depends upon classical conditioning where the words are paired with a stimulus—like being restrained—that elicits a negative emotional response. When the parent attempts to comfort the child while saying "Hurt . . . that hurts," on observing the child bump herself and then cry, this conditions the child to have a negative emotional response to the word *hurt*. When the parent says "Dirty . . . Don't," while grabbing something the child has picked up from the street and started to put in her mouth, the child will experience a negative emotional response from the abruptness and roughness of the parent's actions and from the loudness and urgency of the parent's voice. The child will, in these ways, thereby learn a negative emotional response to the words *dirty* and *don't* and various other words. And this repertoire will be extended by the language conditioning process described in the previous chapter (see Staats & Staats, 1958). As an example, when the child later hears "_____ people are dirty," for example, this will condition the negative emotional response elicited by "dirty" to the name of those people and to the people themselves.

With respect to controlling undesirable behavior, when the words elicit a negative emotional response they will elicit the child's "desisting" behavior. Learning words that control such behaviors is important, for the words can be employed in place of physical punishment. It is possible to raise a child where the use of physical punishment is minimal or nonexistent, by beginning early to create a negative verbal-emotional repertoire such that words can be used to control undesirable behavior when other stimuli would otherwise attract that behavior. It is also possible to use language to get behavior to occur that would otherwise not (because of the effort involved) by the use of words from the positive emotional repertoire.

Moreover, when the verbal-emotional repertoire and the other language repertoires have been well learned the individual may control her own behavior by what she says to herself. A person considered as cautious is, in part, this way because behavior that would otherwise occur is restrained by the things the person says to herself. "The cautious man who 'anticipates' the aversive consequences of certain actions, the socially sensitive man who 'anticipates' socially aversive consequences of certain actions, and so on, would seem to do so, at least in part, because of training that had established for them effective verbal aversive stimuli, as well as the necessary reasoning verbal response sequences" (Staats, 1963a, p. 398). This analysis continued on to say that the timid person may have learned the verbal repertoires in too great an abundance, while the "irresponsible, reckless, wild individual, on the other hand, may suffer from a deficit [in learning] . . . an aversive [negative emotion] verbal repertoire which functions in 'prudent' reasoning" (Staats, 1963a, p. 398).

The Positive Verbal-Emotional Repertoire

As described in the previous chapter, the child also learns a repertoire of words that elicit a positive emotional response. When the child is told "Good . . . Isn't that good," while taking a bite of a delicious food, the child will learn a positive emotional response to the word *good*. After such words are learned through primary classical conditioning they will serve to condition emotional responses to new words. This language conditioning produces a very large verbal-emotional repertoire that also provides the parent with a means of controlling the child's behavior, for example, in getting the child to do things that are effortful that the child would not do on her own. The development of the language repertoires are important in the parent–child interaction, in the child's ability to interact with others on a verbal level, and in the child's own ability to guide her own behavior. These language repertoires are also central in what is called the child's moral development.

The Emotional-Motivational Repertoire and Child Development

In conclusion, it is suggested that an important part of the field of child development should study the learning of the emotional-motivational repertoire. It is important to know to what stimuli the child should learn positive or negative emotional responses, and how this learning takes place. We all want children who have appropriate interests, values, morals, attitudes, preferences, desires, and so on, as well as their counterparts on the negative side. These concerns have not received the systematic study that would be possible and is needed.

The BBRs, Cumulative-Hierarchical Learning, and Experimental-Longitudinal Research in Studying Child Development

The PB position with respect to the need to study complex behaviors in children has already been stated. This must involve studying the nature of complex repertoires, how they are learned, and the role that these repertoires play in the individual's experience, behavior, and learning.

The Basic Behavioral Repertoire (BBR)

The basic study of learning has not provided a conception of or study of *repertoires* of behavior. There have been concepts of habit families (Hull, 1930), a class of responses that is organized by the *fractional anticipatory goal response* (Hull, 1943a), and similarly of response classes (Skinner, 1938), which are responses under the control of the same reinforcer. These concepts, abstracted from the animal laboratory, have not been developed in the analysis of important human behaviors, and they are not appropriate for that purpose. It may be added that the concept of repertoire is used frequently in behaviorism with respect to human behavior, but it has a common-sense definition, with no technical development and no explanatory value.

The PB conception, established in human research, is that there are various repertoires that the individual learns. Not all of them, however, are *basic behavioral repertoires*. When I was a bored adolescent student, for example, I used to drum my fingers on my desk in various ways, forward, backward, right-handed, left-handed, both hands in a synchronized manner, and such. I learned a behavioral repertoire. It was not a basic behavioral repertoire, in the sense that it was the foundation for learning another repertoire, for widely affecting my experience, or for providing me with the elements of behavior for a variety of life situations.

There are, however, repertoires that do have these three kinds of significance. As an example of how a BBR can affect experience, let me describe the verbal-image repertoire. A child who has learned images to many words, including *mauve, tenebrous, twilight, warm, and tranquil,* will have an experience (image) elicited by the words "The tenebrous mauve twilight, warm and tranquil, . . ." A child without the repertoire misses that experience on hearing that passage.

Besides providing the basis for experiences of many kinds, the BBRs also provide the basis for learning. Let us take the learning that may take place through the verbal-motor repertoire. For example, the child may come to the Sunday-school teacher and say, "What does genuflect mean?" The teacher may then tell the class, "Genuflect means to bend one knee in worshipful gesture." Later, before the class ends, the teacher may test the learning by saying to the class, "Before leaving I want you to genuflect by your desk—now, please genuflect." Those pupils who have learned the new element in their verbal-motor repertoire will perform the response, and no reinforcement is necessary (following the principle of higher-order operant conditioning).

The basic behavioral repertoires also provide the child with elements of behavior for the wide variety of situations encountered in the world. Let us take a child who has repertoire elements from having learned to play ping-pong, swim, play baseball, play soccer, dance, skate, climb trees, and from having watched popular TV shows, listened to popular music, and conversed on such topics, as well as from having attended various parties and played various party games. Let us also take another child, raised on a farm, who has had limited learning with respect to these repertoires, spending his time in chores. The two will have different elements in their BBRs. Confronted with different social situations at school, parties, and group get-togethers of various kinds, the two will behave quite differently, because one has many relevant elements in his BBRs that the other does not.

An important part of the field of child development should be devoted to the isolation and study of the basic behavioral repertoires. What are the repertoires that the child needs to be able to respond to the life situations that are presented to her at that particular age? What are the repertoires the child needs to experience life situations in a productive manner? And what are the repertoires the child needs in order to be able to learn well in the life situations that occur? The child's world changes as a function of age, and whether the child will be adjusted or not will depend on whether the child has the relevant BBRs. Having the specification of such repertoires, and how they are learned, would be of inestimable value for parents, and those who help parents in raising their children. And that specification is the knowledge needed to understand what child development is.

It is important to indicate that in PB, when the term basic behavioral repertoire is used, there is a tangible definition. The term is not an intervening variable or an inferred state. This has not been clear to some (Plaud, 1995; Ulman, 1990). Psychological behaviorism calls for the specification of the behavioral repertoires that humans display and children must learn. Some of them have been considered already, but making this a systematic endeavor would yield systematic knowledge that is, at present, not available.

Individual Differences in Learning are Learned

A very central tenet of PB—in contrast to standard behaviorism—is that we cannot understand human behavior and its acquisition solely through knowing the elementary principles of classical and instrumental conditioning. The PB position is that *basic behavioral repertoires (BBRs) are learned that make a human being out of a human organism.* The BBRs give the human being learning abilities that lower organisms do not possess. It is for this reason that a learning theory that is based on animal study alone cannot be complete.

This is not to say that the principles of conditioning no longer apply, as some theories suggest. For example, Gagne (1965) has said that there are fundamentally different types of learning, advancing from basic conditioning to cognitive types of learning. Bandura and Walters (1963) and Bandura (1969) take essentially the same position with respect to modeling. Psychological behaviorism opposes this view and sets forth a different theoretical position; that the conditioning principles are basic to and involved in all learning. However, once children begin learning the basic behavioral repertoires, the individual differences we see in learning are no longer due to individual differences in the ease or rapidity of elementary conditioning. (Those differences do not even account for differences between species; see Staats, 1975, chap. 15). The wide individual differences in human learning depend upon individual differences in the basic behavioral repertoires that have already been acquired.

Child Development in Terms of the BBRs and Cumulative-Hierarchical Learning

What is involved in this conception is the principle of cumulative-hierarchical learning—that it is typical of human learning that acquisition of a new repertoire will depend upon the previous acquisition of a BBR. Human performance cannot be understood without tracing the cumulative-hierarchical learning involved. Child development consists of the acquisition of BBRs. At first these BBRs are simple, composed of relatively few elements. Yet the simple BBR will be a foundation for the acquisition of a more advanced BBR. For example, the child may only have acquired a few verbal-motor elements, yet they can enable the child to follow instructions that will lead to learning in another BBR or in learning additional verbal-motor elements.

The process of child development consists of the long-term cumulative-hierarchical learning of BBRs that are the basis for learning additional BBRs. Child development also consists of learning additional elements in the BBRs, that is, of the enrichment of the BBRs. Two individuals, for example, might have the same basic language-cognitive BBRs—such that tested on a vocabulary test they would both be the same. However, one may have learned extensive verbal-association elements in a special field—for example, in reading a history book. This would constitute the enrichment of the verbal-association repertoire. It is essential to study how BBRs are elaborated and enriched, and the cumulative-hierarchical learning involved. The examples given here have been of elementary BBRs. It should be understood that the child embarks on a very extended cumulative-hierarchical learning voyage. First learning a few verbal-labeling responses, the acquisition of the verbal-imitation repertoire provides a foundation for rapidly adding to the labeling BBR. The child's basic language-cognitive BBR is then the basis for learning to read. And through reading the language-cognitive BBR will be greatly elaborated and enriched (as will the child's emotional-motivational BBR and even the sensory-motor repertoire). Then, on the basis of reading, the child can develop specialized repertoires in science, the humanities, in writing, and so on.

The same is true for the other repertoires. For example, once an individual acquires a positive emotional response to ideas that we might label as conservative (in a political-economic sense), the individual will approach newspapers, news magazines, books, and television programs that espouse those ideas. Contact with those media will produce even more positive emotions to "conservative stimuli," on a wider and more intense basis—as well as produce more knowledge in the area. Indirectly, having acquired some aspects of "conservatism" in the emotional-motivational repertoire sets up conditions that will produce additional development of conservative values (and other things as well). This process of developing the emotional-motivational repertoire begins in childhood. For example, a child led to build an airplane model can thereby receive emotional conditioning that will lead her to obtain another model, and another, and to read about airplanes, and then about subjects related to them, and then to taking subjects in school that will lead ultimately to a career in working as an aeronautic engineer. Another example is that of religious training and an ultimate development of religious values.

The same cumulative-hierarchical learning principles also apply to the acquisition of the sensory-motor basic behavioral repertoires. For example, learning to run, dodge, jump, throw, and hit a ball provides a repertoire of basic behavioral skills that will be the foundation for learning baseball, tennis, basketball, volleyball, or football. Original basic behavioral skills may be learned in one sport—which will produce specific skills that are relevant only to that game—but the BBRs are those having general utility in other sports learning. This, I would suggest is the basis for the conception that there are "born athletes." What is really involved is a person who has engaged in various athletic endeavors and has learned good basic behavioral repertoires of a sensory-motor (and emotional-motivational and language-cognitive) kind. As a consequence this individual when faced with playing a new sport will find her learning, experience, and behavior to be better than someone else who does not have those basic behavioral repertoires.

The study of child development must isolate the BBRs, as indicated, and also *study how they are related to each other in cumulative-hierarchical learning.* Specification is necessary of the "operation" of the BBR in the process of learning another repertoire. Which BBRs are basic, which more advanced? Cumulative-hierarchical learning is fundamental in child development, and must be studied basically as well as in the analysis of the actual process of child development.

The Importance of Methodology: Experimental-Longitudinal Methods

Research methods in psychology have advanced in being able to control irrelevant variables through direct experimental control and by experimental design and statistical analysis. Experimental control may be gained in laboratory studies where, for example, stimulus presentation and response recording are automated and where extraneous stimuli are removed. Experimental design control of individual differences can be obtained, for example, by randomly selecting two groups of subjects, only one of which receives the experimental treatment. As another example, experimental design control can also involve one subject that is alternately subjected to different experimental conditions. Statistical analysis control can be obtained, for example, by removing statistically variations that would affect individual and group performance.

Laboratory experiments deal with simple events and with simple behaviors, for short periods of time. That is necessary for data to be collected quickly and economically. Most research with children in child development is of a short-term nature. The original longitudinal study was modified to deal with groups of children of different ages, also in the interest of time economy. When complex characteristics are studied, as in the case of intelligence, a measure of intelligence is constructed that can be given in a short period of time. If the study is of complex learning, like in evaluating a method of teaching reading, the study is still done in a time-saving methodology. That is, the children's learning will be measured in a brief period following the training—although this does not provide data on the actual process of learning, only on which method generally works better.

But short-term observations do not provide knowledge of child development that consists of the cumulative-hierarchical learning of BBRs. Research is needed that stipulates the complex and variegated stimuli involved and the behaviors that result from experiencing and responding to those stimuli, specifically and in detail. That is what experimental-longitudinal research has been designed to do. The fact is that cumulative-hierarchical learning involves different types of responses and different principles of learning. Experimental-longitudinal methodology handles this by recording everything: the learning stimuli presented, the responses made, the reinforcers delivered. What kind of control and uniformity can be established in such circumstances? There are various answers. For one, the child can be trained in repertoires that will not develop in the child until much later, ensuring that it is the training that has produced the results. Primarily, however, the answer is the explicit detail of experimental-longitudinal research with individual children. When the stimulus materials are recorded in detail, as are the responses made to the materials, the manner in which the child learns can be directly seen, providing the raw data to reveal the process.

For example, a child being trained to write the letters of the alphabet may produce a thousand different responses (many with multiple letters). That raw data shows very generally, for example, that every child in beginning the learning copies poorly, and writes letters sideways, too big, backwards, and with poor form—making the errors characteristic of dyslexia. As straightforward as this seems, the brute fact is that neither traditional nor behavioral research has specified with individual children how such types of learning begin or progress. Our science develops highly sophisticated methods by which many less-than-important things are studied, while neglecting the simple and straightforward study of the child learning essential repertoires.

This is the reason it is widely believed that dyslexic children have some brain deficit, a "perceptual" disturbance, because the learning involved is not known. But the dyslexics' perceptual deficit consists of making the errors that children do who have not yet learned to read and write (see Staats, 1975, pp. 411–413). It is only as learning trials advance that children begin to profit from training. Copying and free writing get progressively better, the responses become smaller, neater, oriented better, right-side up, not backward, and all more in a line. All children demonstrate the same types of errors before the learning occurs; dyslexics' responding is not abnormal at all.

With respect to methodology, the raw data of experimental-longitudinal research can be treated additionally. For example, Staats, Brewer, and Gross (1970) took the first writing response each time a new letter was introduced. The number of learning trials required for each letter could then be calculated. Various analyses could then be made, for example, of whether there was an acceleration in learning as training progressed, as had been suggested in working first with one child (my daughter) (see Staats, 1968a, p. 285). The same result occurred with a five-year-old Mexican-American boy with an IQ of 90 (Staats, 1968a, p. 308), and with additional four-year-old children in reading, writing, and number concept learning (see Staats, Brewer, & Gross, 1970). Findings with one child are general to others. The research also showed that the learning experience overrides age and biological maturation. A three-year-old with brief training did better than five-year-olds when they first began training (Staats, 1968a, pp. 306–318). The same learning acceleration has been shown with adolescent dyslexic children learning to read (Staats & Butterfield, 1965; Staats, Minke, & Butts, 1970).

When every stimulus and every response is recorded in experimental-longitudinal study, the detailed nature of the learning process is there to see. For example, the relative difficulty of parts of complex training materials can be seen. Also the various skills that emerge from the learning can also be seen with detailed study of individual subjects, such as attentional and discrimination (perceptual) skill in examining and comparing letters. Specific aspects of the learning task can be explored, for example, how the child learns phonetic skills (grapheme-phoneme units) that are involved in sounding-out words (Staats, 1968a). Moreover, how one type of training can aid in the development of the next can be studied, as well as how new abilities emerge through each type of training (see Staats, 1975, pp. 396–413).

In the PB methodological conception, experimental-longitudinal research is not the only method to be used. PB research on reading, for example, first explored reinforcement variables (Staats, Staats, Schutz, & Wolf, 1962), sometimes using experimental analysis of behavior methods (Staats, Finley, Minke, Wolf, & Brooks, 1964). But, in the present view, findings established with one child are not enough. It is necessary to generalize the same study with additional individual children. When groups of children can be employed, including a control group (see Staats & Burns, 1981), the findings can be made even more general. When the effects on behavior of experimental-longitudinal manipulations can be supported by the use of standardized tests (see Staats & Burns, 1981; Staats & Butterfield, 1965; Staats, Minke, & Butts, 1970) additional findings are provided. But the experimental-longitudinal research can yield knowledge of learning that traditional group studies (Samuels, 1966, 1973) or experimental analysis studies (Bijou, 1957) cannot.

The essential fact is that a child only acquires repertoires—language repertoires, reading, writing, number skills—over years of time. Without experimental-longitudinal research on the actual learning process traditional researchers are misled. They attempt to characterize what reading is and the personal (biological) factors that "explain" individual differences in reading ability. Without knowledge of the long-term process involved they are reduced to speculation based on the circumstantial evidence of inherited abilities. Short-term studies of relatively simple behaviors do not reveal the importance of learning for the development of human behavior and differences in behavior. Our research orthodoxies must change. As time-demanding as it is, it is necessary to put resources into the study of the cumulative-hierarchical learning process and the child's long-term development of BBRs. We must consider every cognitive or psychological process that is studied in children—for example, the morality of Kohlberg and the cognitive stages of Piaget—in terms of the repertories of which they are composed and study them in experimental-longitudinal detail. *It is the present position that our science and our culture are largely ignorant of the importance of learning in all aspects of child development because the necessary study—centrally experimental-longitudinal study of cumulative-hierarchical learning—has been lacking.*

SOCIAL INTERACTION AND THE
PARENT–CHILD RELATIONSHIP

Psychological behaviorism is based on the multilevel theory construction approach. In this approach social interaction principles are basic to the child development level of study and the other more advanced levels. To illustrate, the principles of social interaction are basic to understanding the parent–child interaction. One of the derivations of the PB analysis is that this is a two-way interaction, with effects in both directions. The emotional response of each to the other affects each individual's behavior to the other, as PB indicated in introducing to behavioral psychology an interest in the effect the child has on the parent (Staats, 1963a, pp. 411–412). Since this PB statement there have been a number of studies concerned with the child's contribution to the parent–child relationship (see Ambert, 1992). A recent developmental psychology study illustrates this clearly, mirroring the PB analysis of attraction; mothers of cute newborns display more positive behavior—such as holding the child close, patting, cooing, talking, caring for the child (as in checking diapers), and in generally interacting with the child (Sawin, Langlois, & Ritter, 1995). This is the same effect of physical beauty found in the social psychology literature.

The parent and child are locked into a long-term, intimate social interaction. That interaction will follow the same principles as other social interactions. When the child in some way brings out positive emotional responding in the parent, the parent learns a positive emotional response to the child. On the other side, each time the parent brings out positive emotional responding in the child, the child learns a positive emotional response to the parent. Ordinarily there will be innumerable such conditioning trials so each will learn a very strong positive emotional response to (love for) the other. This growth of love through learning draws the two close together—each attracts approach behaviors in the other. Doing something that makes the other happy will be reinforced (by the signs of that happiness). This is what bonding consists of.

However, each can also present negative emotional stimuli to the other. Much of the child's positive emotional qualities for the parent reside in the child's behavior. And the child learns that behavior from the experience provided by the parent. If the parent is not a good trainer, the child will not learn behaviors that are liked; rather, the child will learn negative behaviors. That will arouse negative emotional responses in the parent, which will be conditioned to the child. Other things being equal, the parent will be more likely, then, to behave in a negative way to the child, using punishment and abuse or more subtle forms of providing negative emotional stimuli. In this way each can learn negative emotional responses to the other. The social interaction between parent and child can then become mutually destructive.

Because the parent–child interaction is frequent and endures for such a long time there are opportunities for intense conditioning and huge differences in outcomes. In the cumulative-hierarchical process the child will learn very large portions of her BBRs, advantageous or disadvantageous characteristics. The field of child development needs to study in detail the parent–child relationship for the emotional conditioning that occurs, for the behavior that is produced, and for the effects this has upon the child's further learning.

THE PB CONCEPTION OF NATURE–NURTURE

"Maturation (read the genetic program, largely) sets the course of development, which is modified by experience, especially if that experience is deviant from what is normal for the species" (Scarr, 1982, p. 852).

> Can experience retard or speed up the maturation of physical skills? If babies were bound . . . would they walk later than unfettered infants? If allowed to spend an hour a day in a walker chair after age four months, would they walk earlier? Amazingly, in view of what we now know about the effects of experience on the brain, the answer to both questions seems to be no (Dennis, 1940; Ridenour, 1982). Biological maturation—including the rapid development of the cerebellum at the rear of the brain—creates a readiness to learn walking at about 1 year of age (Myers, 1986, p. 68).

It is amazing how tenacious this view is, despite the fact that there is solid evidence to the contrary, and despite the lack of good evidence in support. This view persists because psychology has simply not studied the learning of the child. When learning has been studied it has been of a gross sort—as in the examples above questioning whether being bound or being placed in a walker would affect the development of walking. In the PB view the effect of learning on child development cannot be studied in such a non-specific, simplistic manner.

Psychological behaviorism recognizes the two realms of events that can determine the child's behavioral development, biological events and environmental (learning) events. The PB conception is that the child grows biologically—size, shape, strength, speed, sexual maturity, and so on. These are important changes. The child as a consequence of such growth can behave in ways not possible before. Biological growth also has large effects on the social environment. The child as a social stimulus changes—both in looks as well as in what can be done by the child—and as a consequence behavior of others to the child changes.

It is also the case that there is marked growth in the neural structure from birth. Although the number of nerve cells in the brain is pretty much established by birth, the complex neural networks of interconnections between the cells are very sparse at first and grow progressively more complex. It has traditionally been thought that neural development drives behavioral development—for example, that the child sits, stands, and walks at a certain time because that is when the nervous system (and muscles and bones) have matured. That is why, it is said, behavioral development generally takes place at about the same time in all "normal" children—because they all mature biologically at about the same time.

A contrasting view is constructed in PB, however. We know that the brains of rats undergo anatomical growth as a function of experience (Greenough & Green, 1981; Rosenzweig, 1984; Rosenzweig, Bennett, & Diamond, 1972, 1984). We also know that the neural networks (interconnections among the brain's nerve cells) develop greatly during childhood. The fact is that the child at birth can respond systematically to the environment in very limited ways (which mirrors the child's sparse neural networks). The various reflexes, moreover, other than sucking, are not coordinated actions. Speech is a good example. The infant will vocalize but in a random manner that is not stimulus controlled (except for crying). Responses to stimuli, like a pin prick, are overall responses, not specific in the way that will occur later.

The PB position is that all of the marvelous skilled behaviors (including cognitive and psychological characteristics) the child ordinarily acquires come about through learning. None of them develops as a function of biological (such as brain) development. *Rather, the child's experience results in learning recorded via the formation of the neural networks.* The brain's changes reflect the child's learning, not the reverse. Similarly, the various contemporary studies that relate brain activity to the person's activity—such as thinking—or characteristic behaviors, and interpret this to show how the brain determines behavior, are interpreted quite differently in PB. For example, there is current interest in the fact that musicians with perfect pitch show different patterns of activity in the brain than do musicians without that skill (Schlaug, Jancke, Huang, Steinmetz, 1995). "It has been hypothesized by Lynn Waterhouse and others that such talents may be dependent on the development of a specialized focal neural network or neuromodule" (Sacks, 1995, p. 621). The PB view, in contrast, is that the neural differences result from the different learning experiences that have created the absolute pitch repertoire. This long-term PB view is now receiving support from some of those interested in neural networks.

The child is ready at birth to commence her emotional-motivational learning, her sensory-motor learning, and her language-cognitive learning. The PB conception is that the child is born with receptive organs, response organs, and connective organs (especially the brain), but without much in the way of connections between the first two. For example, the child has few emotional responses to the myriad life stimuli. Prior to the time the child has had experience with the various members of the family, the child will not respond emotionally to them, let alone to stimuli like paintings, pieces of jewelry, beautiful sunsets, movies, football games, music, and so on. With respect to sensory-motor skills, the child can move all of its parts, but not in organized sequences under the control of environmental stimuli. In the language-cognitive area, the child can vocalize, but not systematically, in complex sequences, under the complex stimulus control that will be learned. Moreover, the child cannot respond to language, in the various ways that will later be learned. The PB view is that no complex human behavior is developed through biological maturation, not language, intelligence, morality, temperament, personality, toilet skills, sexual identity, walking, eye–hand coordination, handedness, musical talent, and so on. Rather, the child at birth begins to learn behaviors and repertoires. The environmental stimuli presented to the child are very complex and the learning that results is very complex, long-term, and cumulative. This learning should be the focus of study of the field of child development—that is, the acquisition of the BBRs. Moreover, that study, well begun in PB, is the basis for a learning theory of personality.

CONCLUSION

The PB position is that the traditional field of child development has studied important things, describing important cognitive, emotional, and behavioral characteristics of children that change with age.

But the field *does not* and *has not* studied the causes of child development. The field actually does not have methods for directly studying possible biological causes. Its biological conceptions, as strange as this seems, given their acceptance, rest on assumption.

Likewise, the field has not done anything systematic about studying how learning effects the many phenomena of child development that have been described. Such learning study can only be done in a specific, detailed way.

PB's position, based on specific and detailed research, is that child development—cognitive, emotional, and behavioral—is learned. PB calls for the very extensive study of child learning that is necessary to fill in what is a large framework conception. That study requires a unification of the child development and behavioral traditions, in the behaviorizing-psychologizing methodology that has been proposed.

CHAPTER 5

The Theory of Personality: Basic Structure

Psychology has been described in the unified positivism philosophy as a modern disunified science (Staats, 1983, 1991). Moreover, the various fields of psychology display the characteristics of such sciences. The field of personality is a good example, and it is actually a mess. It has many different theories of varying sizes, many concepts and principles, different methods of study, different basic conceptions of human behavior and personality, hundreds of unrelated tests, and multitudes of studies and clinical applications. These works are created separately and no attempt is made to interrelate them. There is no definitive or accepted definition of what personality is, what the field includes, what types of behavior fall into this interest realm, or how to approach the study of the phenomena of the field. There are no accepted guidelines concerning what should be studied, only the results of past study. It is ironic, for example, that Skinner's radical behaviorism—although it does not address personality phenomena, has stimulated no research in the area, does not incorporate personality study and, in fact, rejects the concept of personality—is nevertheless included as a theory of personality in various personality textbooks. This is because there are no standards concerning what a theory of personality should be, what it should include, what its methodology of construction should be, how it should relate to the other fields of psychology, how it should relate to other personality theories or if this would be important, what parts of the field the theory should and should not cover, what the directions of advancement of the theory should be, and what kind of program should be included to advance the theory. Attempts to build continuing traditions of research are not successful because of these characteristics of the field and of its theory.

"From time to time the interests of researchers are mobilized by themes or areas which appear new and important at the moment; but sooner or later these prove to be sterile or exhausted and they are abandoned" (Moscovici, 1972, p. 32). "These widespread self-doubts about goals, methods, and accomplishments . . . have been expressed recently within . . . personality research" (Elms, 1975, p. 968).

There is a chaotic literature in the field. Thus there is no agreement on what should be taught in the field, that is, what knowledge is to be transmitted to students. Textbooks generally review some of the theories of personality. On the other hand, courses sometimes are organized to sample the many research studies in personality, a separate body of knowledge. What this indicates is that there is not, at present, a framework conception for the field that indicates what its subject matter is, how to go about furthering knowledge of that subject matter, and the theories and methodologies that are appropriate for the task.

The theory of personality to be presented here was developed in a quite different manner than any of the others. The goal of the work that led to the present theory was not that of constructing a personality theory. Rather the work was begun with the goal of constructing a general behaviorism that could comprehensively deal with human behavior. However, the program produced theoretical, empirical, and methodological developments that progressively led to a general theory of personality. As a result of the manner of its development, the PB theory of personality is part of a broad theory that generally applies to psychology.

Important parts of the developmental history of the PB theory of personality have already been given in presenting the first four levels of study on which the theory is based. Several additional steps in this development will be indicated to illustrate how PB concepts and principles were progressively applied to personality phenomena and to constructing the theory itself.

DEVELOPMENTS IN THE PB THEORY OF PERSONALITY

Psychological behaviorism began with a goal of applying learning principles to the study of human behavior. As knowledge collected in this work, new developments were suggested. For example, PB applied learning principles to the analysis of language. Beginning with Watson (see 1930) other behaviorists had analyzed parts of language or considered phenomena like semantic generalization (see Mowrer, 1954; 1960; Osgood, 1953; Skinner, 1957). None of these accounts was based on or led to an empirical program of study. PB's analysis of language, however, began with empirical study of how language is learned. On the basis of such study PB analyzed language into repertoires, which provided the conceptual basis for seeing the relationships of language to other parts of psychology.

Language Principles and Concepts

This work thus produced a conceptual framework that offered new considerations. For example, when analyzing different psychological phenomena—such as communication, problem solving, originality, and scientific reasoning—it could be seen that the language repertoires played a basic role. From this a new concept was derived, that of *language function*. It became important to study not only what language was and how language was learned, but also how language functioned for the individual, and between individuals, in the analysis and *explanation* of different types of human behavior. Problem solving was seen to involve labeling the problem objects, verbal associations to the labeling, and the verbal-motor repertoire that provides problem-solving actions. Communication was analyzed as the functioning of the language repertoires, as was originality (creativity). Scientific work was seen to involve the learning of repertoires, including language repertoires (theory), that resulted from new experiences (observations) for the scientist that, in turn, led to additional developments and new repertoires. Mathematics learning was analyzed in terms of specific language repertoires. These developments, and the more basic analysis of other cognitive phenomena in terms of language function, established a bridge to the consideration of cognition. The PB position became that cognitive phenomena consist largely of the functioning of learned language BBRs. This aim of this unification is characterized in its title *Learning, Language and Cognition* (Staats, 1968a).

The Defense Mechanisms

In turn, the human learning analyses of language function and language repertoires provided new principles and concepts that could be employed as bridging materials in advancing to the analysis of more complex human phenomena. With these bridging materials PB was able to analyze personality concepts in traditional psychology that were derived from clinical observations. An early PB analysis treated Freud's defense mechanisms (Staats, 1963a). His conceptualization was that humans defend themselves from anxiety by developing ego defense mechanisms.

Radical behaviorism considers the ego, including its defense mechanisms, as traditional mentalistic concepts. The psychoanalytic personality concepts are inferred from behavior and then are considered to explain that behavior. They are thus mentalistic in nature. Mentalistic concepts are generally rejected in radical behaviorism, along with the work that has produced the concepts. The PB "behaviorizing" approach, in contrast, is to ask if the behaviors that are involved are important. If so, then the area should be subjected to a psychological behaviorism analysis. The observations underlying the concept of the defense mechanisms are indeed valuable, because Freud was an astute observer of human behavior. In PB terms the defense mechanisms can be seen to involve the functioning of complex language repertoires (largely) in a way that reduces negative emotionality the person would otherwise experience.

For example, rationalization, one of the "defense mechanisms," may be considered as an aspect of the verbal-labeling repertoire. The individual in rationalizing is labeling her actions in a way that increases positive, or decreases negative, social response. The individual, for example, rationalizes her defeat in a tennis match by saying she had hurt her back. There is a general "rationalizing repertoire" that people learn to widely differing degrees. The PB behavior analysis also added another principle with respect to the rationalization repertoire, namely that rationalization behavior determines other behaviors of the individual. "[However,] it must be remembered that the individual's own labeling and verbal response sequences also have an important function in mediating his own problemsolving behavior—and if they are too distorted, the behavior mediated may be maladjustive" (Staats, 1963a, p. 390). If one can rationalize away one's misbehavior, for example, this subtracts from the stimuli that would lead to changing that misbehavior. In the long term this may be maladaptive. Importantly, as will be indicated, this analysis moves PB toward explaining the causal characteristic of the concept of personality.

Similar analyses were also made of the other defense mechanisms. Projection, as another example, involves ways by which we "(1) transfer the blame for our own shortcomings, mistakes, or misdeeds to others, and (2) attribute to others our own unacceptable impulses, thoughts, and desires" (Coleman, 1950, p. 86). PB's analysis—of the language repertoires involved—added to the understanding of how "untrue" language sequences can produce problems in the individual's behavior. "Again, although the behavior [projection] may be considered 'adjustive' because it reduces immediately aversive stimuli (which accounts for the maintenance of the behavior), it may have detrimental consequences if it later mediates inappropriate behavior" (Staats, 1963a, p. 392). To reason and plan well about life's problems the individual's language behavior must be sufficiently truthful or "realistic."

Repression may be considered as the case where certain of the individual's statements elicit in her a strong negative emotional response. Avoiding making those statements—that is, thinking about something else—removes the unpleasant thoughts (statements), and is thereby reinforced. The individual thus learns not to make those statements, even to herself, thus being unaware (unconscious) of them. Eriksen and Kuethe (1956) showed that subjects who were shocked when they made a particular word associate to a stimulus word later did not give that word associate. Since they were not aware of why they no longer had that word associate, it could be said that punishment led to repression. The problem with repression is that one cannot reason about problems if the necessary labels are not available.

The defense mechanism of fantasy was treated in PB as verbal behavior that elicits images that elicit positive emotional responses, and are thus reinforcing. "It is suggested that a life situation in which there are few rein-forcers contingent upon the individual's 'realistic' [verbal] behavior would not be expected to maintain 'realistic' behavior in good strength, and the relatively small reinforcers of fantasy might serve to strengthen fantasy behavior until it becomes much more dominant" (Staats, 1963a, p. 344). In addition, "Fantasy behaviors, however, since they are not problem-solving in nature [in the sense of pertaining to the events of the world], would not ordinarily contribute much to the adjustive behaviors the individual must emit in society. Thus, a preponderance of behavior of the fantasy type would have drawbacks for the individual's adjustment" (Staats, 1963a, p. 394). In each case the defense mechanism is seen as a repertoire acquired via conditioning principles that nevertheless can be maladjustive when it mediates maladjustive behavior.

The Self-Concept

To continue in the development of PB's behavioral concept of personality, the language repertoire (cognitive) principles and concepts were employed to make a theoretical analysis of the self-concept (Staats, 1963a). The self-concept was considered to consist of the individual's *learned* verbal labels to herself. Individual differences in those verbal labels were said to differentially elicit emotional responses in herself and in others, varying from negative to positive. If the individual's self-labels elicit positive emotional responses in others, the individual will have more social power, that is, serve as a positive directive stimulus that elicits positive behaviors in others. The reverse will pertain if the individual's self-labels elicit a negative emotion in others.

> In addition, the statements the individual makes about himself would be expected to function as a stimulus that would control his own behavior. . . . It would be expected that different reasoning sequences would ensue if the individual labeled his own behavior in positive rather than negative terms. For example, the individual who makes derogatory self-statements may "conclude" in a problem-solving sequence . . . not to attempt tasks at which he might otherwise be successful. He may thus not present himself for situations in which he might develop new skilled behaviors. On the other hand, the individual who

makes "confident" self-statements may, other things being equal, attempt the task on the basis of his reasoning and be successful. As a consequence, these two individuals as they progress through life may have different opportunities to gain experience, and their behavior would be shaped accordingly. The self-confident individual might well have many more experiences (again, other things being equal) where he is reinforced for emitting certain skill behaviors. The former individual might not develop those skills in the same measure. The self-confident individual may also, because of his verbal behavior, tend to gain more attention, social approval, and social rewards such as raises and honors. These experiences could reinforce the verbal behavior and [produce] further "self-confident" self-description. (Staats, 1963a, pp. 265–266)

This analysis displays PB's behavioral interaction conception that is integral to its theory of personality, as will be indicated. (This interaction conception was also heuristic for the social learning theory conception of reciprocal determinism; see Bandura, 1968; Staats, 1979c.) That is, in the PB analysis the self-concept verbal behavior is produced by the environment. But it produces emotional responses in the individual that affect other behaviors of the individual. Those behaviors (as well as the self-statements) affect the social environment, which in turn acts back on the self-concept of the individual. The interactions are complex and continuing, and must be taken into account in constructing a conception of personality and human behavior generally. The PB formulation also specified that the self-concept is learned.

> [T]he child [is] trained to make appropriate verbal responses to the stimuli produced by his own behavior. . . . [H]e learns to label his own movements [actions] . . . [and] his own social behavior. . . . [T]he individual's self-statements should to some extent depend upon the physical properties of the individual and the behavior he emits. . . . In addition, however, . . . the child's training to make statements about himself may be to some extent independent of what he is and does. . . . [T]his discrepancy arises when an individual who behave[s] in a certain way has not been trained to describe verbally . . . his behavior in commensurate terms. . . . A child might be reinforced for labeling his skills as low level, . . . whereas they are really very capable. . . . On the other hand, it [is] equally possible to shape . . . verbal behavior that [is] unrealistically flattering. . . .

> Other discriminative stimuli besides those of the individual himself and his behavior seem also to determine statements about the "self." One's statements about oneself [thus] may vary from situation to situation. (Staats, 1963a, pp. 262–264)

The heuristic value of the PB analysis of the self-concept was demonstrated in the development of other behavioral approaches.

In the social learning analysis of cognitive development, conceptions about oneself and the nature of the environment are developed and verified through . . . different processes (Bandura, 1977a). People derive much of their knowledge from direct experience of the effects produced by their actions. . . . However, results of one's own actions are not the sole source of knowledge. . . . [P]eople develop and evaluate their conceptions . . . in terms of judgments voiced by others (Bandura, 1978, pp. 347–348). In addition to the expectancy determinants analyzed thus far, situational circumstances affect [self] efficacy expectations . . . (Bandura, 1977a, pp. 81–83). . . . As a result of such differential reactions, children eventually come to respond to their own behavior in self-approving and self-critical ways, depending on how it compares with the evaluative standards set by others (Bandura, 1977a, p. 133). . . . Social learning theory defines negative self-concepts in terms of proneness to devalue oneself and positive self-concepts as a tendency to judge oneself favorably. (Bandura, 1977a, p. 139)

As another example, Hayes (1987; Korn, 1995) has introduced a behavior therapy that features the self-concept. In PB theory the theory of the self-concept was constructed on the foundation of more basic analyses of language and emotion, and how both can affect the individual's behavior (see Staats, 1963a). However, radical behaviorism has rejected the analysis of how the individual's own behavior (such as language, or emotional responding) can be a cause of overt operant behavior (see Hayes, 1995). This position—if it was consistently followed, which it is not—would rob the concept of the self-concept of its causal (personality) functions.

Intelligence, Interests, and Values

The defense mechanisms and the self-concept in traditional psychology are conceptual developments derived from naturalistic and clinical observations. There are also personality concepts that have emerged in psychometric study. For example, there are psychological tests that measure interests, values, and intelligence. Very early PB analyses began to deal with such topics.

For example, interests were considered in PB in the same framework as attitudes and values, as stimuli that elicit emotional responses—the emotional response elicited then determining whether the stimulus will be positively or negatively reinforcing as well as whether the stimulus will be approached or avoided. Items on the interest test were considered to measure the emotional response the individual had to the stimuli referred to in the items. The interest test was considered to measure aspects of the individual's "reinforcer system" (an early name for the emotional-motivational repertoire) (see Staats, 1963a, pp. 305–306). The same analysis was made of tests of values. Later MacPhillamy and Lewinsohn (1971) composed a test of people's reinforcers that provided empirical definition of the concept of the "reinforcer system."

Another example of PB's early analysis of psychological tests was shown in its incipient theory of intelligence (Staats, 1963a, p. 404–411), based upon my study of children's learning of important language-cognitive repertoires. "[I]ntelligence . . . may be considered to refer to a wide sample of [learned] basic behavioral skills the child (or adult) has acquired which are important to the acquisition of further skilled behaviors." This account continued by saying that, "Intelligence may be considered as a dependent variable (an effect) and an independent variable (a cause) within the same analysis." Another principle was that "we are interested in this basic behavioral repertoire in the first place because we can observe that children who have the constituents of such a repertoire do well in their life tasks and problems" (Staats, 1968a, p. 389).

In addition, consideration of these complex individual difference characteristics also provided the basis for constructing a taxonomy of abnormal behavior. To illustrate, certain types of psychological disorders (such as schizophrenia, psychopathy, and sexual deviations) were considered to involve deficit and inappropriate aspects of the reinforcer system, that is, the emotional-motivational system or repertoire. The individual's reinforcer system was being employed as an explanation of these behavior disorders (Staats, 1963a, chap. 11).

The Elements for a Theory of Personality:
A Beginning Framework Theory

This was the beginning. Two works—*Learning, Language, and Cognition* (Staats, 1968a) and *Child Learning, Intelligence and Personality* (Staats, 1971a) stipulated additionally the concept of the basic behavioral repertoires, the conditions by which BBRs are learned, and made more clear the concept of the basic behavioral repertoire as a personality concept. The concept and principles of cumulative-hierarchical learning were introduced. Analyses were made of the empirical phenomena that define various personality concepts. As occurs in science, the various developments constituted a foundation for and a growing press for a full behavioral theory of personality.

These developments were furthered in the 1975 book *Social Behaviorism* and the conceptual framework was advanced and stipulated. For one thing, the multilevel theory construction methodology was made more formal. The position taken by PB, from the beginning, was that laboratory study of animal behavior can yield fundamental principles of learning. But it does not yield knowledge about personality and complex behavior in general. The realization was deepened that clinical observations and findings, those of psychometric research, and other human behavior study needed to be utilized. Moreover, bridging theory had to be constructed by which to do so. That became a program of PB, the elaboration of a psychological behavioral theory that utilized, among other things, observations of human behavior gained in clinical, abnormal, educational, social, and child psychology.

The concept of the basic behavioral repertoire is an example of a central bridging theory development needed for that program. The concept opened a new way of viewing the schism between traditional psychology and behaviorism. The schism occurs because personality is traditionally seen as a cause of behavior (an independent variable), but behaviorism customarily considers personality only as behavior, as a dependent variable. The basic behavioral repertoire, in being both a dependent variable and an independent variable, provides the element to resolve this fundamental schism. The *BBRs* are learned, but they also help determine the individual's behavior. Thus, language was analyzed as it was learned, as a dependent variable. But language was also analyzed as it functioned as an independent variable in problem solving, intelligence, and the self-concept. Here was a basis for very generally bringing together the *psychological* and the *behavioral*.

PB'S BASIC THEORY OF PERSONALITY

With the behaviorizing goal, the multilevel framework theory construction methodology, and with the accumulating concepts and principles, a personality theory was formed imbedded in a general behaviorism approach (Staats, 1975). Framework theory is intended to develop in successive steps, however, and much remained to be done. The theory needed to formalized, extended more broadly, with deeper and more systematic analyses. Empirical work had to be derived to extend and support the theory. New directions of research needed to be shown. Description of this extension will begin with the presentation of the PB model of personality.

The PB Model

The PB conception is that the infant begins life without the basic behavioral repertoires. That is why the child displays almost no organized behavior. The child has sensory mechanisms—hearing, sight, tactile sensitivity, and so on. And the child has response mechanisms. But the child's responses have no organization with respect to the stimuli that life presents. Child development, as has been indicated, consists of learning organized behavior to life's stimuli.

That learning is complex. The child learns complex sensory-motor, language-cognitive, and emotional-motivational repertoires. As this occurs the child is changed, becoming able to respond appropriately in various stimulus situations. Moreover, whereas at the beginning the child's learning is laborious, involving only the basic principles of conditioning, as the repertoires are acquired the child's *learning* comes more easily, because it now is aided by the repertoires that have already been acquired. Also the way the child *experiences* the world of stimuli depends, in large part, on the repertoires. And the way the child *behaves* depends upon the repertoires that have been learned. It is because the repertoires have those effects on the child that they are called basic behavioral repertoires. As they are acquired they give the child new characteristics.

Traditional psychology has insisted that there are some personal characteristics, some internal biological processes or structures, that are idiosyncratic to the individual, that determine the individual's behavior. Standard behaviorism has no concept that can coincide with that view of personality. The PB conception, however, is that the personal characteristics are provided by the individual's BBRs. *The basic behavioral repertoires constitute personality.* That means that personality consists of the language-cognitive, emotional-motivational, and sensory-motor repertoires the individual has learned. While one individual's BBRs may have commonalities with those learned by someone else, overall the BBRs are never duplicated in two individuals—the complexity of human experience and the complexity of the human BBRs rules that out. Humans indeed have unique personalities.

The PB conception (model) of personality is presented in Figure 5.1. S_1 stands for the experience (environment) the individual has had, up to the present time, that has produced the learning of the individual's basic behavioral repertoires. As indicated, the very complex BBRs constitute the individual's personality; the BBRs are responsible for the behavioral phenomena from which the concept of personality is derived. The environmental situations (stimuli) that go into producing the BBRs contain many elements and are cumulatively very complex. At the time of behaving, which elements of the BBRs the individual will experience or act-out will be determined by the present stimulus circumstances, depicted in the figure as S_2. Thus the present stimulus situation interacts with the BBRs in producing the individual's behavior, which is depicted as B in the figure. B stands for the behavior made in an encountered situation.

This diagram is only a summary representation of the theory. It is useful for describing the basic elements of the theory. As a summary the diagram does not indicate detail or specifics. For example, we might use the model to describe a particular occasion, when S_2 stands for a particular stimulus situation. Or, we may wish to consider behavior more generally, as it exists over a longer span of time than the specific moment. For example, the individual's drinking over a period of months, after a work situation change that includes a new boss, might be considered in terms of the model. In such a case the S_2 would stand for a current life situation that extends over the relevant period, and B (the individual's drinking behavior) would refer to an

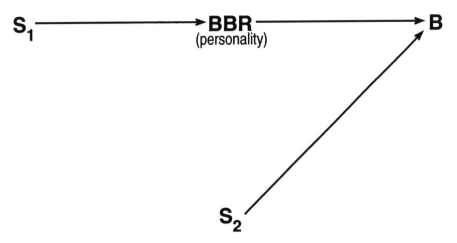

FIGURE 5.1 The psychological behaviorism conception of personality. The individual's environment up to the present (S_1) results in the learning of a basic behavioral repertoire (BBR). The individual's behavior (B) is function of the life situation (S_2) and the individual's BBRs. The BBRs are a dependent variable, because they are the result of learning. But the BBRs are also an independent variable, because they act as a cause of the individual's behavior, and thus constitute the individual's personality.

ongoing, general aspect of the individual's behavior. The figure is not intended to stand for specific circumstances, but only to depict general classes of variables. The model does not constitute a specific behavior analysis, but only a framework for making such an analysis. The conception only becomes an explanatory behavior analysis when its variables are defined in concrete specifics. As is generally the case, the model is only an abbreviation which must be filled in to constitute a real theory. The preceding chapters provide specifications of the theory, as will the rest of the present chapter and that which follows.

BIOLOGY AND PERSONALITY

As in the field of child development, in personality study there has been a long-standing nature–nurture schism—an unfortunate opposition of the biological and environmental positions in the explanation of personality. It is important, thus, in setting forth a theory of personality, to deal with this issue.

Part of the status of biologically oriented conceptions, it should be noted, accrues because they are seen to *represent* the powerful biological sciences.

Most such conceptions, however, do not actually involve biological study. What is involved is that the orientation makes assumptions that attribute personality traits (and human behavior generally) to biological processes—genetics, anatomy, physiology, disease, biochemistry. The expectation is that at some time in the future the biological processes will be found. Such orientations—in attributing complex traits, like intelligence, extroversion, sociability, or dyslexia, to a biological process—have the effect of establishing an obstacle to a behavioral/biological unification. If a trait is laid down in the individual's biological structure, if it is prewired, then that cuts learning out of the explanatory loop.

Biological techniques of study of brain processes have advanced a great deal. This includes many studies that show that brain damage of various kinds will produce behavioral losses and change what is considered to be personality. And there are findings that drugs will do the same. Such studies are considered to support the conception that brain characteristics determine personality characteristics. But there is a theoretical jump here that is not warranted. Let me take intelligence as an example of one type of personality trait. Despite more than a hundred years of belief that some feature of the brain determines intelligence, there is little in the way of direct evidence of such causation. The fact that brain damage can subtract from the individual's intelligence does not indicate that the individual's intelligence had been produced by his brain. The fact is that huge differences in intelligence occur in people whose brains are not different. "You study the brain of a genius, and it doesn't show anything different from the brain of an idiot. Their tissue is the same, their brain waves travel in the same way. No chemical analysis, no electrical presence separates those two individuals. In a . . . [biological science] laboratory, you'll never discover why one person can write so well or paint so well or do mathematics so well, and another cannot" (White, 1967, pp. 112–113).

Because direct evidence has been lacking, many scientific resources have been devoted to gaining "circumstantial" evidence of the presumed genetic determination of intelligence. That is, many studies attempt to "prove" that biology causes a trait, not by direct evidence to that effect, but by ruling out the possibility that the trait could have been learned. For example, a favorite type of study of "genetic" effects on intelligence involves comparing the intelligence scores of identical twins (raised in different homes) to same-sex non-identical twins and to plain siblings (see Bouchard, Lykken, McGue, Segal, & Tellegen, 1990; Herrnsstein & Murray, 1994; Jensen, 1969). The correlation of IQ scores is highest for identical twins and diminishes with lessened genetic similarity. The interpretation of genetic cause in such studies rests on the assumption that being raised in different homes controls the effects of the environment. The logic of the approach will not hold water, however. The position rests on the assumption that placement into adoptive homes has been random—which is not the case. Those who place children try to match the child's characteristics to those of the home, which means children are placed systematically. Moreover, identical twins will be placed in more similar homes than others (Kamin, 1974; Staats, 1970, 1971a). It is also the case that physical attributes of *subjects* constitute an "environmental" variable that influences the results. That is, the individual's physical characteristics affect how people respond to the individual, and that environment effects what the individual learns. Beautiful people face a different environment than do plain or odd-looking people, and big, strong, and fast males face a different environment than small and weak males. Such things affect twin studies—for identical twins *share* any social environment that is produced by their shared physical attributes.

In any event, twin studies (the strongest available evidence) are indirect; they do not show just what biological processes "cause" intelligence or any other personality trait. Such studies can only have an exhortatory purpose that encourages efforts directly to find the biological mechanisms. But exhortation is not needed. Our popular as well as scientific cultures are already convinced of genetic determination of personality. Research to find biological causation of personality has been going on for some hundred and fifty years. What is needed—if there really are biological variations that determine individual differences—is direct evidence of what those biological mechanisms are and how they work their effects. Such evidence is lacking.

The same criticism may be directed at the environmentalist side, it may be added. Its traditional evidence, too, has been lacking. For example, there are studies showing that children exposed to an enriched preschool experience have higher IQ measures (Dawe, 1942; Peters & McElwee, 1944). As another example, Scarr and Weinberg (1976) showed that black children adopted by middle-class white parents had better than average IQs, and those adopted early had more positive IQ effects. Such studies, also, only serve an exhortatory purpose. For in such studies there is no specification regarding what the children's experience was, how it affected their intelligence, what intelligence is, or how it has its effects on behavior. The environmentalist approach, like the biological approach, has been vague. Just what personality traits are has not been specified, the learning conditions and principles that produce them, and so on.

This same weakness, it may be added, applies to behaviorists, like Watson and Skinner. They, too, have not come to grips with the study of individual differences, except by way of suggesting a general environmentalism. And that is not always clear: "A certain gene may fail in laying a proper foundation for the brain; the result will be to produce a feeble-minded individual. . . . It is clearly proved experimentally that diverse [genetic] combinations yield . . . diversities in behavior" (Watson, 1930, p. 51). The same may be said of Skinner. His statements have been taken to represent an extreme environmentalism. But he actually did not formulate such a position, or provide any substance to support one. He did not study the importance of learning in childhood, or call for this study. He did not indicate how in childhood the child learns personality traits. His work does not indicate a conviction that it is learning that produces all of complex human behavior. His position with respect to biological causation was stated in a paper entitled "Phylogeny and ontogeny of behavior" (Skinner, 1966). The position is that biological evolution produces adaptive behavior in the organism. The shaping of behavior, via the principles of reinforcement, is said to take over where evolution leaves off in producing adaptive behavior (Skinner, 1966). This position suggests there is biological determination of behavior and that learning is like evolutionary effects in this way. But that position does not constitute a framework that unifies biological study with learning study, and thereby provide a basis for solving the nature–nurture schism.

The nature–nurture issue is a perennial problem in psychology. The interactionist conception—that both biology and learning determine human behavior and personality—only represents a "let's not fight" political compromise. No interaction approach has actually shown how learning and biological work together to produce individual differences. And, in actuality, studies and theories follow one or the other position. Some studies attempt to establish biological variables as *the* cause in a way that eliminates or trivializes the role of learning. Other studies or theories take a general environmentalist position in a way that leaves out the biological organism. No conceptual framework has been set forth indicating how to consider biology and learning as they jointly determine personality (and human behavior generally).

Evolution and Personality

The PB position is a first step toward establishing the roles of biology and learning as they operate to produce behavior. One consideration is to realize that biology is responsible for learning. Organisms operate according to the laws of classical and operant conditioning, because to do so has been adaptive in evolution (Staats, 1963a, pp. 68–69). One important aspect of unification occurs is establishing the biological basis of learning (see Staats, 1975, chap. 15) and this should continue as an important problem of study. To continue, however, the increase of learning capacity has occurred over species through evolutionary principles. We recognize that certain animals have greater learning ability than others, with humans at the top. Anthropology has also shown us that the human brain has increased dramatically in volume and in other features over the species that preceded *homo sapiens*.

Evolution has also given humans general sensory systems—visual, auditory, taste, smell, proprioceptive, and others. It is noteworthy that evolution in humans has produced acuity in various sensory organs, versus the greater *specialized* developments we see in the dolphin's echo-location sensory system, the smell that is so highly developed in dogs and pigs, and the sight that is so acute in eagles. In addition, evolution has given humans a hand with an opposable thumb, a bi-pedal gait, and a complex of vocal organs that compose a multifaceted, sensitive, and flexible apparatus that can produce a large variety of sounds. Evolution has endowed humans with a sensory apparatus, variously to contact the stimuli of the world, a response apparatus of wide capacity, and an enormous learning ability.

The PB position is that biological evolution also made humans more general than lower organisms in learning. There are no prewired, specific complex human behaviors (in contrast to reflexes). Here PB differs from most approaches. The PB position is that it would be non-adaptive for humans to inherit specific behaviors. Mathematics skill, playing a violin, interest in science, or love of reading would have been non-adaptive 40,000 years ago when *homo sapiens* appeared, as would courtly courtesy, answering intelligence-test items, or risking one's life to make the world safe for democracy. "Rather, such men *learned* to shape rocks, fight savagely, throw spears, club prey, make fire, plan group hunts, stitch furs, carve fishhooks, find and eat insects, discriminate subtle cues in tracking prey, communicate, and so on" (Staats, 1971a, p. 551). In the PB view the traditional belief—that humans respond to complex environmental stimuli with their complex responses because they have inherited a "hard-wired" nervous system—is a poor conception from a biological orientation. Such hard-wiring would be a handicap in an evolutionary sense. The inheritance of specialized behavior patterns limits the organism to specialized environmental niches. Specialization is disadvantageous in variable conditions. A great power of humans is a universal adaptability, a variability in behavior that makes it possible to survive under a great variety of conditions. The PB theory is that the human *learns* all but the simplest (reflexes), the only S–R connections that are hard-wired. The glory of *homo sapiens* is learning ability, and the generality, as well as complexity of behavior that can be acquired. That has made it possible for humans to learn the behaviors necessary to adapt to all of the world's climates and physical features, which no other animal can do. Any position that trivializes the enormous impact of human learning in acquiring personality traits is a poor theory from a biological perspective.

Psychological behaviorism is thus very environmentalist, perhaps more than any other systematic theory of human behavior. Does that mean that PB leaves out biology? Is the role of biology finished after the evolution of learning? The answer in each case is no. Biology does play additional roles, but not as an explanation of particular behaviors or traits of behavior. *Biology provides the mechanisms for the sensing, learning, and performance of behavior.* In the PB view it is learning that explains human traits, but various biological conditions can have an effect on that learning. Figure 5.2 indicates more specifically how PB conceptualizes the relationship of learning and biology, within its model of personality.

S_1 in the figure stands for the original learning circumstances that produce the basic behavioral repertoires (BBRs). O_1 stands for the biological conditions that exist during this original learning. For example, let us take a severely brain-damaged child. Even though the environment is normal, the child will not learn BBRs in a normal manner. Similarly, genetic conditions, such as Down's syndrome, may impair brain development and hence BBR learning. Also the microcephalic child has brain development that is more severely lacking and learning is more severely limited. In a different way, the child with cerebral palsy might be neurologically capable of normal learning, but uncontrollable movement may prevent normal learning circumstances from occurring. Drugs can also alter neurological function and interfere with learning. And Ritalin has been effective in increasing the learning of hyperactive children, probably by reducing the activity, not by affecting the neurological ability to learn. The point is that the biological organism constitutes the mechanism by which learning takes place—and that mechanism can be affected in various ways.

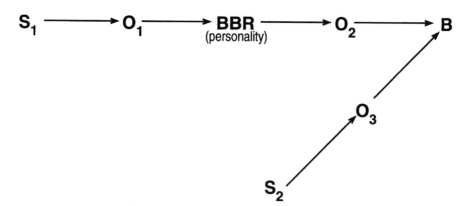

FIGURE 5.2   The psychological behaviorism conception of how the biological state of the individual affects personality, perception, and behavior. The biological organism (O_1) is the mechanism by which the environment (S_1) produces the learning that results in the BBRs (personality). If there is something awry with the biological mechanism, then the learning of the BBR will be affected. In addition, if something happens to the biological organism (O_2) *after* the BBR is learned, the BBR may be affected. A change in the BBR will result in changes in the individual's behavior. Finally, the individual's behavior depends upon sensing the confronting environment (S_2). Anything awry with the individual's sensory organs (O_3) will alter the perceived environment and affect the individual's behavior.

In addition to these effects, biological conditions can also play a role, at O_2, after the personality repertoires have been acquired. For learning experiences may be considered to produce neurological connections between stimulus and response events that persist. The central nervous system "carries" or "stores" the BBRs, for example, by adding neural connections. It is important to consider O_2 as that storage. At a later time, in the current environmental situation, how the individual behaves will be determined by what BBRs have been learned (stored in O_2). Thus, at this later time, the individual's biological state is an important determinant of behavior. A brain tumor, injuries, a stroke, fever, physiological conditions (such as hormone levels), drugs, or toxic conditions can affect the biological mechanism (O_2) in a way that will affect the BBRs that have *already* been acquired. As an example, an individual may have learned a rich language-cognitive repertoire. However, a head injury may literally remove that repertoire, or parts of it. Such an individual in a normal environment may not behave normally in various ways—in problem solving, reasoning, planning, or learning, and on neuropsychological tests—because the individual has lost the necessary BBRs through organic damage. Such losses may be temporary or permanent, depending on the organic condition involved. For example, drug effects will ordinarily wear off, but not loss of brain tissue. In this and other ways biological conditions at the O_2 time can determine behavior and individual differences in behavior.

Organic conditions, in another way, may also exert their effects on how the current environmental situation acts on the individual. By way of illustration, an individual may have fully developed language-cognitive repertoires and an intact central nervous system at O_2, such that an appropriate environmental stimulus—such as a restaurant menu—would ordinarily elicit the individual's reading behavior. Let us say, however, that as a consequence of aging (which happens around 40) the inflexibility of the lenses of the eyes may make it impossible to see the letters clearly enough to read without glasses in the dim light. There are various organic conditions (shown as O_3 in the figure) that can interfere with the individual's ability to respond sensorily to the current environment. The individual may have defective sight, hearing, smell, or taste through a variety of biological problems. In addition, there are other biological mechanisms that may determine how the individual responds to the current environment, without having an effect on the individual's BBRs. As an example, a man with a normal life environment and normal organic conditions has learned the normal language-cognitive, emotional-motivational, and sensory-motor repertoires necessary to make love. However, alcohol or some other drug may impair his "response mechanism," leaving him impotent in a situation in which he would otherwise perform adequately. Removal of the temporary organic condition, however, will return the individual to normal behavior because the BBRs are intact. Thus, there are organic conditions that can interfere either with the individual's ability to respond sensorily to the current environment, or with the individual's response mechanisms. In these ways organic conditions at O_3 can affect behavior. Such conditions may be permanent, as in the sensory or response losses through aging, or they may be temporary, as in illness or drug conditions.

Organic conditions, thus, are important in the PB theory of personality. *But an essential feature of the theory is that organic conditions affect behavior only through affecting learning, basic behavioral repertoire, behavior, and sensory processes.* The theory sets forth how biological study is to be introduced to the endeavor. It calls for stipulation of the organic processes in terms of how they effect how personality is acquired and how personality functions after it is acquired. General illusions to genetic, physiological, anatomical, or other biological conditions—like the concepts of minimal brain dysfunction, genetically induced autism or shyness, learning disability, dyslexia, and the like—do not fulfill the demands of the theory. They provide no stipulation of what is supposedly involved. In the PB view organic conditions by themselves do not produce behaviors or traits of personality of any kind.

In the PB view a biological explanation of personality or behavior is only useful if it provides specification of when and how organic conditions affect learning the BBRs, the retention of the BBRs, and the perception of the environment or ability to respond. A first step in gaining such knowledge is the realization that biological variables can have behavioral effects at the three different sites indicated in Figure 5.2. For example, although we may see that a child cannot read when presented with appropriate stimuli, it would make a great deal of difference whether an interfering organic condition had its effect (1) in early childhood, preventing the formation of the relevant basic behavioral repertoires; (2) later, in the form of brain damage, removing basic behavioral repertoires the child had already acquired; or (3) later, involving conditions (like retinal damage) that leave the basic behavioral repertoires intact, but prevent the child from sensing or responding to current situations in a way that would activate the repertoires and result in adjustive behavior.

Biology Provides the Mechanism, Learning Provides the Content

Biology thus plays its role, not as a "creator" of complex human behaviors or personality repertoires, but as the *instrument* by which those behaviors are learned. Biological problems may "delete" or disturb already learned complex repertoires—traits, abilities, talents, and so on. For example, serious biological problems may produce general behavior effects such as in Alzheimer's or Korzikoff's disease. Biological manipulations can also affect the individual's emotional responding and thereby affect behavior in general ways. But biological conditions do not create complex behaviors.

Biological development, for example, does not create language in the individual, or toilet training, social skills, altruism, ambition, suspiciousness, and reading ability. However, after the individual has learned some complex, general behavior (repertoire) a brain injury may delete that repertoire in whole or part, or disturb the display of the repertoire. Similarly, drugs cannot produce complex human behaviors or personality. However, drugs can affect brain operation and, by so doing, affect the BBRs the individual has learned, thereby affecting the individual's behavior, experience, and learning. Drugs can produce euphoria, or reduce depression, or create anxiety, and thereby affect behavior drastically. This is ordinarily a general effect that is brought on by changing the way the mechanism functions. But in this way the drugs can affect the individual's emotional response to various life stimuli. The result may be change in the individual's emotional-motivational repertoire and various ways of behaving. Changes in the BBRs will be interpreted as changes in personality. Understanding what is occurring demands explication of the mechanisms. The PB conception places learning and biology into relationship in the causal process, but demands specificity.

Additions to the Nature–Nurture Position

In the present view, biologically oriented approaches to personality have been "barking up the wrong tree." The field tries to establish or find the manner in which humans are hard-wired to display certain behavior traits. As has been indicated, this is a poor biological conception, as in eliminating or downplaying the importance of learning. Rather, those interested in how biology affects behavior should approach the task differently. At the basic level, there is a need to study what the biological mechanisms of learning are (see Staats, 1975, chap. 15). There is also a need to study how biology can affect the learning of the BBRs. If mental retardation, for example, involves biological limits on learning, then it is important to ascertain just how this occurs. Do children with Down's syndrome learn basically more slowly? Or does their limitation have more to do with the quantity of learning that can occur? Can they learn early basic behavioral repertoires, but not later BBRs? Or, is it the case that they can learn BBRs but not with as many elements as is usual? What are the mechanisms by which the learning is affected? Conversely, what are the differences of these kinds in people who have very high ability? For example, if we took a large sample of newly born infants and tested their rapidity of conditioning, would it turn out that those who conditioned more rapidly would be the ones who turned out to be better learners? Are there any significant individual difference variations in the basic rapidity of primary conditioning (see Staats, 1975, pp. 546–549)?

In addition, the PB framework calls for research on the manner in which change of the biological mechanism can affect already learned BBRs.

There has been, of course, much study of how brain damage, drugs, and other conditions can affect behavior. But such study is ordinarily used to show that brain characteristics determine individual differences in behavior (personality). It is important to establish *how* brain damage affects the operation of BBRs the individual has learned. There are localization studies that attempt to correlate area of injury with type of behavioral loss. But this study has not been used to bridge biological and learning theories. Psychological behaviorism suggests that brain localization study should be pursued as a means of finding out more about the functioning of the BBRs. For example, is the verbal-motor repertoire localized in a different place than the verbal-labeling, verbal-emotional, and verbal-image repertoires? Preliminary consideration might suggest this as a possibility, since there are emotional and sensory and response parts of the brain. The point is that if biology is involved in personality traits then there has to be a biological-behavioral mechanism involved that must be ascertained.

In addition, however, other questions arise. There is a great deal of research on how alcohol and drugs affect perception and sensory-motor skill and learning. Such study could be conducted in a manner that would tie it into the PB theory of the BBRs. When depression is alleviated by drugs, what BBRs are affected? Is the effect only one of generally making the individual's emotional responding more positive? Or, are there effects on specific BBRs of the three types? When caffeine slightly increases the individual's learning ability, is this through affecting the rate of basic conditioning? Or is the effect due to some action on the functioning of the BBRs in cumulative-hierarchical learning? Or does caffeine have its affect by promoting more rapid responding, or better perception of stimuli? In what way do drugs affect the way the BBRs function, and thereby affect behavior?

In terms of O_3 there are also things to be studied in relating the theory of the BBRs to biological study. Age, drugs, and injury can affect the individual's sensory acuity—in hearing, vision, taste, smell, and so on. For example, changes in behavior as a function of aging could arise in two different ways. On the one hand, biological conditions in aging could result in losses in the BBRs. The individual's behavior losses would then be due to personality changes. Senile diseases appear to obliterate previously acquired BBRs. On the other hand, aging might have no effect on the BBRs. However, sensory losses and response losses (as in physical agility) might be the reasons for the individual's behavior losses. The old person might not be scintillating in conversation because of hearing difficulty, not because of loss of intellectual power, as one example.

The lack of research relating biology to learning, the BBRs, and behavior underlies the behaviorism/biology schism. Traditionally, attempts to use biology or learning to explain personality have been general and vague. Specificity in conception and in study can remove these qualities and replace them with definitive treatment of both types of causes and how they relate. The point is that if biology is involved in personality traits, then there has to be a learning–brain mechanism involved. The PB position, thus, unlike that of radical behaviorism, has been to effect a learning–biology unification. Interestingly there are beginnings now on the neurobiology side (Begley, 1996; Merzenich, Jenkins, Johnston, Schreiner, Miller, & Tallal, 1996) that constitute a recognition of the importance of learning in complex human behavior.

BEHAVIOR AND PERSONALITY

There are other questions that arise concerning the PB theory of personality. For one thing, the basic behavioral repertoires are composed of behaviors. Why, then, is it productive to formulate a theory that has a concept of the BBR (personality) as well as a concept of behavior? Are they not the same? Is it not sufficient to say that personality is behavior, in a Watsonian manner, which dispenses with the need for a concept of personality? The basic question, which arises within a radical behaviorism framework, is a good one. The answer, however, is that the BBR and behavior are not the same thing, in various ways that call for explication.

Differences between Behavior and the BBR

There are various reasons to differentiate the concept of the BBR from the concept of behavior in constructing a theory of human behavior, as will be briefly indicated.

Distal and Proximal Effects of the Environment

One reason is that behavior occurs in the here-and-now. It is the environment acting *now* that is the eliciting agent. The BBRs, however, are determined by the learning conditions that occurred in the past. In this sense the BBRs can be seen to fulfill the role of such cognitive concepts as "memory" and "personality" in traditional theory construction. In experimental psychology, the fact that the environment plays two roles—one distal and one proximal—is included in the traditional *learning and memory* dichotomy. There is the acquisition process and then memory keeps the learning there, waiting for later circumstances that will call it out. This has the drawback of making memory a vague mental characteristic. Standard behaviorism, with only a concept of displayed behavior, lacks a good conceptualization of the past, capable of dealing with concepts such as memory and personality.

In the PB theory the distal environment results in the *acquisition* of behaviors. The proximal environment, on the other hand, constitutes the present eliciting agent for the behavior that is displayed. Of course, the one environmental situation may have both effects, that of eliciting behaviors and of providing experience that results in further learning. This does not, however, change the need to separate the two roles of the environment.

Behavior as a Sample from the BBRs

We may record everything a person says for some extended period. This would be a large sample of the individual's verbal behavior. We would know, however, that this was just a sample. It would not constitute all of the verbal behavior that the individual could display. That can never be observed, for various reasons. Each of us, for one thing, has learned single words that we have never employed and will never employ in speech. No matter how long someone recorded our verbal behavior, the nature of our verbal-labeling repertoire will never be revealed with respect to that word. There are many words like that. Moreover, that example is increased manyfold when we consider the huge number of combinations of words that we could utter, but never have and never will.

The BBR can be considered as the universe of behaviors that the individual has learned. The current situation "samples" from that universe. The behavior the individual displays in the particular situation is a function of the universe and a function of the situation, which is the sampling mechanism. But the individual could meet an infinite number of different environmental situations. Most will never occur, however. Thus the infinite number of responses that could be made to those environmental situations—by virtue of her BBRs—will never take place. For example, my theory represents a large BBR for me that I have, in an incipient manner, extended to various areas in outlining future papers and books. There are many more plans than I will ever have a chance to write. Even those who have the most intimate knowledge of my behavior will never know those plans.

Let me suggest that samples of the individual's life behaviors can reveal less about the nature of the individual's BBRs than would an artificial sample whose goal is the measurement of such BBRs. This is especially relevant for psychological evaluation: the PB conception says that an important part of evaluation concerns measuring the elements of the basic behavioral repertoires. Sometimes measurement of the BBRs will be better than measurements of actual behaviors. Let me suggest that people speaking to each other display smaller differences in vocabulary than will be shown on tests, because everyday speech is made up of common words to common situations. This statement thus provides us with one of the important distinctions between behavior and the BBRs. Behavior is that which occurs in specific life situations. Observations of that behavior constitute the most direct means of assessment, but not necessarily the most complete. The individual's life situations may not sample well the individual's BBRs; the contrived observations of psychological testing may yield more information concerning the BBRs, contrary to Mischel (1972) and Kanfer and Phillips (1970).

Creativity of Personality

Behaviors displayed are actual occurrences. The BBRs are also different from behavior in constituting a *potential* for action, in several respects. One is that the BBRs are composed of elements that can be "put together" in different ways, depending upon the stimulus elements in the situations that are encountered. Novel situations can evoke new, original behavior *combinations* in the individual—behaviors that have never occurred before (see Staats, 1968a, pp. 168–178). Behaviors in that combination will not have been learned, since the situation has never occurred before. Moreover, we might not be able to predict the behavior combination from any recording of the individual's past behaviors. Let us take a simple example. A young child may have just have been trained to say "dog" to such animals, and "running" to the stimulus of the rapidly alternating legs of a horse. Confronted with a running dog, this child may say something it has never said before, and has not been trained to say, that is "running dog," or "dog running." To predict such phenomena we need to have done something else than observe the child's behavior. This is especially the case with people who have acquired exceptional BBRs—let us say an Einstein, Newton, or Freud—and whose life circumstances have elicited combinations of elements that are surprisingly novel (see Staats, 1963a, pp. 236–245).

Since the BBRs have a great number of elements, the combinations that can occur under the action of different environmental combinations are almost infinite. For example, observing the pieces a musician has played cannot be used to predict what she can or will play—for she has the potential for playing an infinite number of new compositions just by being presented with the written music. As another example, the ordinary individual is said to know from 10,000 to 80,000 words. The size of the repertoire makes the individual capable of infinite variation in combinations of words uttered in response to appropriate external and internal stimulus conditions. In these senses this language-cognitive repertoire is a capacity or potentiality, a personality (cognitive) characteristic which cannot be known from observing the individual's behavior.

The Case When the BBR Is Different From the Behavior

Finally, a most important reason for introducing both the concepts of behavior and the basic behavioral repertoire is because in many cases they are different. As background for this point, an early (and continuing) behavior therapy position is that it is behavior that is the problem, in contrast to psychodynamic approaches that consider the underlying psychological problem to be the real cause. There are many cases when the behavior therapy position is correct—where the problem is the displayed behavior itself. But there are many important cases where the problem is not the same thing as the behavior. Let us take as an example a child with a conduct problem in the classroom. In some cases the real problem is not the behavior itself, that is, the sensory-motor behaviors that disrupt the class. To illustrate, let us say the teacher is reading a story to the class, and the other children's attentive behavior is maintained by the reinforcement provided by the images and emotional responses elicited by the words of the story. The language-deficit child, however, will experience no images and no emotional responses, and hence no reinforcement for the behavior of sitting and listening. The result is this child's attentive behavior will not be maintained. Rather, alternative sensory-motor behavior will have been learned because they have been reinforced by disrupting such boring situations. The overt behavior of this child is unimportant, consisting of very usual sensory-motor responses. Attempts to treat the problem by reinforcing the child's attentive sensory-motor behavior and extinguishing the child's undesirable sensory-motor behavior would be ineffective—and would constitute symptomatic (versus causal) treatment. Understanding the real problem lies in understanding the relationship of the BBRs and behavior, that language BBR deficits can give rise to disruptive behavior. For many behavior problems have the BBRs as the proximal cause. The problem behaviors themselves may be very usual, ones that everyone has learned.

The concept of personality was no doubt constructed because much of overt behavior is the result of other behavioral processes of the individual, frequently within the individual where they cannot be observed. After all we experience some of these processes. Traditional psychology made the mistake of considering those internal events in different, non-behavioral, mentalistic terms. As a consequence, behaviorists rejected such considerations *in toto*. What is necessary is to recognize that personality is composed of the same *types* of events as behavior, but that personality is different from displayed behavior itself. Differentiating the two concepts—behavior and the basic behavioral repertoires—allows us to deal with the phenomena that have been of importance to traditional psychologists, but within an objective, unified, explanatory set of behavioral principles and concepts.

Additional Reasons Why the BBRs Constitute a Concept of Personality

There are vast individual differences in BBRs. Moreover, fitting traditional expectations, they are carried within. Behaviorism traditionally has been rejected because of suggesting that the external environment determines overt behavior. This disagrees with our common experience that personal characteristics differ and are causes of behavior. The theory of the BBRs allows us to accept that there are causal personality characteristics without sacrificing behavioristic demand for objective specification.

The BBRs fulfill that aspect of the traditional definition of personality. They are also general, not situationally specific. In the example above, attending to a teacher's story was seen to depend upon having learned verbal-motor, verbal-image, and verbal-emotional repertoires. Those same repertoires will be functional in many situations and affect the behavior displayed by the individual. The BBRs, thus, are the basic reason that individual differences in behavior can be seen across a variety of situations.

The fact that individual differences persist over time has also given support to the traditional concept of personality. Let it be said, thus, that the continuity of personality is due, in part, to the fact that BBRs generally persist over time. This occurs for several reasons. One is that the more elements compose the BBR, the less impact each new experience has on the nature of the BBR, simply because the new element is a smaller fraction of the total. The larger the BBR learned, the more learning is needed to change it.

More importantly, the BBRs provide continuity by maintaining the consistency of the individual's experience. Thus, for example, once the individual has developed a certain aspect of the emotional-motivational repertoire, this itself will determine behavior such that additional experiences will add to what has already been learned. For example, once the individual has learned a positive emotional response to classical music, the individual's behavior will be *reinforced* by such music. So music-relevant behaviors—like turning on certain TV and radio programs—will be maintained. In addition, music-relevant stimuli as incentives will *elicit* approach behaviors. So the individual will buy tickets to announced concerts, buy newly published books on music, enroll for classes on music appreciation, associate with friends who talk about music, and attend musical events. The experiences such behaviors yield will further ensure continuance of this BBR development and consequent behavior. Developments in the emotional-motivational repertoire affect sensory-motor behaviors.

The concept of the BBR also suggests that personality will have continuity and persist over time because one's environment ordinarily has a good deal of continuity. But, since the BBRs are learned, circumstances can occur that will produce change. For example, the music-oriented person described above may have an intense love affair with someone in the field of music that ends catastrophically. That may produce such negative emotional conditioning that the individual avoids musical occasions that may arouse those negative emotions. The avoidance behavior may lead the individual into experiences that condition her emotional-motivational repertoire in a different direction. This is to say, thus, that BBRs once learned will ordinarily tend to persist, but they are not immutable. The PB theory provides specific principles and analyses for considering the way that individual differences can be stable or unstable.

PERSONALITY IN BEHAVIOR CAUSATION

It has been said that the BBR is an independent variable—a cause—as well as a dependent variable—an effect. If the BBR is composed of behavior, how can it be the cause of behavior? The BBR can be a direct cause of behavior in various ways. For example, let us take the case of the child who has learned to attend to what an adult says when requested to do so. This is a part of the verbal-motor repertoire. A child who has this repertoire will attend to what a teacher says in school, will experience the stimuli the teacher presents, and thus learn new things. The child without that aspect of the verbal-motor repertoire will not attend, will not experience the stimuli, and will not learn. The BBR is thus the proximal cause of children's behavior in class, the experience received, and the learning that results.

This conception of the BBR changes one's view of the causation of human behavior and the phenomena of individual differences. We can see that a child with a certain BBR is different from a child lacking that BBR. The two will behave differently, experience things differently, and learn differently. These differences will occur when the children are in the same situation, where the same reinforcers are available, and where the same controlling stimuli are present. That is why non-behavioral psychologists have not accepted radical behaviorism's insistence on considering the cause of human behavior to be the situation that confronts the individual.

Intrinsic to the traditional concept of personality is that it is a cause of behavior. Everyone has personal experience of internal events—commonly called thoughts, images, and emotions—that affect one's behavior. That personal experience is supplemented by all the findings that show that people who measure differently on tests—like intelligence tests and interest tests and tests like the Minnesota Multiphasic Personality Inventory (MMPI) (Dahlstrom & Welsh, 1960)—behave differently. Tests seem to be measuring a cause of human behavior.

The concept of personality causation is thus firmly entrenched in the field of personality and in cognitive psychology. But traditional personality theories have never faced up to the demands of good theory with respect to explaining that causation. If an internal process or structure is said to determine the way the individual behaves, then this statement calls for specification. For one thing, the question of how personality *affects* behavior must then be specified—how and according to what principles. For another, the way that personality determines behavior cannot be specified unless personality itself is first specified. It is necessary to define personality before indicating how it acts as a cause. What are interests such that they cause one individual to behave in a successful manner in a particular job, and another person, with different interests, to fail? And how do interests work these effects, by what principles? What is the extroverted personality trait that makes the individual behave in an outgoing manner with people, and how does the trait function to affect behavior? What is intelligence that it makes the individual behave skillfully in various situations?

Traditional personality theories do not answer such questions. Psychological tests do not provide the definition of the personality traits they measure, or the principles of how the personality traits determine the way the individual behaves. Freud's theory, interestingly, provided some specification of this kind. For example, his theory stated that the stage of psychosexual development determined the individual's needs. Those needs determined in what objects the individual would have an emotional investment (cathexis). Cathected objects became goals to be attained, and thus affected behavior. However, despite tidbits here and there, Freud's theory generally contained little specification of his personality concepts (like the *id, ego,* and *superego*), and of the manner in which they determined behavior.

The PB personality theory lends itself to the type of specification required. Personality is seen to be composed of specified and specifiable BBRs. Some have mistakenly thought that the concept of the BBR is an intervening variable—a logical term that connects the experienced environment with behavior. But personality in the PB theory is not an intervening variable. Personality is considered as something real and substantive. Psychological behaviorism's analyses of personality refer to complex language, motor, and emotional repertoires. These are not logical figments; they are actual stimulus–response constellations that have to be stipulated; what they are, how they are learned, and how they act upon the individual's behavior. The preceding chapters have aimed to indicate that the BBRs have specific contents. Nevertheless, study is necessary to specify fully the behavioral contents of the BBRs, how the BBRs function, and by what principles. PB has begun this task. But it is a very large task, and there is much to do. Additional specification will be provided in the next chapter.

THE ENVIRONMENT IN BEHAVIOR CAUSATION

One of the features of the PB personality theory is how the environment is treated. Systematic separation of the roles of the distal and proximal environments helps provide reasons for introduction of the new concept of the

BBR, for one thing. For another, the concept of the two actions of the environment sharpens the way organic conditions can be considered, as indicated in Figure 5.2. The environment separation makes it clear that organic conditions operate on the individual at different times, in three different ways. Organic conditions must be considered as they affect the learning of the BBRs, the later functioning of the BBRs, and the individual's ability to respond to the life situation. The distinctions should help in studying the way behavioral conditions interact with organic conditions in determining behavior.

How about the other behaviorisms? Second-generation behaviorism has lacked systematicity here. There used to be a difference in the manner in which the second-generation behaviorisms considered learning and behavior. A central concept in Hull's (1943a) theory was habit strength (sHr), which represented learning. And in experimentation, Hull employed situations in which the learning of a response was critical. So Hull thus was interested in learning (as a theoretical concept), and focused on defining his concept of learning and its relationships with other concepts.

But Skinner differed from other behaviorists in this respect. He did not consider himself a learning theorist (Ferster & Skinner, 1957; Skinner, 1938). His experimental worked ignored learning in favor of the reinforcement variables that affected the organism's *already learned* behavior in the operant chamber. His study was of the effects of reinforcement schedules on *behavior,* not learning, with individual animals subjected to successive variations in reinforcement to see the effects on that behavior (Ferster & Skinner, 1957; Skinner, 1938). What that represents conceptually is a focus on the effects of the present situation on behavior.

This characteristic is carried by those who employ Skinner's theory for considering human behavior, as in the fields of behavior analysis and behavior therapy. How about the concept of "learning (or conditioning) history"? Although the concept is used widely in behavior analysis, the concept actually proves the point. For there has been little systematic study in radical behaviorism—or any other second-generation behaviorism—of the learning histories that produce human behavior. The concept is thus scientifically empty. That fact has recently been recognized for the first time in behavior analysis (Wanchisen, 1990).

Skinner's methods were valuable in the study of animal behavior in stipulating how reinforcement schedules could affect behavior. However, in human behavior *past* learning is centrally important. To illustrate, the stimulus circumstances, including the *potential* reinforcement conditions (schedules), in a classroom are largely the same for all. The behavior the children display in that situation is determined by what they bring to class, that is, their BBRs. *In fact, that behavior will largely determine the reinforcement the children receive.* One child with rich BBR development will behave in a way that harvests reinforcement for achievement behaviors, while the child with sparse BBR development will display disruptive behaviors that harvest the teacher's disapproval. Such characteristics of human behavior underlie the traditional rejection of radical behaviorism's focus on explaining how the environment determines behavior, and the concept that the individual is not responsible.

These are reasons why the position that PB takes is fundamentally different from Skinner's radical behaviorism. The PB framework, in separating the distal and proximal environments, provides for the systematic study of the former (and the latter). The human learning/cognitive and child development levels have been explicitly developed for the study of distal learning, and the BBRs that result. Radical behaviorism has lacked these levels of study. Because PB theory treats both a learning environment and a behaving environment, I have referred to it as a learning-behavior theory, not just one or the other.

THE PERSON–SITUATION SCHISM, AND PB'S INTERACTION APPROACH

Watsonian behaviorism was seen as a challenge to the conventional conception of personality traits that determine individual differences in behavior, across situations. Moreover, studies were conducted that appeared to support the radical behavioristic idea that it is the situation that determines behavior, not general personality traits. Thus, Hartshorne and May (1928, 1929) conducted an extensive study of children's "moral" character using a number of different situational tests of honesty. These researchers found a low correlation among the various tests, indicating that a child who was honest in one type of situation might not be in another. Their conclusion was that there are specific habits, elicited by specific situations, but not traits that are general. Newcomb (1929) found the same situational variability with indices of the trait of extroversion–introversion. The issue died down in the 1930s, only to be revivified by Mischel (1968), who again asserted the situationism position of behaviorism. In response, a number of studies were conducted, some in support of the situationism position and some in support of the person (personality) position (Bem & Allen, 1974; Block, 1971, 1977; Epstein, 1979; Olweus, 1974, 1977; Rushton, Jackson, & Paunonen, 1981).

When such contests occur, a resolution may be offered that says, in effect, that both sides are right. This has occurred in the several cycles of the situation–person issue, most recently in what is called interaction psychology (see Bandura, 1977; Endler & Magnusson, 1976; Mischel, 1973).

This interactionist position draws upon studies that suggest there are personality-causal variables and situational-causal variables, as well as an interaction between the two, also considered as a causal variable. For example, Gilmor and Minton (1974) found that, under a success situation, internal locus-of-control personalities attributed success to internal factors more than did external locus-of-control subjects, but such attribution was reversed under a failure situation. The statistical interaction, thus, predicted the attributions better than either the personality variable or the situation variable.

However, the PB view (see Staats, 1980) is that such interaction is a statistical figment of the analysis of variance experimental designs employed. There is no real "interaction"—it is only that people differ in their BBRs and, for that reason, do not respond to situations in the same way. Actually there is consistency in behavior (see Staats, 1980). There are only two types of causal variables in subjects, the personality (BBR) variable and the situation variable. It is suggested that analysis of what internal and external locus of control BBRs actually are would reveal directly why the subjects responded in one way in the success situation and in another way in the failure situation.

Let me exemplify this analytic PB position. Let us say in studying learning ability we select two groups of subjects: one composed of individuals with a highly developed language-cognitive BBR, and a poorly developed sensory-motor BBR, and the other with the opposite BBRs. If we then exposed these two groups to two types of learning—one involving language materials and the other involving learning sensory-motor skills—we would find one group would be the better learners in one situation, but the other group would be the better learners in the other. An analysis-of-variance treatment of the results would produce a large statistical interaction term. That term, however, only reflects the very direct effect of the different BBRs on learning. There is no "interaction causation." It is only because person–situation interaction studies do not analyze the situations, BBRs, and behavior involved that the statistical result is interpreted as some sort of person–situation interaction causation. As PB has pointed out, if we wish to explain behavior it is necessary to be analytic. Vaguely specified studies are fertile ground for unresolved issues (Staats, 1980).

FREE WILL, AGENCY, AND SELF-CAUSATION

In traditional views humans are thought to have free will and self-determination. Originally the concept of free will was that the individual's divinely given soul was responsible for the individual's behavior. And this soul was free, not determined like the material, physical things of our world. When psychology became a science its interest was directed toward the study of natural, rather than supernatural events, and the soul was given up as an appropriate subject matter. Concepts, such as personality, which could be studied using scientific means, were substituted. Still, the general reluctance to view humans as automatons, directed by their environment, was satisfied by including a concept of freedom within the concept of personality.

Radical behaviorism, in its eagerness to deny anything else than natural causes of behavior, has rejected the idea of freedom from environmental causation. Watson maintained that the legitimate subject matter of psychology consisted of the observable environment, as the cause, and observable behavior change, as the effect. The deterministic behavioral philosophy of science has had no place for indeterminate, "free," causative events. Skinner set his position forward on this issue in dramatic fashion, stating that "a person does not act upon the world, the world acts upon him" (Skinner, 1971, p. 211), thus subtracting humans' freedom and dignity. Non-behavioral psychologists have considered that behaviorisms, in general, thus make humans passive responders to the environment.

Psychological behaviorism takes the position that the major problem here is the manner in which the issue is posed. Neither position cares what phenomena and issues the other is trying to consider. This is in contrast to the PB approach, which is to examine what is involved in the phenomena that give rise to the original conception. Then PB's approach is to analyze those phenomena behaviorally, in order to create a unified view—thereby strengthening the behavioral approach, while satisfying the legitimate interests of traditional psychology (see Staats, 1993a, 1994). In this particular case it is necessary to consider what it is that prompts so many, including psychologists, to believe in freedom and spontaneity in human behavior.

There are various phenomena that lead to the belief in personal causation. Centrally, the conception of freedom is based on the many experiences we have of doing what we want to do, what we plan and intend to do, what we have reasoned we should do, and such. And it is based on the experience we have that others do the same and that people who want different things, who plan different things, and such, behave differently from one another. We experience these things in our common experience. Radical behaviorism rejects consideration of such experiences. Psychological behaviorism recognizes them and sees the task of analyzing those phenomena in terms of behavioral principles (see Staats, 1963b). What we experience are our BBRs. We experience their operation as our *self*, our being. We experience the operation of the BBRs in our thinking, planning, and wanting, and how we behave as a result of these activities. We experience that our thinking, planning, and wanting is different from others', as is our purposive behavior. We experience the way our behavior affects the environment, especially the social environment. And we experience the way that our behavior, as it acts on the social environment, in turn, acts back on us. These are the reasons that all of us are so sure that we have had a hand in our destinies, that we have not just passively responded to the environment, that we are responsible for what has happened to us, that we are purposive. And we are right. But it is not necessary to go outside of scientific causality to provide an explanatory account (see Staats, 1963b, 1971a, 1975, chap. 13). PB, not resting on analysis alone, has conducted experiments to demonstrate the principles of its *behavioral interaction* position. For example, Staats, Gross, Guay, and Carlson (1973) showed that individuals who differed in a part of their emotional-motivational repertoire displayed different choice behaviors. Moreover, that choice behavior resulted in the subjects having different experiences that produced different learning in the subjects. Difference in measured interests in this experiment produced an interaction—in the same situation subjects with different personality measures behaved differently and, in doing so, set different causal sequences in motion. The manner in which the individual's behavior is determined by what she feels and thinks can be studied in behavioral research.

The reason that the belief in self-causation and freedom is so strong is because the individual does not know why her thinking, planning, intending, and wanting are the way they are. The extraordinarily complex cumulative-hierarchical learning processes involved are too complex and too removed to be recognized as causes. The BBRs also are too complex to comprehend. It is understandable that the lay person will not recognize these causes; psychology itself does not generally provide the necessary knowledge.

Psychological behaviorism's personality conception, in contrast to Skinner's position, says that the world acts upon the person, *but that the person also acts upon the world and on herself.* That is, the individual learns BBRs which determine how the individual will act in the situations met. But that behavior will affect others, importantly acting upon the world. Moreover, those effects on the world will, in return, act back upon the person. In this way the individual determines the environment she meets, and she determines her own behavior, because that environment will affect her.

A general theory of personality must confront and resolve such issues as this, toward establishing unification of the psychological and the behavioral.

The psychological behaviorism conception of interaction, developed in various analyses, such as the PB theory of abnormal behavior (Staats, 1963, chapt. 11), was begun very early (and was continuously developed in later works [see Staats, 1968a, 1971a, 1975]). In adopting PB's approach to abnormal behavior as social learning theory, Bandura (1968) summarized the PB interaction conception. In further works the social learning position came to be called reciprocal determination. A more detailed comparison of the two related conceptions has been made (see Staats, 1979). It may be added, however, that there are fundamental differences also. As indicated here, the PB conception of the environment/personality/behavior/environment interaction is based on detailed, specific analysis, with explicit theoretical and empirical definition. The conception is founded in the basic learning/behavior principles and is tightly constructed, level by level, through the human learning/cognitive, child development, and personality levels. The theory of personality involved includes specification of the content of personality and is unified with psychological testing, as the next chapter will indicate. These are the characteristics that allow such topics as freedom, agency, creativity, self-direction, and self-determination to be dealt with in a manner that unifies the psychological (and cognitive) and the behavioral.

CHAPTER 6

The Theory of Personality: Content

The radical behaviorism rejection of personality and its measurement has led to a general separation. Contemporary radical behaviorism, and cognitive social learning theory, which took its lead from radical behaviorism, do not incorporate and use profitably products from the field of psychological testing and do not contribute to the development of that field. Since the field is important, behaviorism's position in psychology is thereby weakened. Moreover, behaviorism has been handicapped in its own development because it has not been able to make use of the knowledge provided by the field of psychological testing. One of the primary aims of psychological behaviorism is to produce an approach that can utilize, as well as contribute to, the field of psychometrics, in a synergistic unification.

THE DEVELOPMENT OF BEHAVIORAL ASSESSMENT

To begin, the radical behaviorism/psychological testing schism rests on methodological as well as conceptual grounds. A firm part of Skinner's radical behaviorism has been a methodological orthodoxy that originally included only his experimental analysis of behavior (EAB) methodology (see Sidman, 1960). To illustrate, in 1969 Skinner was still taking the position that his experimental analysis of behavior methodology was the way to study human behavior, and that work based on verbal reports and ratings was useless. Verbal ratings, of course, are integral in the methodology of the field of psychological testing.

Instead of observing behavior, the [psychometric] experimenter records and studies a subject's statement of what he would do under a given set of circumstances, or his estimate of his chances of success, or his impression of a prevailing set of contingencies of reinforcement, or his evaluation of the magnitude of current variables. The observation of behavior cannot be circumvented in this way, because a subject cannot correctly describe either the probability that he will respond or the variables affecting such a probability. If he could, he could draw a cumulative record appropriate to a given set of circumstances, but this appears to be out of the question. (Skinner, 1969, pp. 77–78)

As this statement indicates, the methods of psychometrics cannot be considered meaningfully within Skinner's framework; the valuable data that he recognized were the cumulative records of simple responses in his EAB technology (see Staats, 1975).

It is not only that the force of operant behaviorism, so important in other fields, may never have been very successful in behavioral assessment. It is also true that one has the impression that the developments of behavioral assessment, or at least the major portion of those developments, occurred in spite of operant behaviorism and by assaulting its principles. (Silva, 1993, p. 13)

This lack of development of a conceptual-methodological structure from which to derive a field of behavioral assessment was general to the behavioral field in the first half of the 1960s and beyond, as the following indicates.

. . . [B]ehavioral assessment is relatively recent when compared with psychological assessment in general and with clinical experimental psychology and, more precisely, with behavior modification and therapy. For example, we find no systematic discussion of behavioral analysis in Eysenck and Rachman (1965), Meyer and Chesser (1970), or Wolpe (1969). (Silva, 1993, p. 2)

That was also true of social learning theory. Psychological behaviorism, however, set forth a different behaviorism framework (Staats, 1963a). Intelligence was considered in terms of language BBRs (also Staats, 1968a). The concept of the reinforcer system (the emotional-motivational repertoire) was set forth in preliminary fashion as an individual difference concept and it was said that interest, values, and preference tests measured parts of the reinforcer system. Furthermore, as will be indicated in the next chapter, PB set forth the first general behavioral analysis of abnormal behavior, yielding a taxonomy of the behavior disorders and calling for the development of a "learning psychotherapy" (Staats, 1963a, chap. 11). This theory of abnormal behavior also called for the development of behavioral assessment.

[A] rationale for learning psychotherapy will also have to include some method for *the assessment of behavior.* In order to discover the behavioral deficiencies, the required changes in the reinforcing system, the circumstances in which stimulus control is absent, and so on, evaluational techniques in these respects may have to be devised. Certainly, no two individuals will be alike in these various characteristics, and it may be necessary to determine such facts for the individual prior to beginning the learning program of treatment. Such assessment might take a form similar to some of the psychological tests already in use. . . . [However], a general learning rationale for behavior disorders and treatment will itself suggest techniques of assessment. (Staats, 1963a, pp. 508–509, italics added)

In addition to the above call for a field of behavioral assessment, the PB book introduced the concept of *behavioral analysis* as an approach (Staats, 1963a, pp. 459–460; 1965), setting forth the methodology by which to generally analyze human behavior in terms of conditioning principles. The methodology of behavioral analysis was elaborated in a systematic way using PB's program of research on reading and various new directions of research were outlined (Staats, 1964, pp. 435–449). Behavioral analysis involves first systematic, naturalistic observation of the problem of behavior, including stipulation of the reinforcers and discriminative stimuli that are involved. This may be theoretical, but such analyses have implications for observation and data collection. To continue, demonstrational studies based upon the behavioral analysis are then conducted to experimentally show that conditioning principles apply to a simplified version of the behavior problem. With that verification, the next step is a systematic set of studies testing the principles with the behavior. On the bases of the preceding research, the final step is application of the principles to actually treating the behavior problem. "[I]n order to approach various problems of behavior, the behavior involved must first be carefully observed; then the determinants may be sought and procedures commenced to bring the behaviors under experimental control" (Staats, 1963a, p. 460).

There were no other positions of this kind or analyses of human behavior that called for behavioral assessment, and the elements provided by PB were later considered as foundations for the field of behavioral assessment. Goldfried (Goldfried, 1976; Goldfried & Sprafkin, 1974) considered the PB taxonomy of abnormal behavior one of the four foundations of behavioral assessment. More recently, in a definitive historical analysis of the development of the field of behavioral assessment, Silva (1993) describes the PB contribution as "pioneering" and "prescient," preceding by two years Ullmann and Krasner's (1965) call for psychological assessment in the field of behavior modification.

The Radical Behaviorism Contribution

Following 1963, however, various behavior assessment developments began to arise (as described in Fernandez-Ballesteros, 1994; Silva, 1993). Kanfer and Saslow (1965) published an article entitled *Behavioral Analysis* that was later considered as another foundation of the field of behavioral assessment (see Silva, 1993, p. 3). This analysis also called for assessment of the reinforcer system, as had PB. Another foundation of the field was Goldfried and Pomeranz's (1968) influential article entitled "Role of assessment in behavior modification." These several individuals, however, worked within Skinner's radical behaviorism, and thus helped establish the swing in this direction that was to occur.

Mischel (1968) in that same year published a book that also took the nascent field in that same direction. He resurrected the original radical behaviorism position in denying that there are broad traits of behavior that are general across different situations. The commitment to Skinner's radical behaviorism became progressively more pronounced. Kanfer and Phillips stated that "Behavioral assessment in the future is likely to depend upon elaboration and extension of laboratory analogue or response sampling techniques: (1970, p. 510). The position that behavioral assessment should be based on EAB methods of research was additionally developed (see Patterson, 1967; Weiss, 1968). The following influential analysis further specified, in psychometric terms, the turn toward Skinner's radical behaviorism in the field of behavioral assessment.

> Predictive validity tends to decrease as the gap increases between the behavior sampled on the predictor measure and the behavior that is being predicted. On the whole, research regarding the relative *specificity of behavior* suggests that sampled predictor behavior should be as similar as possible to the behavior used on the criterion measure. (Mischel, 1972, p. 323, italics added)

This methodological-conceptual position, of course, places most psychological tests beyond the pale, since the behavior measured on tests—like verbal ratings—are quite different from the behaviors the tests predict. Thus, as the field of behavioral assessment developed it turned toward the incompatible Skinnerian philosophy. Even by the mid-1970s it was apparent in the PB framework that "Skinner's rejection of the concepts, methods, and instruments associated with traditionally oriented psychometrics, in favor of direct behavior observations, has had a growing [and deleterious] influence" (Staats, 1975, p. 424). But criticizing this position did not stem the tide.

Indicative of the confounding that occurred in the development of the field was that, although PB introduced the methodology of behavioral analysis, that methodology became the most fundamental tenet of the radical behaviorism approach to the field of behavioral assessment. Behavior analysts used the methodology as a standard for the rejection of other types of works, including those in PB. In the PB view behavioral analysis (also called functional analysis) was *one* of the methodologies needed. In the radical behaviorism approach to behavioral assessment, it became the only methodology. It should be noted that there were others (see Fernandez-Ballesteros, 1979, 1981, 1983) who recognized that restriction to direct observation of environmental-behavioral events was a misstep, saying that hypothetical analyses of behavioral and environmental events are generally made prior to collecting empirical evidence. Evans also criticized the simplistic methodology in saying that "It is obvious that behavioral assessment uses constructs and that no science of behavior or model of behavioral measurement could exist without doing so (Evans, 1986, p. 135).

In the two decades that followed introduction of the behavioral assessment conception, the field became a bustling endeavor, because its positive behavioristic elements are heuristic. But the field never achieved what came to be its goal of replacing psychological measurement. In cutting itself off from important phenomena, methods, concepts, principles, and findings, behavioral assessment became limited. Its separation from traditional psychological testing was an egregious error. As a consequence of its limitations, evidence began to accumulate that the approach was losing ground. Several studies showed that only a minority of members of the Association for the Advancement of Behavior Therapy used functional analysis in their clinical practice (Haynes & O'Brien, 1990; Piotrowski & Keller, 1984), whereas a much larger percentage used traditional test instruments, even projective tests. Fernandez-Ballesteros (1988) indicated just as tellingly that even articles published in the major behavior assessment journals involve mostly test development works and only a minority involve functional (behavioral) analysis works. The results also show that restricting the field of behavioral assessment to the analysis of behavior in terms of reinforcement principles was a crucial drawback. So behavioral assessment did not include a sufficient conceptual-methodological foundation. And that brought the field of behavior assessment to a crisis of stagnation and loss of direction (Fernandez-Ballesteros & Staats, 1992).

The PB position from the beginning has been that functional analysis— the analysis of specific problems of behavior by means of reinforcement principles—is important. PB, as indicated, provided one of the foundations for developing this type of study. But functional analysis is just one of the types of valuable works to be done. For example, there are behaviors in which analysis in terms of classical conditioning principles is important. There are cases where the analysis must employ human learning/cognitive principles, child development principles, social interaction principles, personality principles and concepts, and so on. But radical behaviorism does not provide the bases for such analyses. Radical behaviorism is not developed enough to provide the complete framework needed for dealing with complex human behavior, in the area of assessment as well as elsewhere. Moreover, radical behaviorism—still caught in the rivalry of the second generation of behaviorism—is an inward-looking approach that resists the inclusion of elements introduced by other behaviorists. New developments are included only after they are translated to radical "behaviorese" and thus can be considered indigenous.

The social learning theorists, even while retaining basic characteristics from radical behaviorism, later on repudiated their earlier position that was clearly radical behavioristic. For example, Mischel (1973) "reconceptualized" his previous rejection of personality (Mischel, 1968) and accepted that there are cognitive and emotional traits. Bandura (see 1968, 1978) also added a general conception similar to the PB behavioral interaction approach (Staats, 1963a, 1968a, 1975), saying that there is an interaction between the person, the environment, and the person's behavior. However, although these cognitive social learning accounts freed themselves from radical behaviorism in certain ways, they constitute general statements, without the substantive developments necessary to make them usable theories. They do not provide a framework for unifying behavior principles and methods with the field of psychometrics. While Bandura (1977, 1978) has constructed a theory of self-efficacy—a personality concept—this is a specific concept and the approach does not provide general unification with or understanding of the field of psychological testing. The approach does not indicate what personality tests measure, what personality is, how it is acquired, or how it has its effects. Cognitive social learning approaches, thus, do not provide the necessary conceptual or methodological foundations for a general approach to the study of the content of personality or how that content is to be measured.

PROBLEMS WITH THE FIELD OF PSYCHOLOGICAL TESTING

On the other side, the traditional field of psychological testing also has fundamental problems stemming from its basic orientation. That orientation is that observed individual differences in behavior are due to internal, psychological traits, laid down by biological variables as affected by the environment. The task of the field is to measure psychological trait differences, because traits are the determinants of general behavior, across situations. The focus of the field is on measurement. Its methods are made for measurement, not for studying the inferred biological or learning conditions that determine the traits. Moreover, the field's methods are not made for establishing the character of the psychological traits that are found, just for measuring them, whatever they are. The fact that tests can be constructed that are predictive of individual differences in performance in life has been a central support in psychology for the concept of personality.

Let us examine this framework. What tests do, actually, is to measure test-taking behaviors of the individual. The fact that the test predicts life performance simply reveals that behavior measured at *time 1* can be predictive of later behavior that is displayed at *time 2*. Spence (1944) termed such relationships R–R (response–response) laws. While such laws are predictive, the reasons why are unknown. He distinguished these laws from S–R laws—those that show that environmental manipulations produce changes in behavior. S–R laws are cause-and-effect laws, in contrast to R–R laws. As an example, the intelligence test (which measures test-taking behavior) predicts another type of behavior (school performance), but does not cause the performance. Analyzed in this way, the behaviorism position has been that the inference of an internal, *causal* psychological trait (such as intelligence) on the basis of a psychological test is inappropriate; relating test scores and life behavior establishes no cause for either.

This analysis can be elaborated, for there are actually various weaknesses in the foundation of the field of psychological testing. Another weakness is that the field does not define what it is that its tests measure. For example, there are many conflicting definitions of intelligence, and no way to decide which one is correct. For that reason, defining intelligence is no longer a serious research endeavor. However, without stipulating what intelligence is there is little basis for study of the possible causes of this trait, and this applies to the various personality traits. Traits could be biological in nature, or the result of learning, but the field has really developed no means of studying either. Studies that attempt to show that personality traits run in families can only yield circumstantial (indirect) evidence; they do not deal directly with the biological (genetic, anatomical, physiological) variables that might be causes.

The real problem is that the field has not produced or adopted methods by which to study how biology or learning determine personality traits. Since what personality traits are also is not specified, there is no basis for studying *how the personality trait determines behavior.* Because of the vagueness of the traditional personality concept it is not even realized that the personality–behavior causal connection must also be explicated. To illustrate, if there really are biologically based personality traits then psychology must study the biological mechanisms by which those traits affect behavior.

Because the field lacks such specifications, the work in the field lacks guidelines. There are many commonsense conceptions of personality traits that can serve as the basis for the production of new tests. With no restrictions—given the number of investigators, the complexity and variability of human behavior, and the productivity of test-construction methodology—the possibilities are endless for the multiplication of psychological tests. So the field currently contains hundreds of tests. Since there is no definition of what the tests measure, there is also no basis for interrelating the various tests, to indicate what they mean with respect to one another. What is the relationship of tests of readiness to tests of intelligence to developmental tests to reading, mathematics, and writing tests, to a learning aptitude test, to a verbal reasoning test, to a cognitive ability test, to the Bender Visual Motor Gestalt Test (Bender, 1938), to perceptual-motor tests, to object-sorting tests, to a basic language concepts test, to an adaptive ability test? What is the relationship of tests of depression to tests of anxiety, stress, phobias, attitudes, interests, values, and preferences? Without a conceptual structure by which to relate the many tests, the field is amorphous. What constitutes a full battery of tests with which to measure the individual's personality? What areas of personality have not yet been measured? Do two tests that have different names measure different aspects of personality, or are they redundant in whole or in part? What kind of knowledge do we need to answer such questions?

The important thing to realize is that, despite its important substance, the field of psychological testing is not complete as an independent field of study. Whether individual differences in behavior are due to biology or learning, the field of psychological testing is incomplete, because it does not meaningfully connect to the relevant fields of biological science or behaviorism.

THE PB THEORY OF PSYCHOLOGICAL TESTS: PROVIDING CONTENT FOR THE THEORY OF PERSONALITY

This analysis indicates that there are two traditions of study, that of behaviorism and that of psychological testing, each isolated from the other. The traditional field of psychological testing measures personality traits, but has lacked specification of the content of its personality traits. The traditional field of behaviorism studies behavior principles but has lacked specification of the content of human behavior (other than the problem behaviors considered in behavior therapy/behavior analysis). Each, by itself, is an incomplete approach to the study of human behavior and of personality. The PB view has been that the two are complementary and must be integrated into the work of formulating an adequate approach to the interests of each. Moreover, it is the present view that the PB theory of personality provides the means by which to develop such a unified theory.

The fundamental conception is that individual difference phenomena—those from which the concept of personality is inferred—result from individual differences in the basic behavioral repertoires (BBRs). The concepts and principles of the BBRs provide the basic theory with which to analyze psychological tests and the functions of tests in the prediction of individual differences in behavior. This means that the items of the various psychological tests that predict behavior must be analyzed in terms of elements of one or more of the three major BBRs.

The achievement of this theoretical task constitutes an integral part of constructing a theory of personality that is explained by the lower levels of the theory, on the one hand, and that explains the field of personality measurement, on the other. The analysis of personality tests in terms of the BBRs, moreover, is a central means of putting meat on the bones of the theory, that is, of giving content to the PB theory of personality, and hence content to the fields of behaviorism and psychological testing. The manner in which psychological tests can be analyzed into the BBRs—giving content to both behaviorism and the field of personality—will be indicated in the next three sections.

TESTS OF THE LANGUAGE-COGNITIVE BBRs AND THE CONTENT ASPECTS OF PERSONALITY

The first BBR that will be discussed is the language-cognitive repertoire. There are various types of tests that deal with this BBR, including intelligence tests. In conjunction with the PB theory of child development, the following sections constitute the psychological behaviorism theory of intelligence.

The PB Theory of Intelligence and Intelligence Tests

"Intelligence was first used in its modern sense by Herbert Spencer in 1895, although the term itself can be found in use as far back as the writings of Cicero" (Cunningham, 1986, p. 243). The traditional concept of intelligence is based on the naturalistic observations that people's performances in many of life's tasks differ in quality. Some people behave very well, they reason well, they are articulate, they display wide knowledge, they solve problems well, and so on. Others do not do such things so well. Very centrally people show large differences in the quickness, ease, and quality of their learning, as seen clearly with school children. Moreover, the various differences appear to go together; those who display advantageous behavior in one case tend to do so in others. Those who are well informed are those who learn well and easily, and who do other things well also. It is also the case that a child who displays such characteristics is likely to grow into an adult who does so also. Our common experience is that parents who have these characteristics tend to have children who have such characteristics.

Such phenomena very early were interpreted as evidence that intelligence was a biologically based quality of the mind on which there were variations important in an evolutionary sense. Darwin thought psychological traits were inherited and evolved. Drawing from the example of earlier sciences, measurement of the characteristics of the mind became a focus of psychology. The first attempts at measurement of the trait of intelligence were derived from the particular definitions of intelligence employed. For example, on the basis of the idea that intelligence variations depended upon the goodness (quickness) of the nervous system, the speed of conduction of nervous impulses was measured. Reaction time was considered to depend upon the rapidity of individuals' neural conduction (Boring, 1950). However, there was no success with attempts to compose an intelligence test based on organically based definitions.

Another tack, introduced by Alfred Binet, involved the collection of a number of problems of various kinds thought to demand intelligence for their solution. The difficulty of the problem items were found to vary depending on age. Items were selected for each age when half the children of that age would solve the problem. Children who passed the items up to and including their age level would have an IQ of 100. Those who passed fewer would have a lower IQ, and those who passed additional items would have a higher IQ.

Then, very significantly, it was found that the IQ scores of children were correlated with their school grades. The higher the IQ, in general, the higher the school grades. How a child would do later in school could be predicted from knowledge of an intelligence test given at an earlier time. So the intelligence test was a useful predictor of school performance (behavior). The intelligence test, moreover, predicted generally across various school subject matters. Such findings gave a strong boost to the conception of intelligence, for being able to measure "something" lends credence to belief in the existence of that something. Various studies were conducted to show that the trait has continuity over age, that it runs in families, and so on. It is anomalous that, although the field has not been able to define what intelligence is, there are various theories of what determines intelligence.

Focus, however, has been on constructing and using intelligence tests. For example, generally children whose intelligence test scores are low enough do not learn well in a regular classroom. So such tests can be used in decisions regarding special education placement. Intelligence tests have also been used in other types of selection tasks. As another example, since the First World War, soldiers have been accepted or rejected on the basis of intelligence test scores, as is also the case in occupational and educational placement.

This is thus an example illustrating the general case. The field has developed "intelligence" tests that predict behavioral performance, and the tests thus have important uses. But just what intelligence is remains a problem. Perhaps it is a biological-mental process that is inherited. Perhaps intelligence is affected by learning. In either case it would be important to establish just what is involved. But there has been almost no progress in either direction within the field of psychological testing. Moreover, the field does not have the tools for making such progress. Without this type of knowledge the field can do nothing about intelligence or problems of intelligence or, in fact, make any progress in that direction.

This is the type of case that is appropriate for the behaviorizing work that has been described. Traditional psychology has established the field of study of intelligence and has constructed important methods of measurement with predictive value. But much is lacking and much is incorrect. A psychological behaviorism theory of intelligence can supply that which is missing, and serve to delete that which errs, and provide a central unification in doing so.

The Psychological Behaviorism Theory of Intelligence Test Construction

A first step in providing an explanatory foundation for the concept of intelligence is to make a psychological behavioral analysis of how intelligence tests are constructed. So far it has been said that intelligence tests are composed of problem items. The generally held conception is that such items are related to age because intelligence is based on the child's biological development. In contrast, the PB explanation is that this methodology was selected because it worked, and it worked because it involves a central behavioral principle. By selecting items that are age-related, Binet inadvertently selected items that depended upon learning. Children cannot pass an item until a certain age because the repertoires necessary to pass the item generally are not learned until that time. In the present view, the method of test construction was successful because it abandoned the search for some biological process in favor of measuring the child's advancement in *learning* the BBRs.

In addition to selecting items that are age-related, however, Binet also correlated children's scores on the test items with school performance. Thus, items came to be selected for intelligence tests, not only because they are age-related, but also because they predict school success. In the present theory this manner of selection had the effect of ensuring that the items measure important elements of the BBRs. Let me explain. The reason an intelligence item is predictive of good performance in school is because the item is measuring some skill (repertoire) that enables the child to learn well in school. As has been indicated, that is precisely what the BBRs give the child, the foundation for later learning. The child must have learned previous BBRs if she is to respond appropriately, and to learn, when presented with new school tasks. What happened was that Binet (and other test constructors) gathered a group of problem items and gave them to children and then selected those items that predicted school performance. The criterion of predicting school performance guarantees that the items included will measure *repertoires that are important for the child's learning in school.* This psychological-behavioral analysis takes the mystery out of what intelligence is and what intelligence tests measure. Inadvertently, intelligence test construction guarantees that intelligence test items measure elements of basic behavioral repertoires that are foundations for school learning.

It is deceptive that typically the intelligence test items appear to involve different things than the specific tasks taught in school. For example, an item that requires that the child string beads as the examiner has done appears to have little relationship to learning to read or to do arithmetic in school. Such items thus appear to be indices of a deeper *mental potential* for learning that is different from the specific skills involved in school success. However, as will be seen, when the items are analyzed into the behavioral repertoires they actually measure, what is involved becomes clear. The present theory is that it is not the *specific* content of the items that enables them to predict success in learning. It is because the items on an intelligence test, at the same time that they measure specific content, are also measuring general BBRs that apply to various learning tasks (see Staats, 1971a; Staats & Burns, 1981). The test items are not indices of an internal mental quality of intelligence. The items are direct measures of the BBRs. This theory of intelligence can be illustrated by analyzing a few intelligence test items in terms of the BBRs they involve.

The Psychological Behaviorism Theory of the Content of Intelligence

Given that PB has specified in theory and research what some of those BBRs are, there is a framework for examining explicitly what intelligence is. Early analyses of intelligence tests in terms of the language-cognitive BBR indicated the fruitfulness of the approach (Staats, 1963a, 1968a). As can be seen easily at the younger age levels, when the items involve relatively simple BBRs, items that measure the language-cognitive repertoires already described are fundamental on intelligence tests.

The Verbal-Motor Repertoire and Intelligence Items.

The verbal-motor repertoire is a good one with which to begin because it is tested on so many items. This is the case because each item includes instructions to the subject to do something and the child must follow the instruction if she is to succeed. Some items on the Stanford-Binet (Terman & Merrill, 1937) are very clear in this regard. As examples, the young child is told to "Watch what I do" (p. 75), "Show me the kitty [from a group of objects]" (p. 75), "See what I'm making . . . You make one like this [from a group of blocks]" (p. 76), "Give me the kitty," . . . "Put the spoon in the cup" (p. 77)," and so on. For older age groups the instructions become increasingly complex. A child without the verbal-motor repertoire will fail on the test right at the beginning. Unable to respond appropriately to the examiner's instructions the child's attending and participating behaviors will not be directed to the relevant stimuli and the child will not endeavor to make the required response. Such a child only has a random chance of succeeding on the items.

The importance of the verbal-motor BBR on intelligence tests is clear. But there is still the question of why items that measure this BBR are predictive of school success. The reason is also clear; very few learning tasks in school years do not involve instructions that must be followed if learning is to take place. Whether the child is learning to read, to write, to do numbers, to acquire sensory-motor skills, or the like, the child must follow instructions. So children who follow instructions well will—other things equal—score higher on IQ tests *as well as in school learning*. The richer the child's verbal-motor repertoire, the more complex the instructions that can be followed, and the better the child will be at learning tasks.

The Verbal-Image Repertoire and Intelligence Items.

The verbal-image repertoire is composed of the words that elicit an image (conditioned sensory response) in the individual. There are many such words in our language—*sharp, white, round, long, screech,* and *ear* represent samples. Various intelligence test items tap this language repertoire. Take, for example, item 2 at the Superior Adult III level of Form L of the Stanford-Binet (Terman & Merrill, 1937, p. 130), which asks for solving the following problem without use of paper and pencil. *"I drove west for two miles; then I turned to my right and drove north for half a mile; then I turned to my right again and drove two miles further. What direction was I going then? . . . . How far was I from my starting point when I stopped?"* The problem can be solved easily if the first sentence elicits the sensory response of a map (like of the United States) with a line moving left (west) to a distance labeled two miles, with the line then moving up (north) a distance labeled ½ mile, and then a line moving back east for two miles parallel to the first line. The person with the verbal-image repertoire can respond in this way and thus succeed on this item. Other items also depend on this BBR. For example, similarities items require seeing commonalities between named objects. Having a verbally elicited image of both objects can provide the answer. Intelligence tests also frequently test vocabulary, where the verbal-image repertoire is important.

Why is this repertoire important in school performance? As one general example, there are many passages to be read in school that are incomprehensible unless the words elicit the appropriate images. The child with a poor verbal-image repertoire will have to look up many words in the dictionary and will read slowly and learn poorly from the reading. The child with the rich verbal-image repertoire will be able to read rapidly, have a rich image experience, and learn very well from the reading, and be reinforced by the reading as well as by her achievements. The child cannot profit from spoken language, such as stories read by the teacher, without a verbal-image repertoire.

The Verbal-Emotional Repertoire and Intelligence Items. The same thing is true of the verbal-emotional repertoire. That is, as described in Chapter 3, there are many words that function to elicit an emotional response in the individual. For a person with such a repertoire, words may be used to elicit emotional responses that can be conditioned to new stimuli. This type of learning is also important in school, for example, in listening to and in reading stories. It is the power of words to elicit emotional responses that reinforces attending to those words. It is only when printed words will elicit positive emotional responses in the child that the child will read "for pleasure." Much learning of the language-cognitive repertoire will depend upon reading. And the child needs a good verbal-emotional repertoire to provide the reinforcement.

The Verbal-Labeling Repertoire, Concepts, and Intelligence Items. The verbal-labeling repertoire is one of the central language repertoires and it enables the individual to respond verbally to the many external and internal stimuli that are experienced. The individual can label what is seen, heard, tasted, smelled, felt tactually, and so on. The individual can also label the internal experiences that are referred to as consciousness, that is, internally experienced emotions, images, implicit speech, and so on. The verbal-labeling repertoire is central in various human activities such as communication, both in sending and receiving, problem solving and reasoning, and in conceptual thinking. Much is learned in these activities.

It is also the case that the more labeling responses the individual has learned, the more the individual can respond with complexity to the environment that is experienced. Let us take as an example two children, one with a rich verbal-labeling repertoire, and the other with a sparse repertoire. The two children would profit differently from seeing a movie, as could be seen by asking them to describe what they had seen. The first child would do so much more richly than the second, and because of that difference would remember the movie in much greater detail. Various studies have shown that the labeling responses to stimuli will directly affect the perception of those stimuli and their learning and retention (Birge, 1941; Brown & Lenneberg, 1954).

We might expect, thus, that there would be items on intelligence tests for young children that would measure this repertoire, and that is the case. For example, at the 3½-year level of the Revised Stanford-Binet Intelligence Test the child is shown pictures of common objects and asked, "What's this? What do you call it?" (Terman & Merrill, 1937, p. 83). Another item involves asking the child to tell the examiner about pictures that are shown (p. 84).

Another item asks the child "Which stick is longer? Put your finger on the long one" (p. 84). When a child can label such things, we say she has the concept of length. Training the child to such "concepts" is straightforward, although more complex than simple naming. In a study that contributed importantly to the PB theory of intelligence, Burns trained a group of four-year-old children to label objects in different classes. The children also learned the concept name of each object group. Burns then found that these children scored higher on similarities intelligence test items that involved those objects. The trained children's conceptual ability in correctly classifying the objects in categories was also increased (see Staats & Burns, 1981).

Number responses, which occur frequently on intelligence tests, are first learned as verbal-labeling responses. We see tests for this beginning repertoire at the five-year level of the Revised Stanford-Binet. The child is shown four blocks and is asked, "How many?" As has been indicated, however, the child can only learn a limited repertoire of numbering objects via straight labeling training. After learning to label up to about five the child must be able to count, which involves skills in addition to the verbal-labeling responses of number (see Staats, 1968a; Staats, Brewer, & Gross, 1970). Many items on intelligence tests tap the counting repertoire and the other number repertoires that are learned later (the number operations such as addition and subtraction). Number operations are basic to learning mathematics, such as algebra, as involved in more advanced intellective tests. In PB's experimental-longitudinal research a program for training preschool children in number labeling and counting (and number operations as well) was designed. It was found that children who received training in such a number BBR improved in intelligence (see Staats, 1968a). Staats and Burns (1981) showed specifically that children who received the PB number training scored better on intelligence tests on number-relevant items.

A child who has a rich labeling repertoire, of the various types of labels, will learn better, write better, understand better, read better, and, in multiple ways, perform better in school than a child with a less rich repertoire.

The Verbal-Association Repertoire and Intelligence Items. Psychological behaviorism in introducing the concept of the verbal-association repertoire indicated that the repertoire was involved in such psychological activities as grammatical speech, mathematics, problem solving, originality, and communication. To illustrate, the addition and multiplication tables, such as "two and two are four," are composed of word associations, as are other aspects of the mathematics repertoire such as algebraic rules (Staats, 1963a). Grammatical usages, such as "He has gone" versus "He has went," are composed of word associations. Much of what we call knowledge consists of verbal-associations, for example, historical knowledge such as "The battle of Hastings was fought in 1066," knowledge in algebra, such as *a* times *a* equals *a squared,* knowledge in psychology, such as "a reinforcing stimulus strengthens responses it follows."

Based on such an analysis we might expect many items on intelligence tests would measure the individual's word associations—increasingly so as the age level advances. As one example, one Stanford-Binet item asks the subject to complete the statement "Trees are terrestrial; stars are *celestial*" (Terman & Merrill, 1937, p. 178). Answering the item demands development of several verbal repertoires in addition to the verbal-association repertoire. As another example, at the 13-year level of the same test, item six asks the subjects to repeat sentences exactly. Ability to do that will depend, in good part, upon previously established verbal associations.

Repeating sentences is an artificial test. But it is a way of measuring the richness (extent of development) of the subject's word-association repertoire. And the extent of development of this repertoire will tell a lot about the individual's language capability and hence success in various academic (and life) tasks. The verbal-association repertoire is affected greatly by reading (as are the other language repertoires). This means that those who read a lot will develop a richer verbal-association repertoire than those who do not. The richer verbal-association repertoire will result in better verbal memory, reasoning, academic learning, and cognitive abilities in general. Hence individual differences in reading will be reflected in individual differences in intelligence, increasingly with age. Research on this effect should be conducted. Recent studies in psychology, albeit from a cognitivism orientation, already provide support for the PB theory of intelligence. For example, Stanovich, West, and Harrison (1995) found that how much individuals read is correlated with intelligence. It would be important to generally incorporate the many relevant cognitivism studies into the PB theory, and to generate additional research in doing so.

Verbal-Imitation Items and Intelligence Test Items. As has been indicated, the child's verbal-imitation repertoire is an important BBR in the acquisition of the verbal-labeling repertoire (Staats, 1963a, 1968a, 1975). It would be expected in PB theory, thus, that tests of intelligence at the early age levels would contain items that test for this repertoire. This can be exemplified by the Uzgiris-Hunt Scales (see Uzgiris, 1975), which has items that measure the infant's vocal and gestural imitation. The PB analysis suggests that items that measure the child's ability to repeat (imitate) sounds, syllables, and words should be very valuable in infant tests of intelligence (and development and adaptive ability).

The Verbal-Writing Repertoire and Intelligence Testing. The description of the language-cognitive repertoires has focused on some of the basic types. However, as already indicated, additional repertoires are learned on the foundation of the basic types. And those additional repertoires can be basic to further learning, and hence be measured on intelligence tests. The verbal-reading-and-writing repertoire is one such case. Whether or not the child has a beginning repertoire—reading and writing the letters—on entering school has been said to be the best predictor of how well the child will learn to read (Chall, 1967). It would be valuable to include items on intelligence tests that measure letter reading and writing skills. It is thus reasonable that items are included that do the same thing.

Let me begin with an example that occurs at the three-and-a-half-year level of the Stanford-Binet (Terman & Merrill, 1937). The examiner draws a diagonally oriented cross, or X, and tells the child "You make one just like this" (p. 85). The child must be able to look at the stimulus the examiner has drawn, take up the writing implement provided, and make a drawing response that suitably copies (imitates) the X, in an appropriate plane. This item does not test the child's letter-writing repertoire, but rather the basic skills that enable the child to learn that repertoire. That is, PB has analyzed the repertoire the child must have to be able to copy line figures (see Staats & Burns, 1981). This repertoire includes various sensory-motor skills, including perceptual and attentional skills. For example, being able to attend closely to small visual stimuli, to compare them and detect differences, involves fine skills of this type. Other aspects of copying the X lie more in the motor realm, such as making guided lines with an implement, within which there is a wide range of skill (see Staats & Burns, 1981). The child must also become able to write line figures in a particular orientation, spaced in a certain way, and homogeneously of a certain size. Moreover, as on this particular intelligence item, the child must have a verbal-motor repertoire by which directions can be followed. The drawing-an-X item thus involves a general repertoire, because there are various items on intelligence and other tests that are based on the same repertoire.

It is important to indicate here, however, that PB has thoroughly researched this particular repertoire. The work began with the development of experimental-longitudinal methods for training the author's daughter to write letters and words, as described in Chapter 4. This work was extended to other children and a learning program was designed with which to generally train children to read and write the letters of the alphabet, as well as the underlying line-figure-writing repertoire involved. In addition, analysis of two of the ten subtests on the Wechsler Preschool and Primary Scale of Intelligence (WPPSI) (Wechsler, 1967)—the Mazes and Geometric Design tests—showed that these subtests very prominently measure this repertoire. On the first the child is told to trace between a complicated pattern of two lines that constitute paths in a maze. Doing so takes the child to the end of the maze. On the second type of task the child is asked to copy various geometric line figures. The PB framework of analysis and research suggested that children trained to read and write the letters of the alphabet would acquire a general repertoire that would provide them with the skills to successfully perform on the Mazes and Geometric Design intelligence subtests. An experiment with four-year-old children proved this to be the case. Children who had learned the letter writing BBR were significantly more intelligent on these two subtests (Staats & Burns, 1981), usually considered to measure two different intelligence abilities.

Analysis in terms of the BBRs indicates clearly why such items test "intelligence" (why they are predictive of success in school). The answer is that, in early learning in school, many of the things the child has to learn—like learning to write letters and numbers—require sensory-motor and perceptual skills. Those skills can be learned in training to draw, learning to copy line figures, learning pencil mazes, and in learning to write the letters of the alphabet. PB theory states that perceptual and sensory-motor skills of writing are learned. But these skills constitute a BBR, because they are basic to further learning in various tasks.

The Sensory-Motor and Emotional-Motivational Repertoires in Intelligence

Traditionally intelligence is considered to be a cognitive mental ability. The PB theory of intelligence, however, suggests that the sensory-motor and emotional-motivational BBRs are relevant to intelligence testing. These topics will be treated in later sections.

Additional Specifications of Intelligence

There are several additional specifications to be added to the PB theory that intelligence is composed of learned BBRs that are also basic to further learning of the individual.

Intelligence as Combinations and Enrichment of BBRs. The BBRs are acquired in a cumulative-hierarchical way. As already indicated, for example, the verbal-imitation repertoire is basic in the child's acquisition of the verbal-labeling repertoire, and the various language repertoires are basic to learning to read. Children can differ in how *far* they have advanced in such cumulative-hierarchical learning. However, children may also differ in terms of the *richness* of their learning. Two children may both have the various language repertoires and thus be ready to learn to read. But one child can have acquired those language repertoires much more richly than the other.

Ordinarily, the child with the richer repertoire will be able to respond successfully to and learn from a greater number of situations. This child generally will do better than the child with the less rich repertoires, both in the classroom and on an intelligence test. This type of difference can be discerned on the intelligence test that includes a number of items, even when these items measure the same types of repertoires. Let me add that originality and creativity frequently depend upon the individual "putting" elements together in new ways (see Staats, 1968a, 168–178). Ordinarily, the richer the individual's basic repertoires, the more elements the individual has for such combinations, and the more creative or intelligent she will measure and be.

Intelligence as Rate of Learning.   Intelligence has frequently been defined as the ability to learn, with the assumption that learning ability is some inherited quality. Psychological behaviorism, however, introduces the concept that learning ability is itself learned. Humans ordinarily go through a *learning acceleration,* becoming better and better learners *as a function of learning the various BBRs.* As indicated already, PB research has shown that various types of children learning writing, reading, and number skills require progressively fewer learning trials (see Staats, Brewer, & Gross, 1970; Staats & Burns, 1981; Staats & Butterfield, 1965; Staats, Minke, & Butts, 1970). Leduc (1988) has even found the learning acceleration phenomena in experimental-longitudinal study with a wild ("feral") child. The acceleration occurs because the child learns general skills (BBRs) when engaged in specific tasks. For example, as a child learns to write a specific letter she also learns general line-drawing skills, how to attend assiduously to stimuli, how to compare stimuli for similarity, and so on. As those skills are learned, learning additional letters becomes easier and faster. The general skills also will be helpful in other tasks—such as in learning to read words, learning to draw, and such.

Differences in learning ability, rather than revealing some inborn trait, simply indicate how far and richly the child's cumulative-hierarchical learning of the BBRs has progressed. "The quick learner is the one who has acquired already the basic repertoires relevant to the new learning. As soon as the slow learner has acquired the necessary basic repertoire, he or she too will learn rapidly" (see Staats & Burns, 1981).

The Psychological Behaviorism Theory of Intelligence and How It Causes Behavior

The PB theory (Staats, 1971a; Staats & Burns, 1981) is that variations in learning opportunities produce individual differences in the language BBRs, which constitute (largely) individual differences in intelligence. Strong support for these several aspects of the PB theory of intelligence has been provided by radical behaviorists Hart and Risely (1992). Parent–child interactions were observed monthly for two and a half years. The results showed parental training variations were related to the children's language development and to differences in their intelligence test scores obtained after the study. Typical of radical behaviorism methodology, Hart and Risley did not integrate their important work with the PB developments, a unification that would considerably advance both. The following sections add points to the PB theory of intelligence.

Why a Measured Sample of a BBR Is Broadly Predictive of Behavior. Intelligence tests measure a sample of the basic behavioral repertoires that are important for performing well and learning well in school. How can a small number of items on an intelligence test predict behavior so broadly? It should be understood that, when an examiner presents several small objects and asks the child to "Give me the kitty," only a particular verbal-motor element is being measured. But if life conditions have trained the child to this verbal-motor element, likely those conditions have produced additional learning of the same kind. Moreover, parents who are good trainers for one repertoire will ordinarily be so for other BBRs. In this sense the item is sampling (1) the goodness of the child's learning experiences; (2) the repertoires the learning has produced; and (3) the level of learning of which the child is capable in new situations. For various reasons, of course, the sample dealt with on the intelligence test may not be a good indicator of the universe of the child's "intelligence" BBRs. For example, the child may have received specific training that enables her to pass a particular item, while having much less developed BBRs generally. In any case where the performance on items is poorly representative of the child's BBRs—either in an enhancing or diminishing manner—the test will be a poor predictor of later behavior. Any particular item in various ways may be in error for the particular child or group of children.

Basic Repertoires Underlie Multiple Performances. Neither traditional psychology nor standard behaviorism has indicated why it is that personality tests, involving a brief period, an artificial environmental situation, and a small sample of behavior, can predict a much broader universe of behavior across a variety of situations. One concept that is helpful in that regard is that a particular basic behavioral repertoire will be important in multiple, different performances. For example, in one PB experiment the children were given training in copying, writing, and reading letters of the alphabet. Children who had learned the BBRs involved scored higher on *both* the Geometric Design and Mazes subtests, on the WPPSI (Wechsler, 1967), which are considered to measure two different types of intelligence ability.

As another example, Burns (see Staats & Burns, 1981) designed a study in which children were trained in learning the names of the members of classes of objects, as well as the names of the classes. The repertoire that resulted improved the children's performance on a test of sorting objects into classes, considered a test of conceptual ability. In addition, however, as a consequence of the verbal BBR the children had learned they improved on a similarities test involving the items. Similarity items are widely used on intelligence tests, involving such questions as, "In what way are a cat and a mouse alike?" Seeing relationships has been said to be the essence of intelligence. Let me suggest that the language repertoires underlie seeing relationships as well as many other performances, such as composing prose and poetry, speaking well, having a good sense of humor (which includes drawing relationships between objects and events), problem solving, and so on. The point is that, traditionally, we consider each of these human behavior phenomena to involve a different mental ability, whereas they are all related by the fact that they depend on the same underlying BBRs. Analysis of "cognitive ability" in terms of the BBRs produces a more parsimonious theory.

Let me add one more point here. This PB theory of intelligence is a cognitive as well as a behavioral theory. Intelligence is treated as a dependent variable, a function of past learning. But intelligence is also treated as an independent variable, as a cognitive structure that determines behavior. Traditionally theories of personality, including behavioral theories, are vague, general, without specification. Such "intervening variable" definitions are of little use for projecting research or treatment. A useful, heuristic theory must be specific, give content, indicate what personality is, how it is learned, and how it has its effects. The PB theory of intelligence provides that specification. Intelligence consists of language-cognitive (and other) BBRs. Some of those BBRs have been specified by analysis of intelligence test items. And the theory has been used to project studies showing how the BBRs are learned and how they function.

Other Intellective Tests

The language-cognitive BBRs are measured on various tests other than intelligence tests. There are tests of language ability, cognitive ability, cognitive styles, readiness, learning aptitude, conceptual ability, verbal reasoning, scholastic aptitude, academic achievement in various areas, and others that measure the language-cognitive BBRs. It is important that the various instruments be analyzed in terms of the BBRs they measure—to enrich the theory as well as to understand better the field of psychological testing and the tests it contains.

It should be noted that PB theory does not accept all of the conceptions that exist in the traditional field of psychological testing. For example, some theorists do not consider intelligence to be a part of personality, which makes no sense in PB analysis. Another division is made between achievement and aptitude tests. The latter, including intelligence tests, are considered to measure potentiality for something, rather than knowledge that has been achieved. But, in the PB view, the difference between these two types of tests resides in the way the tests have been constructed, not in the nature of the BBRs being measured. Aptitude tests are *composed* for prediction of how the individual will learn; achievement tests are *composed* for measurement of what has been learned. A BBR like the reading repertoire may be measured on an achievement test, in evaluating what a child has learned, or what a school program has taught. But reading skill is also an "aptitude" (BBR) in that reading is basic to much additional learning.

Psychological behaviorism's theory of intelligence has been outlined to exemplify the general approach. The same type of specific behavioral analysis must be made of other intellective tests.

TESTS OF THE EMOTIONAL-MOTIVATIONAL BBRs AND THE CONTENT OF PERSONALITY

There are various concepts that refer to emotional and motivational elements of personality such as interests, attitudes, values, preferences, cathexes, and needs. Particular theories of personality include concepts of emotional-motivational processes. For example, Freud's theory of psychosexual development as the determinant of personality gives a prominent role to emotional development. The child's four stages of development centered on emotional processes, since a stage determines what the child needs emotionally and by which the child is satisfied. For example, in the oral stage the child's emotional needs were satisfied by oral gratification. Failing to get that satisfaction, the child's emotional development is fixated at that level, and oral gratification remains as a primary form of emotional satisfaction, and the individual continues to pursue avenues of oral satisfaction. The stages of development are supposed to be biologically determined, with the individual's emotional characteristics determined both by biology and by personal experience.

The fact is, the situation is similar with respect to the measurement of emotional processes as it is with the measurement of cognitive processes. "The construction of a personality inventory often begins . . . by writing items that appear to bear a relationship to the trait being measured" (Brown, 1983). This means test construction in this area typically begins with commonsense notions of an emotional trait. After composing a fund of items, the test constructor conducts a study to see if the items predict the behavior of interest in the first place. Sometimes a conglomeration of items are simply gathered and submitted to research to find out what some of the items predict—such a test is considered to be empirically constructed, rather than to be based on prior conception of a personality trait.

As in the case of intellective tests, emotional tests have been composed that are useful for predictive purposes. Examples will be given and subjected to PB analysis.

Interests and the Emotional-Motivational Repertoire

The interest test may be used as an example in illustrating the traditional approach's strengths and weaknesses. There was once an effort to theorize about interests, for example, that interests arise as a result of the individual's practical adjustment to the environment (Carter, 1940), that interests are closely linked to personality development (Darley, 1960), that "interests are the product of interaction between inherited neural and endocrine factors, on the one hand, and opportunity and social evaluation on the other" (Super & Crites, 1962, p. 410), or simply that interests are determined by genetics (Campbell, 1971). It is interesting to note that, although these are considered to be definitions of interests, they describe conjectured causes of interests, and do not specify what an interest is. The fact is the field has had no way of systematically specifying what is involved, what interests are, how interests come about or, indeed, how interests determine behavior.

Perusal of the Strong-Campbell Interest Inventory (SVIB-SCII) (Campbell, 1971, 1974; Campbell & Hansen, 1981) reveals that it contains various items which ask the individual to indicate in one manner or another what is liked. Some items ask whether a particular stimulus object, event, or activity is liked, disliked, or neutral. Some items ask the subject to indicate relative liking for a stimulus compared with other stimuli. There are over three hundred such items. Centrally, however, interest test results have been valuable in predicting who will be successful in different occupations, in selecting individuals for training programs, and thus in counseling psychology in advising individuals concerning what careers are appropriate to pursue.

Analysis of Interest Test Construction

Those uses derive from the manner in which the SVIB-SCII was constructed. That is, the SVIB-SCII was given to various occupational groups. The various results were analyzed by group and it was established what are the common ways of answering some of the test's items within each of the groups. It was found that there are some items that a particular occupational group answers in a characteristic way, either liking or disliking them. Only some of the items are valuable in identifying a particular occupation, and different items pertain to different occupational groups.

It is this information that provides the predictive value of this interest test for the individual. When a subject takes the test his responses are compared with those of all the other occupational groups. If the individual responds to a cluster of items in a way that is similar to that of a particular occupation, research shows she will do better in that occupation than will someone whose responses do not match that of the occupation. But why does the individual do better in some pursuit if his "profile" of liked and disliked items closely resembles those of individuals who have been successful in that pursuit? More specifically, why is it that answering items on an interest inventory has any predictive value for the quite different behaviors that make for success in an occupation.

That is a question that has not been systematically considered or answered within the traditional psychology framework. But it is a question that is very central in making a PB analysis of interests (and other personality tests).

Behavior Analysis of Interests

There has also been no analysis in behaviorism of what interests are, how individual differences occur, how they determine behavior, and why interest inventories are predictive of behavior. The reason is that behavioristic research and interest test research are too widely separated—so neither can be understood in terms of the other. The PB view is that this separation must be bridged by empirical, methodological, and theoretical study to see the relationship. At the basic level, PB established the classical conditioning principles by which emotions are learned and by which they affect behavior. At the human learning/cognitive level, PB study showed that emotional stimuli can be learned by humans through language, that there are many emotional words, and that humans learn many emotional responses to life events through words.

As this research and theory advanced, it defined the concept of the emotional-motivational repertoire, the vast complex of stimuli each individual learns that constitutes a BBR uniquely different from anyone else's emotional repertoire. Once two individuals have learned different emotional-motivational BBRs, they will emotionally experience life situations differently, their behaviors will be differently reinforced in those situations as a consequence, and they will be attracted to different kinds of life situations. These principles, thus, define the individual's emotional-motivational BBR as an aspect of personality, because the BBR helps determine what the individual experiences, how the individual behaves, and what the individual learns.

What is the connection to interest tests? Well, in the PB view people in different occupations have different emotional responses to some of life's stimuli. And people in the same occupation have the same emotional responses to some of life's stimuli. Interest tests are seen to measure a part of individuals' emotional-motivational BBRs. The PB theory of interest tests is that they measure subjects' emotional responses to the words in the items of the test. In doing so the interest test measures the subjects' emotional response to the life events that are denoted by those words. Thus, interest inventories measure the extent to which the individual has an emotional-motivational repertoire that, in certain respects, is similar to the emotional-motivational repertoire of people in a particular occupation.

But certain methodological questions arise concerning the assumption that how the individual responds on an interest inventory measures a part of the individual's emotional-motivational repertoire. To justify that assumption, it is necessary to show there is a relationship between personality test items (involving responses to words) and life behavior. After all, Skinner (1969, pp. 77–78) said that an individual's verbal reports cannot provide information concerning the variables that affect the individual's behavior. Based upon the radical behaviorism position, various behaviorists have rejected the use of tests with which to measure the reinforcement value of stimuli (Patterson, 1967; Weiss, 1968).

Psychological behaviorism, however, has established the necessary foundation for understanding why tests like the SVIB-SCII can measure behavioral variables. The psychological-behavioral analysis states that we all have extensive histories of learning, in which if we say what it is we want or do not want (that is, how we feel emotionally), we are reinforced by getting what it is we want. We learn a rich verbal-labeling repertoire to our internal physiological emotional responding, because emotional responses have stimulus properties. That verbal-labeling-of-emotion repertoire provides ways of indicating verbally whether we like or dislike any stimulus that elicits an emotional response. We learn not only to label actual objects and events in terms of the emotions they elicit in us, but we also learn to do the same for the words that stand for those objects and events, since they elicit conditioned emotional responses of the same type. Thus, when someone asks us if we like vanilla ice-cream we can do so by virtue of experiencing the emotional response those words elicit in us. We can compare relative strengths of our emotional responses to the words denoting other flavors also.

This analysis is based on empirical research. Subjects conditioned emotionally to stimuli correctly rated the "pleasantness–unpleasantness" of the stimuli to which they were conditioned (Staats & Staats, 1958; Staats, Staats, & Crawford, 1962). Finley and Staats (1967) found also that subjects could reliably rate the reinforcing value of stimuli. Word stimuli rated as positive would *function* as positive reinforcers in strengthening operant behaviors they followed. And Staats, Staats, and Crawford (1962) showed that subjects could rate correctly the intensity of the physiological emotional response to which they had been conditioned. These findings indicate to us basically how it is that interest test items actually measure emotional responses. The subjects in indicating likes and dislikes are indicating whether they have positive or negative emotional responses to the items listed on the test (Staats, 1963a, p. 305).

Behavioral Analysis of Interests as a Cause of Behavior

But *why* does the individual's interest test predict his success on the job, since that involves complex behaviors quite different from those involved in taking the test? The PB view is that there are many stimuli associated with one's work, and these stimuli differ over different occupations. Following this rationale, it would be possible to construct an interest test composed of items that describe the kind of stimuli that are confronted in the different occupations. If the individual had positive emotional responses to those stimuli, that would be an appropriate occupation for her. Constructing such a test would be a very large task. Those constructing interest tests got around that task in a very clever manner. What they did, instead, was to construct the kind of occupational "profiles" of likes and dislikes that have already been described. By virtue of the test construction, these profiles involve important emotional stimuli that are characteristic of groups of successful people in the occupations.

If an individual's profile is like that of an occupational group, why will that individual be likely to be successful in that occupation? The answer is that people in different occupations are confronted with different stimuli. Individuals who have been successful in those occupations have been successful, in part, because the stimuli encountered in those occupations have elicited (in good part) a positive emotional response in them. Mechanics are faced with certain kinds of tasks (stimuli); salesman, accountants, librarians, and professors with different kinds of tasks. It is important to maximize the extent to which the stimuli that are faced in the different occupations elicit a positive emotional response in the working individual. When that is the case the individual will experience positive emotions on the job—that is, will be happy with work.

Moreover, the individual's behavior will be affected in other ways. When the individual has a positive emotional response to a task his behavior in doing the task will be reinforced. The individual consequently will attend well during work hours, work hard, take few breaks. Job stimuli and related stimuli, because they elicit a positive emotional response, also will be positive incentive stimuli that will attract behavior. The "interested" mechanic who sees an article on a new piece of equipment will "approach" the article and read it and gain useful information. The salesman who loves his work will read books on salesmanship. We will also see that the job itself, because it elicits a positive emotional response, will attract the individual's approach behavior. The individual will show up for work on time, stay until late, and display little absenteeism.

The individual who does not have a positive emotional response to the situations that occur on the job, however, will have quite the opposite experience. This individual's work behaviors will not be reinforced and strengthened. The individual's work behavior will not be eager, there will be dawdling, inattention, frequent visits to the restroom, water fountain, and such. We will also see that the job is not a positive incentive. The individual will display avoidance behavior in the form of absenteeism. Moreover, the individual will not do things off the job—such as reading, and attending lectures—that will enhance job skills.

Empirical Evidence and Implications

Various empirical expectations can be drawn from this analysis of interests. For example, it would be expected that subjects with different profiles would find occupationally relevant stimuli to have different emotion-eliciting, reinforcing, and incentive values. Psychological behaviorism substantiated these expectations in three experiments (see Staats, Gross, Guay, & Carlson, 1973). Subjects were first given a Strong Vocational Interest Blank (Strong, 1927). In the first experiment positive, negative, and neutral items were selected for each subject. Positive items (consisting of a word) were paired with a stimulus in a classical conditioning procedure. Negative items were paired with another stimulus, and neutral items with a third stimulus. The results showed that subjects were conditioned to have a positive emotional response to the stimulus if it was paired with positive interest items, and a negative emotional response to the stimulus paired with "negative interest" items. So the interest items did elicit emotional responses, in a different manner for different subjects.

In a second experiment subjects' positive and negative interest items were again selected. Later, in another situation, the items were used as reinforcers for the subjects, in a task involving learning two motor responses. One response was followed with a positive interest item; the other response was followed by a negative interest item. The subjects learned to make the first response, showing that positive interest items served as positive reinforcers, and "negative interest" items served as punishments.

The third experiment tested whether interest items had directive (incentive) value. One group of subjects was selected to be high on one occupational interest profile (e.g., music teacher) and low on another (e.g., chemist). Another group was selected with the opposite interest profiles. These subjects, under the guise of measuring their physiological response to reading materials, were asked to select an article to read from a stack labeled MUSIC or a stack labeled CHEMISTRY. The question was which word stimulus would elicit approach behavior in the two different groups. The choice behavior of the subjects was 100 percent predictable from the Strong Interest Inventory results. This indicates the powerful incentive value of interests. Furthermore, in the experiment half the subjects were given the type of article to read they chose to select and half were given the other type of article. The results showed that the subjects learned more when they read the article of their choice (interest). We can infer that the chosen material elicits stronger emotional responses and thus reinforces the behavior of attentive reading more—resulting in learning more. This inference is supported by the fact that subjects who read in their interest field reported the article to be more pleasant, that is, to be more positive emotionally.

The three experiments showed that interest test items elicit an emotional response, and thus will serve as reinforcing stimuli and as directive stimuli. Response to the interest items indicates whether the stimuli encountered on the job will have positive emotional value, negative emotional value, or neutral value—and hence whether those job stimuli will act as positive or negative reinforcers and incentives. These experiments support the PB analysis of interest tests. In addition, it should be indicated that these experiments constitute a new and powerful type of validation. That is, the experiments demonstrate the *behavioral function* of interest items and why personality tests can be predictive of behavior. We need to conduct many such studies in a manner that will give behavioral (psychological) meaning (validation) to what are now psychological tests that provide prediction but no understanding of what is involved.

Psychological behaviorism's theory, thus, is a theory of what interests are, how they are learned, how they work their effects, and why they can be measured by interest inventories. In the process the concept and psychometric specification of interests are drawn into a very general theory, adding to the specification of the content of the BBRs and to an understanding of personality.

Values, Needs, and Other Parts of the Emotional-Motivational Personality Repertoire

If interest tests measure only a part of the emotional-motivational repertoire then there may be *various* personality tests that measure other parts of the repertoire. Some of the most prominent psychological tests can be seen to do just that. Let me introduce another example:

Needs

Need theory is a major approach to personality revolving around the concept that humans have various needs, that people differ on these needs, and that their behavior is determined by their needs (Maslow, 1954; Murray, 1938). Murray constructed his personality theory—one of the major approaches in the field—on the basis of a systematic description of various human needs, including the needs for achievement, order, defendence, and rejection.

Murray's need descriptions—which mix observations of behaviors people display with those of stimuli for which they strive—are not definitions in terms of more basic principles. Nevertheless, without being able to define needs, the Edwards Personal Preference Schedule was designed to measure the Murray Need System. What Murray refers to as needs may be considered in the present theory really to involve parts of the learned emotional-motivational repertoire—that is, stimuli that elicit emotional responses and are thus reinforcers and incentive stimuli (see Staats, 1963a, pp. 293–312).

The term *need*, thus, involves the same principles and concepts that interests do, but the stimuli involved are different, as are the behaviors the stimuli affect. And the items are not normed with occupational groups. As one example, Murray's achievement need is defined as follows: "To accomplish something difficult. To master, manipulate, or organize physical objects, human beings, or ideas. To do this as rapidly and as independently as possible. To overcome obstacles and attain a high standard. To excel oneself. To rival and surpass others. To increase self-regard by the successful exercise of talent" (Murray, 1938, p. 154). The items of the Edwards Personal Preference Schedule are designed to measure the various needs that were defined by Murray. As an example, the items ask the subject to select from two alternatives such as "I like to tell amusing stories and jokes at parties" versus "I would like to write a great novel or play" (Edwards, 1953, p. 2). This Schedule, thus, indicates where the individual has high or low "needs."

The present theory (see Staats, 1963a, pp. 287*ff*.; 1975, pp. 430–439) is that the Preference Schedule also measures life stimuli that differentially elicit emotional responses in people, and hence are reinforcers and incentive stimuli. So people with different needs will experience things differently, will behave differently, and will learn differently. This analysis could be tested, and the Preference Schedule validated, by seeing whether its items elicit emotional responses and serve as reinforcers and directive stimuli in the expected ways, using the methodology developed in the types of studies described above.

Values

Let me continue with the analysis of another aspect of personality—values. As usual, the traditional concept of values is not clearly stipulated, but has a commonsense motivational definition. The expectation is that a person's values affect the person's behavior. For example, a person with high values for education should strive to be educated, support expenditure of public money for education, and so on. In contrast, a person with economic values should strive to obtain economic goods, be in interested in economic issues, and read about such things. The *Study of Values* (Allport, Vernon, & Lindzey, 1951) is a test that measures different types of values, including religious, economic, asthetic, and political values. The following are examples of items on this test, constructed to tap the particular values: No. 9: "Which of these character traits do you consider the more desirable? (a) high ideals and reverence; (b) unselfishness and sympathy." No. 29: "In a paper, such as the *New York Times Sunday Times,* are you more likely to read (a) the real estate sections and the account of the stock market; (b) the section on picture galleries and exhibitions?" No. 4: "Assuming that you have sufficient ability, would you prefer to be (a) a banker; (b) a politician?"

In the PB view such items measure the emotional-reinforcing-incentive value of the types of stimuli described in the items. To illustrate, a person who scores high on religious values is a person who has a positive emotional response to religious stimuli, of which there are many. Consequently, the behaviors of participating in religious events—including attending church, reading religious literature, and listening to religious broadcasts—are reinforced for this person and they are thus high in frequency. Moreover, religious stimuli exert control over approach behavior—for example, the individual responds positively to requests for donations to religious causes, invitations to religious meetings, and requests to subscribe to religious magazines, because such stimuli elicit a positive emotional response and serve as incentives (positive directive stimuli).

In support of this last expectation, and the general analysis, Staats and Burns (1982) conducted a study that established that subjects high in religious values—as measured on the Allport–Vernon–Lindzey—did indeed display a stronger approach response to religious stimuli than did subjects who measured low on that scale. Those with religious values learned a task more readily than those without those values when the task involved making an approach response to a religious word. When the task involved learning an avoidance response to religious words they did more poorly than non-religious people. Thus, the religious stimuli—the words—did indeed have more directive (incentive) value for religious subjects.

We can thus see that a person's values are an important part of the individual's personality. Individual subjects, placed in the same learning situation, performed differently—depending upon the nature of the personality (emotional-motivational repertoire) they brought with them to the situation. Again, the experiment validates behaviorally the Allport–Vernon–Lindzey *Study of Values* (Allport, Vernon, & Lindzey, 1951), putting psychological substance into a test that is only vaguely defined.

Additional Aspects of Emotional-Motivational Personality

The PB theory states the emotional-motivational repertoire constitutes a complex, multifaceted, multi-acting part of personality. There are various tests that measure different types of emotional stimuli that, hence, elicit behaviors that are relevant to different life concerns. Interest tests deal with occupationally relevant stimuli; tests of needs and values deal with other types. Other classes of emotional stimuli are dealt with on tests like the *Attitude to School Questionnaire* (Strickland, Hoepfner, & Klein, 1976), which involves school stimuli; the *Creativity Attitude Survey* (Schaefer, 1971), which involves stimuli relevant to creative achievement; the *Multiple Affect Adjective Check List–Revised* (Zuckerman & Lubin, 1965), which includes a scale measuring "sensation seeking," involving this particular type of stimuli; and the *Coopersmith Self-Esteem Inventories* (Coopersmith, 1981), which deals with stimuli descriptive of the individual taking the test.

The actual responses demanded by the items on different tests may vary. For example, the items on the *Attitude to School Questionnaire* require the child to respond by drawing a circle around either a happy, neutral, or sad face. The *Campbell-Strong Interest Inventory* employs several different types of items, one being where the individual responds to the item by indicating "Like," "Dislike," or "Indifferent." The items on the *Coopersmith Self-Esteem Inventories* differ in that the subjects respond by selecting "Like Me" or "Unlike Me." In each case, regardless of the specific form of the item, the items measure emotional responses to verbal stimuli.

It should also be indicated that any of the three functions of the stimulus can be measured on a test. Most tests measure the subject's approach or avoidance response to an item, that is, the directive (incentive) function. But, one could use physiological instruments to measure the actual emotional response to the stimuli—as is done with penile plethysmography (Freund, 1967), which is a laboratory method for diagnosing predominance of physiological emotional response to homo- or heterosexual stimuli. Patterson (1965) used an operant conditioning type of task to assess the relative reinforcing value for the child of pictures of peers or parents, following the radical behaviorist view that what are effective reinforcers for the individual can only be measured with EAB technology (see also Weiss, 1968).

It is important to show, in clear-cut experimentation, that the emotional response to a stimulus can be measured in the three ways that derive from the three functions that emotional stimuli have (see Harms & Staats, 1978; Staats & Burns, 1982; Staats & Hammond, 1972; Staats, Minke, Martin, & Higa, 1972). Moreover, the word denoting the stimulus may be employed, rather than the stimulus itself, for the reasons supplied by PB (Staats & Fernandez-Ballesteros, 1987). This understanding is fundamental in the PB theory of emotion-motivation, in constructing emotional-motivational tests, and in dealing with human behavior. It is also fundamental to effecting a unification of psychometrics and behaviorism—for behaviorists in general, as well as behavioral assessors, at present do not understand that psychometric measures can be subjected to behavioral analyses.

The Concept of Emotion in Psychological Testing

There are many psychological tests that are based on common language definitions of unrelated concepts of emotions. In the common language there are many different individual emotions (joy, love, excitement) and there are various more general emotional concepts (attitudes, values, interests, and needs). Generally, the many different emotions are considered as separate psychological entities. And, since tests are constructed on the basis of such concepts, there are many tests of general emotional processes. The present position is that such psychological tests and their relationships to each other can be understood within the PB theory of emotion.

In the PB theory of emotion there are not a large number of different emotions that operate via different principles. Rather, there are only two kinds of emotional response—positive and negative (Staats, 1975, chaps. 4, 15; Staats & Eifert, 1990). (Lang, 1995, in constructing a different theory, has come to employ some of the same basic principles, including this one.) PB theory states that what is referred to in enumerating different emotions is that different stimulus situations are involved and different types of behavior. It is suggested that different tests are constructed to address these different situations and behaviors. We call the emotional response an interest when a work-related stimulus is involved and our concern is with variations in occupational success (work behavior). We consider the test to address the emotion of self-esteem, however, when the stimuli involved are those of one's own behavior or physical characteristics. We speak of tests of love when a particular person is involved, and of attitudes when groups are involved. But, in these and other cases, the same emotional response is operating—a positive emotional response.

There are various tests that measure different aspects of the emotional-motivational repertoire. Although these different tests have been constructed around different concepts and theories, and are considered unrelated, the bridging analysis places them into a unified theory framework. This provides a framework for organizing and simplifying our understanding of the emotional aspects of personality. The framework theory needs to be employed in a systematic analysis of the various tests of emotion.

The Emotional-Motivational Repertoire in Intelligence

Another weakness of the field of psychological testing is that it does not address phenomena that are important. As an example, although intelligence primarily involves language-cognitive and sensory-motor repertoires, aspects of the emotional-motivational repertoire are relevant to the individual's intelligent behavior. To illustrate, the classroom situation is a social situation, as is the individual intelligence test. For the child the most significant person in the social situation of the classroom is the teacher. How the child responds emotionally to the teacher will help determine how the child learns, for the emotional response will help determine the child's classroom behavior, such as whether the child pays attention or not, and the extent to which the child participates and works. A child who fears the teacher will respond differently than the child with a positive or neutral emotional response.

The same conditions will affect the child's intelligence test score, for the child can also have a positive, neutral, or negative emotional response to adults generally, including the test examiner. This will affect the child's test-taking behavior. If the emotional response is positive, the child will follow the examiner's instructions better, attend better, and so on. If the emotional response is neutral, those behaviors will not be as strong. If the emotional response is negative, the child will not follow instructions, and will attempt to escape from the situation in various ways. The more strongly anxious child may be incapacitated in other ways. Such behavior can result in the child receiving a lower intelligence test score than would otherwise be possible. One PB study dealt with the principle that children who had experienced school failure underachieved on tests because of avoidance behavior. Such children were reinforced with two pennies for each item passed and lost one penny for each item failed (Staats, Minke, Goodwin, & Landeen, 1967). Under this condition the children scored better on intellective tests. We can consider certain minority groups in these terms, for many black and Hispanic children in the United States will have different emotional responses to white adults (including teachers and testers) than white children do, emotional responses that do not elicit good learning behaviors.

It is important, thus, to realize that emotional-motivational conditions constitute part of the reason why intelligence tests are predictive of classroom performance. *The person's emotional response to the learning situation helps determine behavior and performance in that situation.* The field of psychological testing would do well to consider how to measure the way such emotional-motivational factors operate during test taking. Sometimes those factors are different during the test than would be the case in everyday life. Not measuring them detracts, in that case, from the accuracy of the test prediction.

THE EMOTIONAL STATE AND NEGATIVE EMOTION: A CRITICAL ELABORATION OF THE EMOTION THEORY

The traditional field of psychological measurement has not had a clear conception of emotion and thus of the relationships of the various tests that measure emotion. Thus, what values, interests, needs, preferences, and attitudes are is not made explicit, nor are their relationships to one another. That statement pertains even more to psychological tests that deal with negative emotions. The relationship of such tests to those that measure positive emotions is not indicated. The emotions measured in such tests as those of stress, fear, anxiety, prejudice, negative mood, and depression are not well defined, and the tests are not related to each other. Typically, a test of one of these emotions will be constructed and validated in the usual way, by being able to predict certain types of behavior. What is measured, and why the test has predictive properties, if considered at all, is done so speculatively.

Because the PB theory extends to negative emotions as well as to positive, tests of interests, values, and needs are considered within the same theoretical framework as those of the negative emotions. In the PB conception all of the negative emotions—stress, fear, anxiety, prejudice, negative mood, and depression—involve the same central negative emotional response. In addition, PB's theory of emotion (see Rose & Staats, 1988; Staats, 1975, chap. 4; Staats & Eifert, 1990; Staats & Heiby, 1985) introduces the concept of the *emotional state,* as a technically defined term, as well as the concept of the emotional response. The concept of the emotional state is very central in considering various behavior disorders, such as depression (Staats & Heiby, 1985) and the various anxiety disorders (Staats, 1989; Eifert, Evans, & McKendrick, 1990). It becomes important in elaborating PB's theory of the negative emotions to define the emotional state, along with the related concepts of the emotional response and the emotional-motivational BBR.

Emotion, the Emotional-Motivational BBR, and the Emotional State

One reason it is difficult to bridge basic study of emotion and the emotional aspects of personality involves the lack of differentiation of the basic emotional phenomena involved. To begin, there is the simple emotional response (which includes brain activity). Such a response is elicited by a stimulus and ceases following withdrawal of the stimulus. The emotional-motivational BBR is not the same as the ephemeral emotional response. The BBR represents all the stimuli that—through past learning—if presented will elicit an emotional response in the individual. There are huge individual differences in this "personality trait," as has been described.

In addition to these two emotional-motivational concepts, there is a third, the *emotional state.* PB derives the concept of the emotional state from the elementary concept of the emotional response, plus an analysis of the BBRs and the complex life stimuli confronted by the individual. The emotional state is a resultant of the individual's BBR *and* life situation variables. To illustrate, the individual is in a life situation that consists of large multitudes of stimuli. Many of them elicit emotional responses, both positive and negative. The individual is exposed to myriad stimuli that elicit an emotional response in one single day, even at any particular time. Just the words of others that are experienced in one day—from friends, family, colleagues, the newspaper, TV, and so on—include a multitude of emotion-eliciting stimuli. Our own words, moreover, supply a rich source of emotional stimuli. As an example, take the pornographic images and emotions that people experience by virtue of their verbal-image repertoires; or the fear responses evoked by verbal worrying. Sometimes these language, language-image, and image ways of responding have persistent effects. For example, the person with a long-term ambition—perhaps to become a doctor or to get on the Olympic team—may repeatedly image about the topic for years, and in so doing produce an abundant supply of emotion-eliciting stimuli that have a thematic property in an emotional sense.

An anger that persists for some hours, or longer, may be used to illustrate the concept of the negative emotional state. Let us say a negative emotional response has been elicited by an insulting social remark—at first a single response. Then, the experienced emotion, in turn, may elicit strings of verbal behaviors that negatively describe the character of the insulter, that go over the negative interactions with that person in the past, that project the negative purposes of the insulter, that describe the effects on others who heard the remark, that describe the injustice and outrage involved, and so on. All of these responses will continue to elicit negative emotional responses in the individual. Relatives or friends who are told these things may then contribute additional remarks that further elicit a negative emotional response in the individual. The resultant of such complex stimuli can be a complexly determined, strong, persisting emotional state. This is much more than a simple emotional response.

The *algebraic sum* principle is that the many emotional stimuli to which the individual is exposed will be both positive and negative and, during a period, will yield a resultant emotional state (see Staats & Heiby, 1985; Rose & Staats, 1988, for early forms of the concept). The basic principles involved in emotional states are the same as the principles involved in single emotional responses. But, because the emotional state is made up of multiple emotional responses resulting from various types of stimuli, the emotional state has properties that single emotional responses do not have. For example, the single response is ephemeral while the emotional state has greater duration.

While the persistence of the emotional state distinguishes the state from the simple emotional response, ephemeral emotional responses may nevertheless briefly affect the persistent or chronic emotional state. As an example, a person may be experiencing a negative emotional state (a dysphoria or depression), but receiving a very nice compliment from a revered person could elicit a positive emotional response that would displace the dysphoria for a time. But when this emotional response is gone, if the conditions producing the dysphoria still exist, that emotional state will return. In this way the emotional state may function as a background condition that more ephemeral emotional responding may temporarily make more positive or negative.

The stimuli that determine continuing emotional states tend to be general, ubiquitous classes—like a negative work situation. These stimuli tend also to be less explicit because of sheer number, such that the individual frequently cannot be aware of what they are. Because the causative stimuli are unknown, the individual may be left with an emotional experience that cannot be explained, which can lead to an interpretation that unconscious mental processes are involved, that emotional states are inexplicable, or that they are due to some personal (biological) problem.

Because emotional states are responses to combinations of stimuli, they may be intense. When they are in the positive direction they are called being euphoric, even manic; and when in the negative direction they are called such things as anxiety, panic, dysphoria, stress, and depression. Continuing intense emotional responding can be undesirable for medical reasons, as in the case of stress. The intense emotional state may also affect the individual's behavior in ways that are not desirable, as will be indicated. Moreover, the negative emotional state is something whose reduction will be reinforcing—so the individual will learn things that escape from it. For example, the individual can learn to consume alcohol or drugs that reduce the negative emotional state. This effect has now been shown in important studies with animals (Blanchard, Flores, Magee, Weiss, & Blanchard, 1992; Blanchard, Hori, Tom, & Blanchard, 1987).

It should be understood that an alteration in the emotional state produces other effects that also act back on the individual's emotional responding. For example, generally the individual who drinks will thereby experience a more positive emotional state. As the emotional state is affected, so is the individual's behavior—more smiling and laughing occur, the individual is more outgoing, affectionate, and open, speaking with less constraint. These are engaging behaviors for others and they respond in a more positive way which adds to the drinker's positive emotional state. There is thus a snowballing interactional effect.

With the concept of the emotional state it is also possible to relate organic conditions with behavior principles. For example, drugs can enhance or diminish the individual's positive emotional or negative emotional responding. Since such drugs have their effect over a period of time, they have the ability to affect emotional responding over that period, and thus the individual's emotional state. Alcohol, for example, can induce a euphoric state, either by increasing positive emotional responses or diminishing negative emotional responses, or both. It is hypothesized, also, that drug treatment of manic disorders have their effect by placing a lid on the intensity of positive emotional response the individual can experience. A drug that decreases the intensity of negative emotional responses—as used in treating depression—may be seen to have its effect by swinging the algebraic sum of positive and negative emotional responding in the positive direction. This theoretical context provides the basis for empirical study. For example, measures of emotional responding to (or reinforcement or directive of) stimuli with and without drugs could distinguish an effect. Physiological conditions of other kinds could also effect the emotional state.

In conclusion, the PB theory of emotion-motivation includes three concepts, constructed in a hierarchical manner, one on the other. There is the emotional response to a stimulus, the fundamental emotional process. There is the emotional-motivational basic behavioral repertoire which is composed of the stimuli that for the individual will elicit an emotional response. And there is the emotional state, the multiples of emotional responses that result from the interaction of the environment with the individual's emotional-motivational BBR. A fear response to some stimulus is an emotional response—which occurs when the stimulus is there and disappears when the stimulus is gone. The individual's vocational interests exemplify a part of the emotional-motivational BBR. The interests are characteristic of the individual, are enduring, and have general effects. Depression illustrates the emotional state. It is experienced, is lasting, it has variations, and affecting the state has behavioral effects. These concepts and their distinctions are fundamental and call for a program of systematic research.

Measurement of Negative Emotions and Emotional States

With these concepts in hand we can now consider psychological tests that in terms of the present theory measure negative emotional responding and negative emotional states and, hence, aspects of the negative emotional-motivational BBR.

Fears (Phobias)

A fear may be considered a negative emotional response to a specific type of stimulus—such as snakes, cockroaches, dogs, and the insides of airplanes or elevators. When these emotional responses are intense enough they are called *phobias*. Tests of fears or phobias may be considered to measure emotional responses to specific stimuli. The *Fear Survey Schedule* (Wolpe & Lang, 1964) involves subjects rating their degree of fear toward different stimuli. This test has been widely used to stipulate phobias. Within PB theory it can be seen that the items measure specific emotional responses to specific stimuli; what is being measured is part of the emotional-motivational BBR. Each fear one has provides the potential for a transient negative emotional response, should the environment present the stimulus involved. However, the more stimuli toward which the individual has a negative emotional response, the greater the individual's potential for experiencing a negative emotional state. For this reason it might be expected there would be a correlation between the number of fears that a person has (an aspect of the emotional-motivational BBR) and tests that measure general anxiety.

Anxiety

In PB theory anxiety is an emotional state. Anxiety results when many stimuli elicit a negative emotional response. The stimuli may be common in everyday life, such as those involving relationships to family and friends, conditions in the workplace, the problems facing one's children, financial conditions, as well as the verbal worrying the individual does about all of these things. When there are many negative stimuli, the algebraic emotional sum can be a continuing negative emotional state, which may be described as anxiety.

There are various tests that tap the anxiety state. The *State-Trait Anxiety Inventory* (Spielberger, Gorsuch, & Lushene, 1970) specifically accepts a traditional distinction in concepts of anxiety. On the one hand it is said there are transitory states of anxiety, that is, momentary or short-lived fears and worries. On the other, there is a stable tendency of some individuals to respond anxiously to stressful situations to a greater extent than do other individuals. Put in terms of PB, the shorter-term processes that Spielberger, Gorsuch, and Lushene refer to concern specific emotional responses. However, it is suggested that anxiety does not consist of a stable tendency to respond anxiously to stressful situations. If that were the case the phenomenon would involve overreacting to the negative stimuli, but not a continuing emotional state. Rather, anxiety tests measure some combination of the individual's negative emotional BBR along with a complex environmental situation that results in a continuing negative emotional state that is labeled anxiety.

There are various, more specialized, tests of negative emotional responses to more specific types of situations. For example, the *Test Anxiety Inventory* (Spielberger, 1980) measures students' anxiety toward the test-taking situation. The *Adolescent Separation Anxiety Test* (Hansburg, 1972), as another example, aims to measure the extent of negative emotional response to a variety of "separation" experiences or situations. We can see here that the stimuli eliciting the negative emotional response are more complex than is the case where the individual has a fear or phobic response to a simple stimulus. To the extent that such anxiety tests measure response to a wide number of stimuli, they move in the direction of measuring emotional states rather than single responses.

Depression

As will be indicated in the next chapter, PB includes a theory of abnormal behavior (see Staats, 1963a, chap. 11; 1975, chap. 8; 1989). One of its theories of the behavior disorders deals with depression (see Heiby & Staats, 1990; Staats & Heiby, 1985). Depression involves an interaction between the individual's BBRs and the life environment. In a clinical depression, as a consequence of the interaction, the individual experiences such a preponderance of negative emotional stimuli that the individual experiences a strong negative emotional state (dysphoria) of a duration of more than two weeks. (The full theory makes a more complete analysis.) There are many intermediate intensities of the dysphoria that individuals can experience, which tests of depression have been developed to measure. One such test is the *Beck Depression Inventory* (BDI) (Beck, Ward, Mendelson, Mock, & Erbaugh, 1961). Validated as a diagnostic instrument, it is thought to measure how negative the individual is about herself, the world, and the future—which in the present terms involve many important stimuli.

Stress

Another concept is that of stress, the extent to which situations induce a physiological stress pattern of responses in the subject. In the present theory, stress is another term for a negative emotional state. We may ask what is it that differentiates stress from other negative emotions or states. In the present view the stimuli involved in stress, while they are more general than those involved in phobias, are nevertheless more explicit than those involved in anxiety. Stress tends to be more clearly linked with environmental "stressors," such as those that occur in the workplace or other specific situation. And the concept of stress has emerged more in the context of concern with the individual's physiological conditions. For example, the term stress would be more likely to be used when the concern is with the individual's hypertension or other health problem (Holmes & Masuda, 1974).

One traditional conception of stress is of situations that require adjustment on the part of the individual. For example, one test of a specific kind of stress is the *Parenting Stress Index* (Abidin, 1983). This test aims to measure the amount of stress induced in the parent by the parent–child interaction, as well as to specify the particular aspects of that interaction that produce that stress. Another example is the *Social Readjustment Rating Scale* (Holmes & Rahe, 1967), which obtains ratings on the extent of readjustment required for life's changes, both positive and negative. However, what is considered positive and negative in a commonsense analysis may be quite different from a PB analysis. Although the birth of a baby is ordinarily considered to be a positive life change, the person's life situation and BBRs may make the birth of the child a complex of negative emotional stimuli. The types of life changes included on the test are death of a close family member, of a close friend, divorce, personal injury or illness, and so on.

Moods

I have said that emotional states last, they are not ephemeral like individual emotional responses. Nevertheless, there are variations in how long an emotional state will last, as well as in how intense the emotional state is. Moods—which can be positive or negative—may be considered as emotional states, but they are more transitory than continuing states, such as trait anxiety or clinical depression. Moods also are less intense than clinically relevant states, like a depression, on the negative side, or a manic state, on the positive side. The *Profile of Mood States* (McNair, Morr, & Droppleman, 1971) aims to measure subjects' present mood state. The mood is viewed as a changing emotional state, in response to a changing environment—as distinguished from long-term moods that reflect enduring personality traits. This view, although it is based on commonsense concepts, can be fit into the present general theory. The moods that are assessed are tension-anxiety, depression-dejection, anger-hostility, vigor-activity, fatigue-inertia, and confusion-bewilderment. There are more dimensions here than are included in the positive–negative dichotomy of PB. In the PB view these additional dimensions actually involve variables other than the positive–negative dimension of the emotional response.

Relationship of Negative Emotions

In the world of abnormal psychology, clinical treatment, and psychological measurement, it is generally accepted that such things as depression, anxiety, phobias, stress, prejudice, and negative mood exist as more or less separate problems. Some of these—especially stress, anxiety, and fears—are identified as specific physiological processes within the person. In addition, all of them would be considered to be some type of emotional process, but there is little attempt to specify what that relationship might be, to construct a theory that makes that specification, or even to be concerned about relating the tests that have been constructed to measure the various problems involved.

Within the PB framework, however, there is impetus to consider the several psychological conditions in a related way. To illustrate, in discussing interests, values, attitudes, self-esteem, and so on, it was valuable to realize that the tests in these areas measured aspects of the emotional-motivational repertoire. That indication provides a general theory that relates the separate tests to each other. The PB analysis carries unification also into the realm of abnormal behavior, as will be indicated in the next chapter. As a brief example, however, in the PB view parasthesias are considered when inappropriate stimulus objects elicit a sexual emotional response in the individual (Staats, 1975, chap. 8). Manic disorder, as another example, may be considered to involve an inappropriately positive emotional state. The major point is that the PB theory serves to unify these various phenomena within a theory of emotion-motivation with consistent concepts and principles, in closely reasoned theory construction.

It is important to perform the same type of conceptualization for the negative emotions. The present position is that depression, anxiety, phobias, stress, prejudice, negative attitudes, obsessive–compulsive disorder, and post-traumatic stress syndrome, are related, in that they all involve significant negative emotions. A theory of emotion must be concerned with the commonality as well as with the differences that define the disorders.

In short, the PB position is that the same brain structures are involved for the various negative emotional conditions. The differences among the negative emotions arise from the differences in the stimuli involved and the types of variables distinguishing responses and states. What differentiates fear, anxiety, jealousy, and anger, as examples, is not the emotional response itself, but the various other characteristics that the eliciting stimuli can have, as well as the other behaviors those stimuli can elicit. To illustrate, the individual reports jealousy when a loved one has run off with someone else, and grief when the loved one has been killed. The negative emotional response elicited is similar, and there is a similar stimulus, the loss of the loved one. But there are other stimuli involved that are different. And the individual's and others' language behaviors to the two different events are different in ways that affect the individual's emotional responding. Schacter (1970), showed that induced emotional states are interpreted differently, depending upon the situational stimuli and what the subject is led to believe. Although he did not analyze his results in behavioral terms, these findings contribute support to the present theory of emotion.

This view has implications in the present context. Many tests have been constructed to measure human emotions. They have been constructed largely in isolation, typically using commonsense notions of emotion. Thus, the knowledge in this area is not organized and meaningful. To understand human behavior we need an organized conception of emotion (and one that is further interrelated with other concepts that explain human behavior). In this task it is important to specify what the variables are that lead us to differentiate the different emotions in the field of psychological measurement. PB provides a prototypical beginning in this very large task.

TESTS OF THE SENSORY-MOTOR BBR AND THE CONTENT OF PERSONALITY

There are personality concepts that refer to motor skills. For example, the concept of the "natural athlete" is that some individuals have a special biological quality that enables them to be good at any sport, without much learning. There is also a similar concept of "talent" that is used to "explain" exceptional ability in music, dance, art and other fine performances. These are informal concepts. Traditionally in the field of personality the overt behavior of the individual is not considered the focus of study. Rather, personality is considered to be the underlying structure or process that *determines* behavior. This orientation has been made very clear in psychoanalytic theory, sometimes in opposition to behaviorism. Likewise, even when overt behavior is actually measured in psychological tests, it is typically done to index an inferred personality process. Thus, copying a geometric design is considered important as an index of "intelligence," not as an important behavior in and of itself. It is anomalous that traditional personality testing has studied, at least in part, the content of human behavior, but its theory generally does not make that behavior an important object of study. Behaviorism, on the other hand, although conceptually emphasizing the importance of the study of behavior, has not systematically studied the content of human behavior or used the knowledge provided by personality testing.

There have been in psychology, however, several areas of research concerned with aspects of sensory-motor behavior. A specific example in experimental psychology was study using the "pursuit rotor," with which to investigate perceptual-motor skills. The pursuit rotor is a rotating disk with a point on it that the subject must track and attempt to contact continuously with a stylus. The stylus and point, when in contact, complete an electrical circuit, so the amount of time the subject is on target can be precisely recorded. Quality of perceptual-motor performance, then can be studied with laboratory precision over different variables (such as drug ingestion). The effects of such variables have been studied with other types of perceptual-motor performance. Knowledge of sensory-motor skills and the effects of drug substances is important, for example, in adjudicating automobile accident claims. The findings produced are very valuable as applied to accident litigation.

Another finding is that perceptual-motor skill performance on different tasks is correlated, giving rise to the following position. *"The term basic ability refers to a general trait of an individual which determines the limit of performance he attains on many different tasks. . . .* Basic abilities represent stored *general* potentialities which can facilitate the learning of a variety of *specific skills"* (Gagne & Fleishman, 1959, p. 94). This approach, thus, represents the extension of the concept of personality trait to sensory-motor performance. Some personal (biological) quality is thought to establish individual differences in the learning and display of sensory-motor skills.

Another interest in the study of motor skill has been analytic, for example, in ascertaining the kind of stimuli that function in motor learning. One view has been that kinaestheic cues (those arising within the muscles themselves) are involved in learning sequences of responses, and an opposing view states that the learning is centrally mediated. As illustration, reproduction accuracy in a finger-positioning task was examined when some subjects were deprived of kinesthetic stimulation and other subjects had the usual sensations (Kelso, 1977). Closely related to these types of study has been human factor research that studies particular performances of individuals for a variety of purposes. Thus, human engineering has been concerned with designing equipment—for example, an airplane cockpit—so the human operator can use it most effectively.

There is another, completely separate study of motor (and other) skills as they develop with age in childhood (see Gesell & Thompson, 1938). Detailed tables and charts were constructed of what children will typically do, at what ages. These materials, commonly employed by pediatricians and others working with children, actually serve in the manner of psychological tests, as standards against which the behavior development of the particular child can be gauged. Moreover, as will be indicated, this tradition of research has been elaborated within the psychometric tradition, and there are many psychological tests that, in whole or in part, involve the measurement of sensory-motor skills.

It should also be added in this context that behaviorism—especially of the modern radical behaviorism variety—traditionally had its focus on motor behavior. The principles of reinforcement were established with motor behaviors. Skinner's experimental analysis of behavior methodology, which includes the operant conditioning chamber, was designed for the study of reinforcement effects on motor behavior. This research stipulated systematically how schedules of reinforcement determine the characteristics of motor responding. Although the acquisition (learning) of motor behavior has not been the focus, the operant approach introduced the concepts of the response class and successive approximation (commonly called *shaping*), which is a method for conditioning responses that would ordinarily occur infrequently or never. The methods of reinforcement and shaping have been used widely in training animals in sensory-motor skills (see Breland & Breland, 1961).

Each of these approaches has studied aspects of sensory-motor behavior. Interestingly, however, they are not related to one another in the service of producing a general conception that deals with (1) stipulating the important human sensory-motor repertoires; (2) how these repertoires are learned to individually different extents; and (3) how these repertoires function as personality processes and determine individual differences in behavior, experience, and learning. The various approaches separately, or in combination, do not yield a personality theory that includes human sensory-motor behavior concerns. Notwithstanding this state of affairs, many psychological tests include items that measure sensory-motor skills. And some tests *focus* on sensory-motor skills. This is done, however, without benefit of an over-arching conception by which to consider what these tests represent.

Psychological Tests of the Sensory-Motor Repertoire

As with the other two BBRs, psychological tests are important for the manner in which they contribute knowledge about the content of personality by measuring different parts of the sensory-motor BBR.

Developmental Tests of the Sensory-Motor Repertoire

There are various tests that deal with sensory-motor performance as a means of judging the child's developmental level (which is generally taken to reflect biological maturation). The Gesell Developmental Schedules was the original, introduced in 1925 (see Ames, Gillespie, Haines, & Ilg, 1979). This scale, measuring developmental progress in gross motor, fine motor, language, personal-social, and adaptive behavior in four-week-olds to 36-month-olds, introduced items that have been widely used on infant tests. For example, the *Ring and Peg Tests of Development* (Banham, 1975) includes tests for the development of sitting, walking, balance, throwing, and catching, depending on the child's age range.

The *Minnesota Child Development Inventory* (Ireton & Thewing, 1974) tests the child for gross motor skills employing 34 items measuring locomotion, strength, balance, and coordination. For example, whether the child can do a forward somersault is an item at the 30-month level of the scale. In addition, fine motor skills are tested by 44 items that measure different visual-motor coordinations, such as the ability to copy circles (at the 36-month level). (It is interesting to note the various types of tests that include this type of item.) *The Bruininks-Oseretsky Test of Motor Proficiency* (Bruininks, 1978) is devoted entirely to measuring motor ability. It is divided into eight parts: running speed and agility, balance, bilateral coordination, strength, upper-limb coordination, response speed, visual-motor control, upper-limb speed, and dexterity (Harrington, 1985).

Sensory-Motor Tests for Special Education

Measurement of sensory-motor (adaptive) skills has importance also in tests designed for detecting children who are candidates for special education programs. The *AAMD Adaptive Behavior Scale, School Edition* (Lambert, Windmiller, Cale, & Figueroa, 1975), for example, tests for behaviors associated with daily-living tasks, such as eating, dressing, and shopping, as well as behaviors related to social situations such as damaging property and disrupting class activities. Like other measures of adaptive behavior, the test does not involve direct observations of behavior. Rather, the observations are gained through use of someone who has had an opportunity to observe the behavior, like a parent or teacher.

Another test with similar goals, the *Comprehensive Test of Adaptive Behavior* (Adams, 1984), measures various areas of sensory-motor skills, including such things as the following: self-help skills (toileting, grooming, dressing, eating); home living skills (living room, kitchen-cooking, kitchen-cleaning, bedroom, bath and utility, yard care); independent living skills (health, time-telling, vocational); social skills (leisure skills); sensory-motor skills (sensory awareness, motor skills).

Sensory-Motor Repertoires and Intelligence

In the field of intelligence the items selected are those that predict school performance. Many of those items, especially at the lower ages, involve sensory-motor skills. The underlying assumption is that "intelligence" can be "expressed" in sensory-motor problems as well as in "cognitive" problems. As an example, at the two-year level of the Stanford-Binet (Terman & Merrill, 1937, p. 76) the child is asked to build a four-block tower like one the examiner has built. More complex problems of the same type are introduced progressively, at the succeeding age levels. On the same test there are items that require that the child complete a line drawing of a man (p. 87), discriminate forms (p. 88), tie a knot (p. 93), trace a maze (p. 96), fold and cut a paper a certain way (p. 102), and so on. Infant tests of intelligence are heavily composed of sensory-motor items.

Occupational Sensory-Motor Tests

There are various sensory-motor repertoires of specialized sorts that are relevant to occupations. And there are tests constructed to measure some of the common occupational skills, such as typing skills. For practical reasons such tests tend to be of a paper-and-pencil type that measure knowledge of a job rather than the sensory-motor skills themselves. Work samples are the most direct way, however, of measuring occupational sensory-motor repertoires. In general, the work sample is just that, a standard task that samples the skills demanded by the job. For example, a typing test is a direct way of measuring this type of skill. Campion (1972) describes a very good work sample for testing the sensory-motor skills of mechanics.

Psychological Behavioral Analysis of Psychological Tests of Sensory-Motor Abilities

There is a general belief that individual differences in sensory-motor skill are due to underlying traits. Particular traits account for particular types of skills. For example, the "natural" athlete is thought to have an inborn personal-biological structure or process that confers special ability to learn and to perform athletically across different sports. Different traits are thought to be involved in such things as musical skill, artistic skill, and mechanical skill. This conception is reflected in the concepts of perceptual-motor "abilities," "aptitudes, and "talents." Artists are thought in some way to have better visual apparatus, musicians to have better auditory apparatus. A related conception is that the sensory-motor characteristics typical of men and women are due to a masculinity–femininity personality trait.

This general conception of motor personality traits has various shortcomings. For one thing there is inadequate evidence to support the concept of internal biological-personality processes that determine sensory-motor skill. As large as the differences are in sensory-motor skill, it might be expected that brain differences would be detectable. There are attempts to show that the cortical representation of the fingers of string players is larger than for non-playing subjects (Elbert, Pantev, Wienbruch, Rockstroh, & Taub, 1995). But these results support the general PB position that *learning experiences* produce changes in the brain. Those brain changes are the biological means for storing the BBRs learned.

Dimensions of Sensory-Motor Behavior

Are there different underlying abilities in different sensory-motor performances? Is there an internal biological difference between a virtuoso violinist and a National Football League quarterback? Or is there a set of principles that applies to the various types of sensory-motor skill? In the PB view there are common principles by which to understand different sensory-motor skills, but also by which to distinguish among those skills.

What is necessary in understanding sensory-motor behavior—and the personality traits that are inferred from this behavior—is a detailed analysis of the repertoires involved. Only in this way can similarities and differences in various skill performances be understood. To illustrate, for the pathologist in differentiating normal and abnormal tissue samples the sensory-motor skill involves less the motor response, centering, rather, around sensory skills. The opposite is true of the weight lifter, where external stimulus differentiation is unimportant. Rather the skilled performance lies in having developed precise, and precisely sequenced, movements while exerting maximal power. Unlike the weight lifter, the watchmaker's skill heavily involves making very fine, delicate motor movements. A basketball player or a running back in football has a complex, changing stimulus array with which to respond in a complex manner. The solo ballet dancer has very complex and fine motor skills, but the stimulus array plays a lesser role. Sometimes it is the sequence of responses that constitutes the skill. As with the dancer, in some cases a very important part of the sensory-motor skill can involve having acquired unit responses that can be combined into sequences. The quarterback has to combine running and dodging skills, with perceptual skills of tracking receivers and reading defensive players' locations, with throwing skills. Similarly, the musician has basic playing skills that can be rearranged easily in the acquisition of new pieces.

The stimuli in different skills involve differences in complexity. The stimuli can also involve different senses, and this is another way of differentiating skills. The artist learns a repertoire of responses to many visual stimuli. The musician learns a repertoire of responses to many auditory stimuli. (There is no evidence that exceptional skill in these areas rests on special sensory acuity.) On the response end, some repertoires involve fine muscles and delicate movements. Others involve larger muscle groups. Some repertoires require quick movements, others emphasize precision, and others involve power movements. Sensory-motor repertoires can vary in complexity of the muscle groups involved. And sensory-motor skills differ in the amount of learning and other types of preparation that are required. It takes years of learning to become a concert musician. It takes years also to strengthen the muscles of the weight lifter, in addition to learning the sensory-motor skills involved.

Sensory-Motor Skills Are the Same

The PB position, thus, is that there are various ways that sensory-motor skills can differ without involving anything that is different in principle, or different in terms of some underlying personal-biological trait. But the PB position is that sensory-motor skills (including perceptual skills) are all fundamentally the same. Performing musical skills are not different in principle from artistic skills, from athletic skills, from the perceptual skills of a pathologist, from the imitative skills of the professional impersonator, from mechanical skills, from surgical or watchmaking or typing skills, from dancing skills, from the skills of street-fighting and wife-beating, or from the everyday skills of living. All complex human behavior that is made up of sensory-motor skills involves the same behavior principles.

Sensory-Motor Characteristics Are Learned

Moreover, the position is that the same learning-behavior principles underlie the acquisition and display of human sensory-motor behavior, in all the forms that are displayed in humans. As has been indicated, humans are not born with complex human behaviors, including coordinated sensory-motor behaviors. The neonate at birth begins to *learn* repertoires of sensory-motor behaviors, as the child development norms indicate so clearly. From that beginning all of the skills that humans acquire, even the most marvelous, are learned. What this means is that sensory-motor performances—including those that are thought to index special talents—are acquired and operate according to the same principles. When the skill involved is developed to a high level—whether in tennis, guitar playing, ballet, or brain surgery—

the repertoires involved are learned via cumulative-hierarchical learning. The more complex the skill the longer the learning process necessary. Extraordinary skill means extraordinary learning conditions, years of cumulative-hierarchical learning. Differences among children on items that test sensory-motor development arise from differences in how advanced they are in the cumulative-hierarchical learning of the repertoire that is being tested.

Intraindividual Differences in Sensory-Motor Skill. Various questions arise in this context. The explanation of great skill by learning conditions is hard to accept. Acceptance requires the ability to analyze how learning conditions can create great skill, and such analyses have not been made yet. It is much easier, and is traditional, to assume that the explanation lies in some biological process. For example, two siblings may both be given training in piano and one becomes a concert pianist and the other only becomes a good piano player. Such cases are widely assumed to give evidence that talent in the piano results from special biological gifts, but these cases do not provide evidence of that kind—whether learning or biology is involved is not shown.

The same is true of differences that occur within the same person. An individual may be a world reknown cellist, yet be a clumsy athlete and dancer. Does that not indicate that different biologically based abilities are involved? Not at all. Such a finding does not in itself tell us whether the intraindividual difference is due to biology or learning.

The Personal-Biological Factor in Sensory-Motor Differences

Are there no biological differences that themselves produce differences in sensory-motor skill? The PB position is that biology does have a role that is clear. Body form, strength, and speed characteristics (although affected by body use) can be biologically determined in a way that is an important factor in individual differences in sensory-motor performances. The seven-footer has advantages in basketball the five-footer does not. The individual without color vision is handicapped in becoming a painter. The very large-boned, stocky individual will not break high-jump records. Having long and powerful fingers is an advantage to a pianist. Body structure differences are critically important in a variety of sensory-motor repertoires.

However, world-class tennis players range from five-feet-six-inches to six-feet-eight, with a variety of body builds. Give any normal individual the intensive training regimen of a world-class tennis player like Jimmy Connors (which began at the age of four), and the result will be an outstanding tennis athlete, very different from the man-in-the-street in that sensory-motor realm. The differences in skill due to biological factors that exist among those given that special training will be comparatively small, when considering the range of skills in the general population. But when considering the group of highly trained individuals, those "small" differences may nevertheless be very large, as in the difference between being the number one tennis player in the world and being number 400. But in the present view those do not stem from brain differences.

How the Sensory-Motor Repertoire Is Part of Personality and Determines Behavior

Given this position, in what way does PB consider tests of sensory-motor behaviors to be measures of the content of personality? For one thing, the sensory-motor repertoire provides many of the elements from which the current environment samples. Thus, the nature of the individual's sensory-motor repertoire stamps the nature of the individual's behavior. The individual cannot perform a behavior that she does not have in her repertoire. An individual who does not have the skills of being physically violent, will not evidence violent behavior, even in a situation in which others do. A person who does not have the feminine repertoire of making common movements—as drinking from a coffee cup, walking, gesturing, rearranging disheveled hair, and so on—cannot behave like women do.

The sensory-motor BBR also affects the individual's later learning and in that way, has the character of a personality trait. For example, the child who has been given drawing materials and has learned to hold a crayon or pencil in making lines in a particular way in coloring in a book, in making drawings, and such, will learn a basic set of perceptual and motor skills. That child will do better in learning to write the letters than a child without those experiences and without those skills. As another example, in tennis instruction an individual will learn to jump up lightly on the balls of the feet in receiving a serve, to bend the knees and skip sideways rapidly in getting to the ball, and to jump up to hit an overhead. These, however, are component sensory-motor skills that will be basic also to learning other sports such as volleyball, basketball, and soccer. This individual will learn these sports more quickly than an individual who does not have the component skills. The person who has acquired a wide repertoire of such components, to a high level of skill—from concentrated experience in several sports—will be a "natural athlete," that is, will be able to learn new sports quickly, easily, and gracefully, without going through the awkwardness of the non-athlete. The concept of the natural athlete is a personality concept, but it is explained by the sensory-motor BBR and the enhanced learning it yields.

Another reason that the various sensory-motor items on tests are predictive of later learning in other spheres is because the child's score on such items is a measure of the general quality of the learning experience the child is receiving. That is, the rate at which the preschool child has learned the sensory-motor, including perceptual, skills depends largely on the quality of experience (training) the child has received. If that training has been good in producing some particular repertoire, it will tend to be good in all spheres. If the training has been poor in one sphere, it will tend to be generally poor. There are exceptions, of course, but the items that measure specific repertoires tend to be generally predictive to the extent that they indicate the general quality of the child's training.

Finally, the sensory-motor repertoire has a general effect on the individual's characteristic behavior by virtue of indirect processes. For example, sensory-motor repertoires have a social and environmental value. A person with fine repertoires in athletics, art, music, dancing, carpentry, or whatever, will be responded to by others in favorable ways that will affect the emotional-motivational and language-cognitive repertoires—including those we refer to as the self-concept, or self-esteem. A fine athlete, for example, will have experiences generally that enhance self-esteem.

In such various ways the sensory-motor repertoire is a BBR that affects the individual's experience, learning, and behavior—filling the roles designated for aspects of personality.

Empirical Implications of the PB Analysis of Sensory-Motor Tests

Before leaving this topic it should be indicated that the PB analysis of the sensory-motor BBR has implications for new directions of research. There are many psychological tests that measure sensory-motor skills. They are used to predict important types of performance and thus are useful diagnostically. But there is an absence of understanding the relationships of the tests. Moreover, the tests are limited to predictive-diagnostic uses. When a child is measured and found wanting in some area of sensory-motor skill this does not indicate what should be done to treat the child for the deficit.

The present approach has made analyses of various sensory-motor skills in terms of what repertoires are involved and in terms of how those repertoires can be produced in the child through training. This type of analysis, including experimental-longitudinal research, is needed for the various sensory-motor repertoire elements that are measured on tests. The fact that those sensory-motor repertoires appear on psychological tests that have significant uses indicates that the repertoires are important. That means they should be studied so the repertoires can be dealt with in learning treatments, not just measured.

"PURE" AND "MIXED" CLINICAL DIAGNOSTIC TESTS

Paradigmatic behaviorism categorizes personality into three general repertoires or behavioral systems. The categorization scheme is helpful theoretically in various ways, one being the connection of the theory to existing concepts and studies. But there is no suggestion that there are differences in principles involved or that the BBRs are clearly separable processes. Overlap is common, for example. Thus, the verbal-motor subrepertoire that is categorized in the language-cognitive repertoire could be considered as well in the sensory-motor repertoire. Moreover, as has been indicated, the repertoires are in constant interaction. It is also the case that the BBRs are elaborated in very complex ways. For example, the individual not only learns language repertoires involving single words, but also very complex conglomerations we call opinions, beliefs, schemas, conceptions, ideas, and the like.

In analyzing psychological tests in terms of the BBRs it is important to realize that none of them has been constructed to be pure measures of one, or parts of one, of the basic behavioral repertoires. Some tests—like intelligence and interest tests—do focus on aspects of one BBR, however. Others are much more mixed. For example, the *Minnesota Multiphasic Personality Inventory* (Dahlstrom & Welsh, 1960) includes items like the following: "I enjoy many different kinds of play and recreation," "I enjoy detective stories," "I like school," "I feel uneasy out of doors." These items measure positive and negative emotional responses to different stimuli and, hence, are measuring aspects of the emotional-motivational repertoire. An item like "I love to go to dances" would measure an aspect of the emotional-motivational repertoire and, probably, also measure indirectly the sensory-motor skills of dancing and social skills as well. Items like "I have several times given up doing a thing because I thought too little of my ability," on the other hand, measures the individual's emotional response to his own skills—which relates to the self-concept, a part of the language-cognitive and emotional-motivational repertoires—as well as the individual's past observations of his behavior of giving up on tasks. The same is true of an item such as "I am an important person" (see Dahlstrom & Welsh, 1960, pp. 57–78). The point is that some tests contain a mixture of items that measure aspects of the three basic behavioral repertoires. And some tests contain items that involve complex combinations of the BBRs. In both cases, however, making a PB analysis of test items is central.

NEUROPSYCHOLOGICAL TESTING

One other type of psychological test will be mentioned, because this type illustrates PB's biological/behavioral unification. That is, there are various instruments that have been developed for the detection of neurological damage. For example, the Wechsler Adult Intelligence Scale (WAIS-R) (Wechsler, 1967) was early proposed as an instrument for use in diagnosing brain damage (Wechsler, 1958). Some "performance" subtests—for example, immediate memory for a sequence of numbers, and constructing a specified block design—were said to suffer more from brain damage than other "verbal" subtests—such as general information and vocabulary measures (see also Groth-Marnat, 1990, p. 144). The Bender Visual Motor Gestalt Test (Bender, 1938) has also been employed for neuropsychological damage diagnosis. The Bender Gestalt Test has subjects copy designs and measures errors such as rotation of the figure, lack of completion, and misjudgment of space for drawing (Groth-Marnat, 1990, p. 144).

More recently, specialized psychological tests have been designed for use in the diagnosis of neurological damage. One of them is Reitan's adaptation of a battery of tests that were developed by Halstead (Reitan & Wolfson, 1985). The battery includes sensory-motor tests, like depressing a key as rapidly as possible for ten-second periods, and fitting different shaped blocks into appropriate holes while blindfolded. The battery also includes tests of a number of language abilities like naming objects (including body parts), naming numbers and letters, reading, writing, following directions, and so on. The Luria-Nebraska Neuropsychological Battery (Golden, Purisch, & Hammeke, 1985) has 11 sections, including measuring basic and complex motor skills, rhythm and pitch abilities, tactile and kinesthetic skills, verbal and spatial skills, receptive and expressive language, writing, reading, arithmetic, and memory. Differential abilities on the various types of items on these tests have been found to be correlated with different types of brain damage. In some sensory-motor tests both hands will be compared in terms of skill and, if the difference is greater than usual, that can indicate damage to one side of the brain.

These tests include the same types of items as those that are used on other tests, both of language-cognitive and sensory-motor nature. But additional information is provided by the manner of construction of the tests. For one thing, the different kinds of items are grouped. Then differences in the relative scores of the groups of items can be correlated with knowledge of the actual neurological damage the subjects have suffered. The performance of brain-damaged individuals can be compared with those not so damaged.

In any event, these tests incorporate very well into the PB conception of the organic-behavioral interaction. That is, brain damage at O_2 in Figure 5.2 can, in essence, delete BBRs that have already been learned. Depending on the brain damage, different BBRs will be lost. Since some of the general types of BBRs are "stored" in particular parts of the brain, when those BBRs are absent this indicates that those parts of the brain have been damaged. The fact is, however, that the value of such tests for indicating location of damage is not very accurate, suggesting that there are not precisely fixed places for BBRs to be located.

The suggestion is it would be very productive to apply the PB conception to research on neuropsychological tests. Localization could be studied in the context of analyzing the BBRs involved. There are various interests to be explored through use of the analysis of the BBRs. And it is suggested that analysis of the composition of the various types of items (and subtests) in terms of the BBRs measured would provide a more detailed conception for the construction of neuropsychological tests.

TOTAL SCORES VERSUS INDIVIDUAL ITEMS: A DIFFERENCE IN CONCEPTION

In the traditional approach the test constructor's interest is in measuring some trait of personality that seems to affect a dimension of observable behavior. The items that are used to make the measurement are not of interest in and of themselves, but only as they help index the trait. Items, thus, are not analyzed for what they are. They are analyzed only as they can contribute to the overall instrument that can measure the trait. The measure of the trait is a *total* of the various items.

In contrast, the PB position is that, by virtue of the way tests are constructed, that is, to predict behavior, items are selected that are parts of BBRs that *determine* how the individual behaves. For example, the intelligence test item measures a part of a BBR that determines how the child will behave in school, and thereby the extent of the child's success. The important point is that the *PB perspective makes important the individual items of psychological tests.* The items provide information on the state of the individual's BBRs. It is the items on the psychological test that provide knowledge of the individual's personality and, hence, how the individual should be treated in the event there are problems. This is a large conceptual change with various implications, as will be discussed.

CONCLUSION

The PB theory of psychological measurement is a framework theory. It lays out an approach based upon the multilevel theory of personality. It analyzes various psychological tests within the unified theory. In doing so it elaborates and provides content for this new type of theory of personality. The theory says that psychological tests measure aspects of the BBRs. The manner of constructing good tests guarantees that the elements of the BBRs that are measured are important, because validation studies show test performance predicts important life performance (behavior). The validation methodology, thus, is a very valuable development in a behavioral sense as well as a psychometric sense. But the reigning conception in the psychometric field leads to speculation concerning what biological-mental process or structure within individuals determines both the test performance and the life performance. That is a misleading part of the field, for it lessens interest in, and development of, the study of how learning determines personality.

If personality consists of BBRs, and if the BBRs that are measured by psychological tests are important, then a theory is needed that guides researchers to new directions of study that will deal with such things. PB sets forth such a theory of personality. The theory calls for theory and research to analyze and specify what tests measure in terms of the BBRs involved. When that analysis has been made, and the repertoires have been specified, the PB theory calls for research to study how those repertoires are learned. Furthermore, the theory calls for research that indicates how the BBRs that are measured on psychological tests affect the life performances that are the concern of validation studies. The PB theory of personality thus sets the directions for large programs of theoretical, methodological, and empirical research.

CHAPTER 7

The Theory of Abnormal
Personality and Behavior

In one of the early chapters it was said that the various levels of study are linked together such that each level is both basic and "applied." The advanced levels draw upon more basic levels. But these levels are also basic to yet more advanced levels. The PB theory of personality derives from preceding levels of study, on the one hand, but serves itself as a basic theory for application to other more advanced fields, such as personality measurement. In the present view, in constructing a theory of personality, it is as important to characterize its applications as its foundations. This chapter and the next will constitute applications of the PB theory of personality; in the present case to the construction of a theory of abnormal behavior.

THE FIRST PB THEORY OF ABNORMAL BEHAVIOR

As indicated already, PB presented the first behavioral theory of abnormal psychology (Staats, 1963a, chap. 11). Abnormal behavior, like normal behavior, was considered to be learned. It had been proposed by Eysenck (1960a) that the neuroses consisted of surplus conditioned reactions or deficient conditioned reactions. However, the concept was not employed in a theory that analyzed the behavior disorders. The PB theory developed a concept of the deficit or inappropriate dichotomy as a dimension of abnormality, but several basic dimensions of behavior were added in constructing the general theory. One dimension was that, although the behavior itself might not be abnormal, it will be considered as such if the stimulus control of the behavior is deficit or inappropriate. An example of deficit stimulus control occurs in date rape, when a women's pleas to stop have no effect. The sensory-motor behaviors of intercourse are not in themselves abnormal (although they may be if forceful behaviors are involved). Normal behavior will also be considered abnormal when inappropriate stimuli control the behavior, for example, when the sight of someone in pain controls approach behaviors, rather than eliciting behavior that decreases the stimulus.

Aside from how the behavior is controlled by stimuli, behavior can also be deficit or inappropriate in and of itself. For example, the individual may never have learned a reading repertoire—a deficit. Conversely, the individual may have learned a repertoire of inappropriately brutal physical aggression. Another category of abnormal behavior was said to involve a deficit or inappropriate reinforcement system. For the person with a deficit reinforcement system stimuli that should be reinforcing are not. In the second case, the individual may have learned inappropriate reinforcers. (The term *reinforcer system* was later changed to *emotional-motivational BBR*, as more appropriate to the theory.)

This early taxonomy and theory of abnormal behavior was set forth when the field of behavior therapy was just beginning (Staats, 1963a), and its concepts and principles affected the development of the field and were incorporated into it (see Bandura, 1968; Craighead, Craighead, Kazdin, & Mahoney, 1994; Silva, 1993). The PB account was intended as a framework theory for the field of abnormal psychology, with development planned in several directions. For one thing, the theory was expected to be empirically heuristic, to open new types of research. To illustrate, the theory called for the development of behavioral assessment instruments with which to measure deficits and inappropriacies in the several categories of abnormality (Silva, 1993). Moreover, the framework theory itself was considered to be a beginning, needing development along various dimensions. One dimension involves taking advantage of the advances in the various levels of study basic to the theory. For example, as PB's personality theory was developed, this provided the basis for advanced construction of the abnormal psychology level of theory.

THE BASIC PB THEORY OF ABNORMAL BEHAVIOR

At the time of its introduction, there were no other behavioral theories of abnormal behavior—in radical behaviorism or social learning theory or the nascent behavior therapy. The first PB theory of abnormal behavior was largely a theoretical projection—a derivation from more basic PB theory, PB research, the use of PB analysis in clinical and personal experience, along with the PB analysis of traditional literature and the few behavioral works of others.

The first PB theory focused on the analysis of behavioral symptoms in the disorders that were addressed. But the PB concept of the individual's reinforcer system actually introduced the first behaviorally defined personality concept. The concept stated that each individual learned a large and different set of stimuli that were positively reinforcing for her, as well as a large set of negative reinforcers. The theory also said that the individual's behavior was affected widely by the nature of her reinforcer system, producing individual differences in the control of behavior, as well as in learning new behaviors. Moreover, abnormal behavior was seen to arise because the individual's reinforcer system was deficit or inappropriate. Although this was a personality concept, its most general implication was not generally understood—namely that a behavioral approach to abnormal behavior needed a behavioral theory of personality.

Twelve years later the overarching PB theory had been advanced along various dimensions (see Staats, 1975). One was in the development of an explicit theory of personality. This theory set forth the language-cognitive, emotional-motivational, and sensory-motor BBRs as the constituents of personality (Staats, 1975), a trichotomy that is widely used today. And the theory was then employed as the foundation for constructing a framework theory of abnormal behavior. In summary form, this PB conception dealt with how behavior disorders result from deficits and inappropriacies in the language-cognitive, emotional-motivational, and sensory-motor BBRs. Table 7.1 is taken from that account (see Staats, 1975, p. 247).

Table 7.1 characterizes the conception, with its two dimensions composed of deficits and inappropriacies, on the one hand, and the three BBRs on the other. The symptoms of various behavior disorders are then shown to fall into the six cells created by the two dimensions. There are disorders, for example, that involve deficits in the emotional-motivational repertoire, as is the case with the flat emotionality in schizophrenic patients, and the autistic child's lack of affection for parents. Deficits in the language-cognitive BBR are characteristic of mentally retarded children, autistic children, schizophrenics, and criminals who display a high incidence of non-reading. Deficits in the sensory-motor repertoire are characteristic of certain schizophrenics, as well as retarded and autistic children.

With respect to inappropriate BBR developments, the anxiety disorders involve inappropriate emotional-motivational characteristics—for example, the person with a phobia has an inappropriately extreme negative emotional response to some type of stimulus. On the positive side, a paraphiliac has learned a strong sexual emotional response to an inappropriate sexual object, as in the case with pedophilia, sexual sadism, and masochism. The language-cognitive repertoire can also be inappropriate and result in symptoms of various behavior disorders, as is the case with paranoid delusions, pathological lying, an unrealistically negative self-concept, and such. An inappropriate sensory-motor repertoire is exhibited in cases of rape and

TABLE 7.1 The PB Conception of Behavior Disorders

	Symptoms	
	Deficit behavior	Inappropriate behavior
Basic Behavioral (Personality) Repertoires		
Emotional-Motivational Repertoire	Flat emotionality of schizophrenia Lack of motivation of neurasthenia Lack of achievement motivation of cultural deprivation Childhood autism deficits in affection for parents	Psychosomatic disorders Sadistic pleasures Phobias Sexual disturbances involving aberrant sex objects; fetishes Autistic children's preoccupation with self-stimulation
Language-Cognitive Repertoire	Mental retardation deficits Autism deficits Lack of verbal-motor control in psychopaths Cultural-deprivation deficits	Paranoid delusions Defense mechanisms Antisocial conceptual systems like racism Stuttering, gesticulation substitutes for language in nonspeaking children
Instrumental Repertoire	Lack of social skills Lack of approach behavior to the opposite sex Lack of work skills Enuretic lack of toilet skills Lack of recreational skills Lack of imitational and observational skills	Violent social behavior (rape, beatings) Aversive social behavior (arrogance, cruelty, overly demanding, selfishness) Bizarre actions of psychotics Self-stimulation, repetitive behavior, self-destructive behavior of autism

other types of assault, the bizarre motor behaviors of some psychotics, and the self-stimulation and repetitive behaviors of some autistic children.

This second-generation formulation of the PB theory of abnormal behavior was a considerable advancement but it was still a beginning framework theory. It presented the principles and concepts of the theory-construction endeavor, and gave examples, but it needed development. Even at that point, as with the first PB theory, the theory had some things traditional theories of abnormal behavior lack. For one thing, although the PB theory of abnormal behavior was only of chapter length it was part of and drew upon the multilevels of a much more elaborate theory. Advancement of the PB theory of abnormal behavior was to come from advancement of the overarching behaviorism. But there were advancements to be made within the abnormal behavior level itself. One was in elaborating and stipulating the PB theory of abnormal behavior. A step in this direction was made in constructing the PB model of abnormal behavior and its causes (see Staats, 1977, 1979) as shown in Figure 7.1.

In the model shown in Figure 7.1, the basic concept of deficit and inappropriate was developed in several directions. For one thing, the conception is that the individual's past environment, S_1, may be either deficit or inappropriate. That results in deficit or inappropriate learning of the language-cognitive, emotional-motivational, or sensory-motor BBRs. Since the BBRs help determine the individual's behavior, when the BBRs are deficit or inappropriate they will result in a deficit in necessary behavior or in the occurrence of inappropriate behavior, both of which are abnormal.

The model indicates, in addition, that the individual's current environment (life situation), S_2, also helps determine the behavior the individual displays. If the current environment is deficit, other things equal, the behavior the individual displays will be deficit and, hence, abnormal. If the current environment is inappropriate, other things being equal, the behavior the individual displays will be inappropriate and, hence, abnormal. Thus,

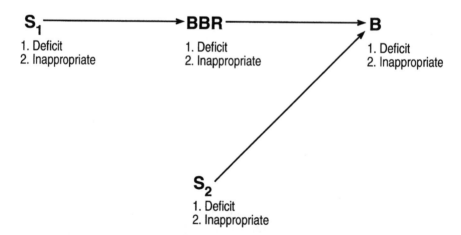

FIGURE 7.1 A model of the psychological behaviorism conception of abnormal psychology. Each site of causation of behavior (B) can be deficit or inappropriate, in which case the behavior will be deficit or inappropriate, and this defines abnormal behavior.

the various sites of causation of abnormal behavior are specified in the model, with various implications.

Thus, separating the distal and proximal environments made it possible to address the several roles of biological factors in abnormal behavior. The greater stipulation of the theory provided for greater stipulation in this area. As shown in Figure 7.1, giving the environment two separate roles makes explicit that biological conditions can play a role in three different ways in the causal chain. That is, biological conditions can be awry at the time the individual is learning the BBRs (as in cases of microcephaly or Down's syndrome), even though the learning environment is quite normal. In Figure 7.2 the biological conditions operative at this time are depicted as O_1. Such abnormal biological conditions can result in *learning* abnormal BBRs, either deficit or inappropriate.

In addition, however, after normal BBRs have been learned, abnormal biological conditions (like brain damage, or drugs) can destroy or distort those BBRs, resulting in deficit or inappropriate (abnormal) behavior. Such biological conditions are represented as O_2 in Figure 7.2. Moreover, abnormal biological conditions may distort or create deficits in the individual's ability to sense and respond to the current environment, S_2—even though the individual's BBRs are normal. For example, the individual may lose hearing in old age and the deficit in auditory stimuli may affect behavior. As another example, a man taking drugs for hypertension may be unable

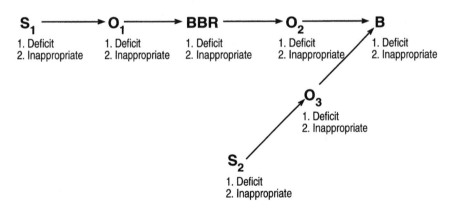

FIGURE 7.2 The PB model of abnormal behavior elaborated to include the places where organic conditions can act as a determinant. The biological organism can be deficit or inappropriate when the BBRs are being learned (O_1), or after they have been learned (O_2). Or the biological organism (O_3) can be deficit or inappropriate with respect to the individual's ability to sense and respond to the current life situation (S_2). Each of these biological abnormalities can produce abnormal behavior.

to obtain an erection in what would ordinarily be a sexual situation. Such biological conditions are represented as O_3 in Figure 7.2.

The conception recognizes that biological conditions can result in abnormal behavior. However, PB methodology requires empirical-theoretical specificity in biological as well as learning explanation. Biological factors in causation must be shown directly, not inferred or assumed. *Moreover, the conception requires that specification be made of how the biological condition affects the learning of the BBRs, the functioning of the BBRs, or the ability of the individual to respond to the current situation.* It is not enough to find that a higher percentage than usual of people with some behavior disorder display an overdeveloped or underdeveloped part of their brain, or show greater activity in a part of their brain. *The unusual part or activity of the brain may result from the individual's behavior, rather than cause it.* Such a biological finding, thus, is only the beginning. For it is necessary to indicate how that anatomy has affected the learning of the BBRs, the BBRs after they have been learned, or the ability of the individual to respond to current situations. Until the biological phenomenon has been extended by the necessary behavioral stipulations its meaning and value are unclear. PB states, thus, that research must be done to establish the manner in which environmental events, organic conditions, and behavioral variables interact in the determination of abnormal behavior. This has to be done specifically; generalities are not useful. This applies especially to studies that show the person with abnormal behavior has parents or siblings who have the same disorder. Such studies assume too much and are too "circumstantial," ignore behavior principles, and do not establish what, if any, biological conditions are involved.

The PB theory and model provide a framework for a broad, unified, explanatory theory of abnormal behavior. This is a framework in the sense that it calls for more specialized treatments of the various phenomena within its purview. In the theory of abnormal behavior (Staats, 1975, chap. 8) the analyses of various behavior disorders were beginning theories of those disorders, intended as heuristic calls for more detailed, complete, and profound theories of the different behavior disorders. That program, actually, had begun very early (see Staats, 1957a)—PB's analysis of the developmental disorders (especially reading) introduced this area of study to behavior analysis and behavior therapy—and the PB theory of reading disorder (see Staats, 1975, chap. 11; Staats & Butterfield, 1965; Staats, Finley, Minke, & Wolf, 1964) constituted one of the foundations of its general theory of abnormal behavior. The rest of this chapter will be focused on presenting several of PB's theories of behavior disorders, beginning with reading disorder, mental retardation, and childhood autism. The adult disorders treated will be limited to depression and the anxiety disorders. (A more complete treatment of the PB abnormal psychology has been drafted; see Staats, 1989, but needs to be completed.)

DEVELOPMENTAL DISORDERS

One of the early focuses of PB was on developmental disorders, especially problems in academic performance. The history of this program, and how it provided one of the foundations for the development of behavior therapy (behavior modification, behavioral assessment, and behavior analysis), will be described in the next chapter. Here I will be concerned only with the PB theories of developmental disorders, beginning with Learning Disorders, especially reading disorder.

Reading Disorder

In our culture dyslexia, or developmental reading disorder, is a devastating deficit. Its impact can be gauged by the fact that a large proportion of prison inhabitants cannot read.

DSM Description

The *Diagnostic and Statistical Manual of Mental Disorders,* called the *DSM-IV* (American Psychiatric Association, 1994), refers to reading disorder only when there is interference with academic achievement and daily living.

> The essential feature of Reading Disorder is reading achievement (i.e., reading accuracy, speed, or comprehension as measured by standardized tests) that falls substantially below that expected given the individual's chronological age, measured intelligence, and age-appropriate education . . . . If a sensory deficit is present, the reading difficulties are in excess of those usually associated with it. . . . In individuals with Reading Disorder (which has also been called "dyslexia") oral reading is characterized by distortions, substitutions, or omissions . . . . (American Psychiatric Association, 1994, p.43)

The *DSM-IV* goes on to describe how reading disorder tends to be associated with various other problems such as dropping out of school, difficulty with employment, Conduct Disorder, Oppositional Defiant Disorder, Attention Deficit/Hyperactivity Disorder, Major Depressive Disorder, and such. With respect to etiology, "There may be underlying abnormalities in cognitive processing (e.g., deficits in visual perception, linguistic processes, attention, or memory, or a combination of these) . . . [and] genetic predisposition, perinatal injury, and various neurological or other general medical conditions may be associated with the development of Learning Disorders . . . (American Psychiatric Association, 1994, p. 47). This coincides with the general belief that there are inherited brain deficiencies—other than those thought to cause mental retardation, sensory handicap, or specific neurological defect—that can cause specific learning disabilities such as reading disorder. This conception represents a vague theory, however, since it does not indicate the specific organic problem and how the child's learning to read is affected. The theory also does not include specification of what reading is, how reading is learned normally, and what is involved when learning to read has gone awry. What is it that the child with reading disorder cannot do that normal children can do? The fact that a theory of that vagueness can be so widely held indicates the low standards that operate.

Reading

When reading is analyzed in PB's behavioral terms—to indicate what repertoires are involved, how they are learned, and how they function in the act of reading—then there is a context for considering what reading disorder is and how it comes about. Essential in the psychological behavioral analysis is that reading is a specialized, advanced development of the individual's language repertoires. Let me exemplify the position by taking the verbal-labeling repertoire. In the ordinary acquisition of language the child has to learn to label many objects and events—that is, to make particular vocal responses to particular stimuli. In learning to read the child must learn to make those same vocal responses to printed or written word stimuli. The child must learn a very large repertoire of speech responses to visual verbal stimuli. The same is true with other repertoires. The child learns motor, image, and emotional responses to different spoken words. To be an expert reader the same words in visual form must elicit those same responses.

Reading Disorder Is Not Biologically Caused

Even this abbreviated behavioral analysis of reading provides the basis for stating that dyslexia does not have a biological cause. First, a diagnosis of dyslexia is only made when the child's intelligence measure is normal (or above that of the reading level). But in PB terms normal intelligence indicates that the dyslexic child has normal language. And the PB theory of language shows that no different ability is demanded in reading than that which is demanded in spoken language. When we examine language and reading we see that the visual stimuli that elicit verbal-labeling responses in natural language are no different in kind than the visually presented words that elicit reading responses. Whether an *ant* itself elicits the word "ant," or whether the printed word *ant* elicits the response, does not involve any different biological structures. Two small visual stimuli are involved. The same is true for the verbal-image, verbal-motor, verbal-emotional, and other repertoires—no different biological structures are required whether the stimulus is an object or an auditory word, as in spoken language, or a printed word, as in reading. There is no biological reason why children with normal language do not learn to read. As will be indicated, children with reading disorder have been successfully treated with PB's training methods, which have been widely used in behavior therapy (Walker, Greenwood, & Terry, 1994). What is clear is that the accepted explanation of non-reading in terms of biological (learning ability) deficit is as errant as it is vague.

Reading Learning

Why is it then that children of normal intelligence do not learn how to read? One of the things that leads to the belief that dyslexia involves some *specific* brain dysfunction is that children who learn to read always have language, but not all children with language learn to read. If the same brain development produces reading as produces language, then children who acquire language should acquire reading skill. So a different "ability" is assumed to be involved for reading. The problem with such reasoning is that it looks for explanation in the inner (biological) characteristics of the child rather than in what the different "abilities" consist of and in how those abilities are learned.

To realize why children can display normal language but no reading, based solely on learning, it is necessary to have an analysis of what the two repertoires consist of and how they are learned. And to generally answer questions regarding reading disorder it is necessary to understand what normal language and reading are and how they are learned and function for the individual. The PB theory of language has already been presented. The language BBRs are acquired in a cumulative-hierarchical learning process. As a consequence, different classes of spoken words come to elicit different types of responses in the child, and the child learns also to produce spoken words herself. These repertoires undergo a progressive elaboration, and thereby become very complex.

Reading involves, essentially, learning the same repertoires that are made to life objects (and spoken words) to printed (and written) words. On a simple level we can see how this learning can take place. Let us say the child already has the verbal-labeling response "cat" under the control of a cat as the stimulus. We could print the word on a card and show it to the child and say this is the word for cat, and ask the child to say the word while looking at the cat. If we did this a few times (with reinforcement) the child would come to be able to read the printed word. (Also, the image elicited by the spoken word would be conditioned to the written word.)

While this type of learning is involved in learning to read, the complexity of what must be learned is great (see Staats, 1975, chap. 11), much more than the above training multiplied by the number of words. For one thing, the example has involved having an adult tell the child the name of the word that is to be read. But there are too many words to be learned to have an adult present to give the name in each case. What must be done, therefore, is to teach the child a system by which the child can teach herself. This involves teaching the child to say the names of letters and syllables, as well as the skills of sounding-out the letters and syllables when new, unknown words occurs. (This is called phonics learning.) The child this way can supply herself with the new names of words so they can be learned. Through innumerable learning trials of this kind, in the expert reader a very large number of printed words must come to elicit spoken words, as well as the image responses, motor responses, and emotional responses the spoken words elicit. Various repertoires must be learned in becoming an expert reader and this requires an exceedingly large number of learning trials (see Staats, 1975, chap. 11, for a more complete theory of reading).

Learning Language Compared to Learning Reading

With this brief analysis in hand it is possible to answer some of the questions concerning reading disorder. First, it is possible to understand why it is that some children with normal IQs (language) nevertheless do not learn to read. Centrally, although reading learning depends upon language, learning language and learning reading have some essentially different characteristics.

For one thing, reading learning is based on already having language, not the reverse. The fact that the first learning has taken place normally does not guarantee the second will also. For example, language training is based on sporadic learning trials. Reading training is done formally in set periods, which means massed learning trials. Massed trials are effortful—work—demanding attention and active participation. The spaced learning of words in the home requires no such effort. Moreover, and this is important, typically there is a reinforcing event involved. When the parent says "Cookie?" and the child answers "Coog," and is given a cookie, there is immediate, personally delivered, and effective reinforcement.

Those elements—spaced training trials, little effort, quick and effective reinforcement—are very good, and they pertain during the learning of the basic language repertoire. Centrally also, from the beginning the child learns language responses that have immediate utility, that is, will enable the child to gain reinforcers more generally in social interaction. For example, as soon as the child learns to name the parents and other objects and actions, the child can call for those things—much more effectively than using only an undifferentiated cry. And, importantly, there is no "failure." Using the above example, if the child does not respond when the parent says "Cookie?" life simply goes on; there is no admonition, no exhortation, no implication of stupidity.

None of those advantageous conditions are involved in learning to read. The training is not gradual for many children, but begins abruptly in school. There are formal teaching periods during which the child is called upon to attend and to scrutinize and compare stimuli, and to make designated responses. Especially for the unprepared child this is effortful, as can be seen in teaching a young child to read the letters of the alphabet (see

Staats, Finley, Minke, & Wolf, 1964). Without some form of reinforcement a child of four will remain voluntarily in such training for ten or so minutes (Staats, Staats, Schutz, & Wolf, 1962). Without reinforcement the young child will begin fooling around and not attending. Even if there is reinforcement, but it is not rich enough, attention and participation will deteriorate (Staats, Finley, Osborne, Quinn, & Minke, 1964).

When the child's attention wanders, and the child begins doing other things, the child is no longer participating in the learning task. That the child is in the classroom means nothing; without participation there are no learning trials. When that happens early, and continues, the child will become dyslexic. What is it that ensures that many children do attend, do participate, and do learn, making normal progress toward acquiring the complex and difficult reading repertoire? Let me suggest that, in general, this depends upon two types of condition: (1) that the child is already so well prepared for the task, by having necessary basic repertoires, that the task is sufficiently easy and the indications of learning provide reward; and (2) that the child has learned work habits such that she remains in the task for adequate periods even without strong forms of reinforcement. This can be elaborated.

Why Do Only Some Children Learn to Read?: Etiology

The Learning Prepared Child. Why are there individual differences in learning to read, from not at all to spectacularly well? For one thing, many parents provide training in the home that yields some of the preliminary, basic skills that are foundations for the beginning part of reading instruction. The child is introduced to coloring books and learns to hold a crayon and colored pencils. The child is read to, and individual words and letters are indicated. The child is also trained in easy, but somewhat formal, circumstances to read the letters of the alphabet and to write some of them.

What does the child acquire through this experience? Whether or not the child knows the letters of the alphabet has been considered the best predictor of whether or not the child will succeed in learning to read (Bond & Dykstra, 1967; Chall, 1967). Why is that? For one thing, the child who has learned to read the letters of the alphabet has learned that important repertoire. But the child in so doing has learned much more. The child has learned to scrutinize small line drawings (the letters), to make vocal responses to those stimuli, to compare the letters, to distinguish them by their differences, to follow instructions, and to engage in a task demanding these things. There are thus perceptual skills involved. In addition, the various skills help compose another repertoire that has general import, that of "work habits." Staats, Brewer, and Gross (1970) showed that children exposed to the task of learning the letters become better and better workers, making more and more responses within a given amount of time.

PB research has also shown that, as children are presented with such training, they progressively become better (quicker) learners. Some children in the home learn the basic repertoires involved, and for them the task of learning to read in school does not require unusual effort.

The Unprepared Child. Some children, whose parents have not tried to teach the children much, will not have learned the repertoires. Thus, they will not respond well when they begin school and, as a result, they will not learn well. Some children will enter school with an even greater handicap. That is, in some cases the parent is not a good trainer. Then the parent may notice the child is not advancing as rapidly as other children, and attempt to more formally train the child to some skill. This is likely to go poorly, since the child has not been prepared properly, and the parent is not a good trainer. As a consequence, the child will then not do well in the learning task and will want to withdraw. Then the parent is likely to attempt to force the child to participate, and the child will learn an inappropriate learning repertoire. That is, the child will learn behaviors to escape the learning situation, and will learn a negative emotional response to learning situations. As a consequence, the child will come to avoid learning situations and, if caught in them, will not attend and not participate as instructed. This child generally will now learn poorly whenever there is formal instruction. Thus, at the time children enter school some will have a good learning repertoire, some will have none, and some will have a negative learning repertoire. The learning ability of the three groups, other things being equal, will vary as a function of the type of learning repertoire the children have.

The School as a Learning Situation for the Developing Dyslexic

The child's own learning repertoire is so central because of the nature of the school training situation. The effortfulness of the formal training situation is one drawback. Another thing is that the sources of reinforcement are not good. Children are taught in groups, so response-contingent reinforcement is not possible, and it is also impossible to monitor the child's attention and participation. Whatever reinforcement is administered comes later, by the teacher or the parent, so it does not strengthen the central behavior of attending and participating. Moreover, there is no intrinsic utility of the reading responses the child learns at the early stages. For example, learning to name the letters of the alphabet is a very large and effortful task, but the responses themselves have no utility—unlike the case with learning language—other than in displaying them to the teacher or the parent. Thus, the traditional expectation that "Learning is its own reward," does not apply for many children.

In beginning school this adds up to effortful learning behavior for long periods when, for many children, there are poor sources of reinforcement, insufficient for maintaining moment-to-moment attention and participation. Under such circumstances, some children do not attend and participate at the very beginning of reading training. When the child falls behind another set of learning circumstances occurs in school. That is, *not learning* does not just produce a deficit. For, in school, how the child learns is the measure of success—both for pupil and for teacher. *Not learning* is failure. Blaming the pupil's "learning ability" relieves the teacher, and the parent. The child is aware of such things. Even a child of six has already learned that doing well at anything constitutes a positive emotional stimulus, and doing badly is a negative emotional stimulus. The negative emotional response elicited by doing badly will be conditioned to the learning situation of the school. The learning situation, as it comes to elicit a negative emotional response in the child, will be avoided. There are various types of avoidance behaviors. When I was a clinical student at UCLA I worked with a child whose avoidance response was to disrupt our learning trials by conversational gambits of various kinds. Avoidance behavior can take the form of classroom disruptions, daydreaming, or truancy. In schools where failure to learn is rather general, the avoidance behavior may also involve setting up a student atmosphere that derogates scholastic achievement and esteems rebelliousness, physical prowess, and social domination through that prowess.

Ordinarily, the child who fails in learning to read will become very "sensitive" because of the negative emotional conditioning. Such a child, as soon as she or he does not do well on some item, will have a negative emotional response that will elicit the child's characteristic avoidance behaviors. In one of my reading studies, for example, there was a volunteer trainer (a former teacher) who did not rely on the token reinforcer system. She exhorted the child to do better, but that was an indication of failure. The child's negative emotional response was reflected in the child's behavior. Attending and participating—which had been maintained very well by token reinforcement—deteriorated, and acting-out behaviors began to appear. The child who has failed in classroom learning will learn inappropriate emotional responses to learning situations, and will be a more difficult learning problem than a child who is yet to begin the learning task. This is a central aspect of dyslexia.

Three PB Concepts Important for the Developmental Disorders

The Learning Repertoire.   At this point it is relevant to introduce three of PB's primary concepts in its theory of learning disorder. In addition to BBRs that constitute recognized abilities (like the language repertoire), the child can learn BBRs that constitute a "pro-learning repertoire." This repertoire consists of such things as attending when an instructional situation arises, following instructions, looking at the stimuli as requested, and making the responses requested. The pro-learning repertoire also includes a "work tolerance," which is being able to continue at a task that demands effortful behavior. And it includes having learned a positive emotional response to learning situations, such that such situations are approached, not avoided. A child with a well-developed pro-learning repertoire, other things being equal, will generally learn better in school than a child whose repertoire is weak.

In considering learning disorders there is a counterpart to the pro-learning repertoire that is equally important. The concept is that of the "anti-learning repertoire." For children can learn a basic behavioral repertoire that interferes with their learning in instructional situations. Elements of that repertoire have just been described. A central element is the negative emotional response to learning situations, for it produces the avoidance responses the child has learned. The avoidance responses are part of the "anti-learning repertoire," for they interfere with learning, or take the individual out of the learning situation. Like the pro-learning repertoire, the anti-learning repertoire is a BBR, for it helps determine how the individual experiences learning situations, how the individual behaves in those situations, and how the individual learns (see Staats, 1971a).

It is important here, however, to add the principle that connects the pro-learning and anti-learning BBRs. They are in a competitive relationship. When the individual has a strong anti-learning repertoire it will prevent experiences from occurring that would produce a pro-learning repertoire in the individual. And the converse is also true.

Learning Ability and the Learning Repertoire.   A general conception in our culture is that there are individual differences in learning ability. This conception is that some people, by virtue of the quality of their nervous systems, have exceptional learning ability, either in the positive or negative direction. The PB conception is that learning ability is composed of the individual's learning repertoire, either pro- or anti-, as well as the other BBRs that are necessary as a foundation in the specific learning task.

Perceptual Development and the Perceptual Repertoire.   Dyslexic children do poorly on tests of visual perception. This is generally taken to prove such children have a biologically determined perceptual deficit. However, tests of visual perception do not measure a biological condition. They measure the perceptual skills the child has learned—and the skills are learned *in the process of learning to read.* Collette-Harris and Minke (1978), using PB's training materials, showed that dyslexic children given training in reading improved on their perceptual test scores. PB research with preschool children has shown that all children start with poor perceptual skills—they write letters sideways, upside down, of unequal size, backwards, and such.

What improved such skills were additional learning trials in writing letters (Staats, Brewer, & Gross, 1970). Dyslexic children miss the usual learning trials, and thus have poor reading skills as well as poor perceptual skills.

Learning ability, perceptual development, readiness, and other concepts that are inferred to be inner processes of a biological nature are seen in PB to consist of learned repertoires.

Additional Points in the Theory of Reading Disorder and Other Academic Skills Disorders

In the PB view, analyses of what reading consists of, the repertoires on which the learning of reading is based, and the conditions that can go awry in the learning process, produce a true theory of reading disorder. The theory indicates the causes that need to be manipulated to prevent the problem. And the theory indicates how to treat reading disorder (see also Leduc, 1984, 1988a, 1988b; Ryback & Staats, 1970; Staats, Minke, & Butts, 1970; Staats, Minke, Goodwin, & Landeen, 1967). The Sylvan Learning Centers today employ methods that, in some essential features, are like those developed in the PB program of research, with similar results.

Attempts to show that reading disorder is inherited by showing that it runs in families, that more boys have the disorder than girls, and the like, do not constitute the same type of data. It is circumstantial, based on inference. It does not yield a theory that stipulates just what the disorder consists of, and that isolates the causes of the disorder. It does not indicate variables that can be manipulated to prevent the development of the disorder or to treat the disorder after it has arisen. The biological theory of learning disabilities has not even shown that particular brain injuries will subtract specific academic skills, like reading and mathematics, while leaving normal language intact. PB has taken the position (see Staats, 1975, chap. 11) that if a child has learned a normal language that child is completely fit neurologically to learn to read. The fact that dyslexic children can be trained to read indicates additionally that there is nothing neurologically wrong with the children in the first place. Now even those in neurobiology are beginning to recognize the logic of this position, as can be seen in the following conclusion, made after finding that children can be successfully treated, through learning, for a particular language deficit. "[T]here may be no fundamental defect in the learning machinery in most of these children, because they so rapidly learn the same skills at which they have been defined to be deficient (Merzenich, Jenkins, Johnston, Schreiner, Mill, & Tallal, 1996, p. 80). For 40 years PB has been developing a learning approach in contrast to the traditional "biological" explanation, and now neurobiology is generally developing a supportive position (see Begley, 1996).

Like reading, writing and arithmetic are BBRs learned in a cumulative-hierarchical manner on the basis of the language-cognitive BBR. Deficits in writing and arithmetic are considered learning disorders (see American Psychiatric Association, 1987, pp. 41–43) in children with normal intelligence. PB research has analyzed what basic writing and arithmetic skills consist of and how they are learned (see Staats, 1963a, 1968a; Staats, Brewer, & Gross, 1970; Staats & Burns, 1981). Writing and arithmetic also are additional learned elaborations of the language-cognitive BBR. Such disorders do not reflect disturbances of learning caused by an underlying biologically based condition. For the children's normal intelligence (language) guarantees they have all the abilities that are needed for successful learning.

Traditionally it is thought that skill in mathematics depends on individual differences in a special ability, located in the brain. The psychological behavioral analysis rejects that speculation (see Staats, 1963a, pp. 219–236). No new abilities are necessary for arithmetic-mathematic learning, save a great deal of learning experience. And there are great individual differences in learning opportunity, for the types of reasons that have been described, as well as others. The sex difference that is found in the development of mathematics in the PB view is to be explained by learning factors, not biological differences.

Mental Retardation

Mental retardation is one of the major classifications in the developmental disorders. As the *DSM-IV* description indicates, it is a more severe disorder than those that have been described.

DSM-IV Description

> The essential features of Mental Retardation is significantly subaverage general intellectual functioning . . . that is accompanied by significant limitations in adaptive functioning in at least two of the following skill areas: communication, self-care, home living, social/interpersonal skills, use of community resources, self-direction, functional academic skills, work, leisure, health, and safety . . . . (American Psychiatric Association, 1994, p. 39)

Another criterion is that the onset must occur before age 18.

The PB Theory of Mental Retardation

Various biological problems—O_1, in Figure 7.2—result in mental retardation. The *DSM-IV* lists children with Down's syndrome, Tay-Sachs disease, and other gene and chromosomal abnormalities that are inherited that cause mental retardation. These are said to account for 5% of the cases. Early embryonic changes are said to account for another 30%, and pregnancy and perinatal problems for 10%. Infections, trauma, and toxic conditions account for 5%. In addition to these biologically produced cases of mental retardation, environmental influences and mental disorders are said to account for 15%–20% (American Psychiatric Association, 1994, p. 43). But mental disorders are generally thought to involve some type of biological problem. So the proportion of cases of mental retardation that are due to environmental-learning problems is thought to be quite small. "In approximately 30%–40% of the individuals seen in clinical settings, no clear etiology for the Mental Retardation can be determined despite extensive evaluation efforts" (American Psychiatric Association, 1994, p. 43).

There are several reasons to raise questions in this area. The first is that, while biological causation in mental retardation is very explicit in a certain percentage of cases, in other cases biological causation is only inferred. When a child is mentally retarded, if case histories reveal there have been problems in pregnancy and perinatal conditions, infections, trauma, and toxic conditions, these will be considered to have caused biological damage that is responsible. In such cases, however, this is an assumption, as it is when "extensive evaluation efforts" reveal no biological causation.

In the PB view the general interpretation that mental retardation is caused by biological defect is overdrawn. In addition to the very strong biological orientation in explaining human behavior in our culture, a counterbalancing learning explanation has been weak. There has not been an accepted learning theory of intelligence and of the lack of intelligence. For this reason it is typically difficult to see how cases of mental retardation could have arisen just from lack of learning opportunity, unless the environment is dramatically deficit. And the fact that there are identifiable biological defects that in many cases lead to mental retardation is, in contrast, impressive. For these reasons it is easy to assume that biological causation exists, even when there is no direct evidence to that effect. This is abetted by poor logic. For example, when a mentally retarded child comes from a home where the parents are of below average intelligence, it is assumed that the child has a poor genetic inheritance. On the other hand, when such a child comes from an advantaged home, especially if there are other normal children, this is assumed to be proof that there must be something wrong with the particular child. The *assumptions* that are made erroneously favor the accepted belief, the biological explanation.

In the PB view, any case of mental retardation for which there is not an identifiable biological cause *may* be due to biological cause or it *may* be due to environmentally caused learning problems. That may involve a majority of the cases of mental retardation. Moreover, a biological explanation of mental retardation is not complete until the biological defect has been identified, as well as how the defect interferes with the learning of the BBRs. For the psychological behaviorism approach states that *mental retardation consists of deficits in the intelligence BBRs that have been described, the language-cognitive*

BBRs and the sensory-motor BBRs, especially, and, to some extent, aspects of the emo-tional-motivational BBR. Having a theory of what intelligence is provides a basis for defining mental retardation. And this stipulation of intelligence must be interwoven with biological study to provide a full theory of mental retardation and its etiology.

The PB position is that the BBRs that constitute intelligence are learned. Biological defects can interfere with that learning. But deficits can occur in the learning conditions necessary for the acquisition of intelligence, and this will result in mental retardation. A theory of mental retardation must indicate the ways the learning process can go awry in childhood to yield retardation. Only with extensive study of this type will the necessary evidence be obtained. In terms of what is known about normal learning of intelligence and the ways that learning can go awry (see Staats, 1989) it can be seen that deficits can occur in many different scenarios. There are the dramatic cases of "feral" children (see Leduc, 1998a, 1988b), who have been raised in different conditions (sometimes with animals) that provide no or little exposure to language. There are the much more widespread cases of children raised in ghetto conditions by parents with little education with poorly developed language and other skills, exposed to a social group that is similarly lacking. There are cases where the parents' problems—criminality, drug and alcohol abuse, depression, and such—so seriously interfere with parenting that the child has a severely deficit environment. But, there are also cases where there is nothing clinically deficit in the parents, even where the parents' achievements are high, that nevertheless involve a cumulative-hierarchical learning process for the child that has gone awry and that results in mental retardation. How can deficits in learning conditions occur, in a way that produces devastating deficits, without being noticed? How do those deficits occur in homes that appear normal? What is not understood is that parents can be highly educated and very intelligent, good parents in terms of the care they give and the love they have for their child, and yet things may occur that very early set the cumulative-hierarchial learning process on a downward path. The parent, for example, may not provide good training conditions for the child's language learning.

The child who does not develop normal repertoires—like the language-cognitive repertoires—when other children do will soon be faced with abnormal experiences. One case with which I dealt involved a child who had no language at the age of four. The child's speech was delayed due to several circumstances including the fact that the parent herself was not vocal and did not speak much to the child. This was observable in the way she was treating another year-old infant she had who had no language and was very passive. With the older child, when the parent recognized the delay in speech development she began attempting to teach the child to speak by trying to get him to repeat nursery rhymes. However, repeating sequences of unknown words has no function—in this case it only produced a few poor echolalic elements. Trying to force the child to endure such training, moreover, is aversive. The most prominent result in this case was to teach the child that learning situations are unpleasant, and to avoid them with anti-learning behaviors.

It should be noted that there may be various types of "skills" in a child's anti-learning repertoire. The child may learn, for example, that passive "dumbness" in the face of learning tasks will be rewarded by the cessation of the effortful and bothersome learning situation. The parent after a number of such interactions simply becomes convinced that the child is unable to learn—is retarded—and abandons the effort. When this occurs sufficiently the parent no longer presents the needed training to the child. I was once asked to evaluate a child of three years of age who the parents (both trained professionals) thought was retarded. I did so primarily by observations in the home. The little boy was a middle child with a very aggressive brother a year younger and a sister several years older. The aggressive younger child had learned to bully the three-year-old—possibly originally because the younger was protected by the parents—and both siblings, in their striving for attention, pushed the "retarded" child away from interacting with the parents. If the "retarded" child did something to attract the attention of the parents, the other two, especially the younger brother, would be aversive to the "retarded" child. The "retarded" child had thus learned to be unresponsive, not to try for the parents' attention but, rather, to spend time alone. In this way he was involved in less rivalry and was picked on less. The other children displayed more skilled behavior, interest, and striving and thus appeared "brighter." The child's behavioral development, including language, was indeed behind the other two. The parents had seen a psychologist, described the behavior of the child, and had him tested, and their concerns had been confirmed. So the parents had come to the conclusion the three-year-old had some biological deficit and was retarded and they had begun treating the child as though he were.

I explained what was happening among the three children and the parents and the effect it was having on the child in question. I also showed the parents how the child could be interested and responsive—that is, intelligent—in play, when there was no competition from the other two children. I instructed the parents how they must provide for interaction with the child and positive learning experiences, where the child could not be pushed aside by siblings. This analysis and the very capable actions of the parents resulted in a complete turnaround in what otherwise was developing into a downward cycle of learning leading to retardation. The child is now in medical school! Had the downward cumulative-hierarchical learning process continued, the child would have been a retardate in a family of accomplished children and parents.

In general, the parent typically learns how to respond "appropriately" to the child who displays the repertoire of non-responsiveness in the face of a learning situation. There is much research that indicates that parents speak to their children differently depending upon the child's ability (see Rondal, 1985; Staats, 1971b). The parent of the child who demonstrates deficits is only a special case. This parent learns not to present learning tasks to the child that will produce awkward and unpleasant experiences for both the child and the parent. The parent does not want the child to experience failure. What that means, however, is that the child has been placed in a "special education class" at home, where the learning opportunities are much less rich than for other children, even for other children in the same home. Pretty soon the whole family, parents, siblings, and other relatives and friends, begin to treat the child as retarded. They are kind and forgiving and undemanding. So the child is happy, is reinforced for the behavior, and continues to develop the "dumb" anti-learning repertoire. That is the child's adjustment. But the result is that, for such a child, learning opportunities are inferior, and that is reflected in the child's "retarded" learning of the BBRs.

This can happen under very benign family circumstances, where everyone has the child's best interests at heart. Deficit learning conditions can also happen in less benign family circumstances, of course, even though the home, on casual examination, appears to be normal. What these examples are intended to indicate is that the human environment is very complex, with an infinite number of variations, and many opportunities for cumulative-hierarchical learning to predominate in developing the anti-learning repertoire that can be central in mental retardation.

Implications of the PB Theory of Mental Retardation

The PB theory of mental retardation may be stated very simply. Mental retardation consists of the absence of the BBRs that are measured on intelligence tests, as well as the absence of the types of repertoires that are measured on tests of adaptive functioning, both of which were analyzed in the preceding chapter. It should be remembered that the intelligence test measures BBRs that are essential to later learning, so the child who is low in intelligence will have difficulty learning "adaptive functioning repertoires." These deficits can occur because of limitations on learning imposed by biological conditions. We need to know much more about these conditions and, especially, how these conditions translate into deviations in the child's learning. At present we do not have a good handle on what takes place biologically during learning. We need to know that. And we need to know how the anatomy of the brain affects complex learning. For example, the brain of a Down's syndrome child is simpler, less convoluted than the brain of a normal child. How does that abnormal condition affect learning? Is it primarily to limit the number of stimulus–response elements the child can learn, and thus the richness of learning possible, and even the rapidity of learning when it depends upon the richness of past learning? Does the condition mean that the child is capable of learning the various human characteristics (BBRs), but more slowly and more sparsely? Or, does the biological conditioning affect specific types of learning? Just what are the learning effects of the condition? That is the knowledge that is needed. This type of knowledge, of course, is fundamental when it comes to treatment of the types of deficits we label as mental retardation. Such knowledge, for example, might tell us that we have to provide the same type of learning opportunities for the child, but introduced more gradually, dealing with less complex material. Or, there may be other directives that will result when our knowledge is more complete. Or, it may be that children with Down's syndrome, as one example, vary greatly in brain structure as well as learning possibilities. In that case it would be necessary to establish *behaviorally* just what it is the child can do, for example, by providing excellent and rich learning conditions in order to see what type of progress the child can make.

In any event, it must be emphasized that the deficits in the BBRs can also arise solely from complex learning circumstances involving deficits in learning conditions. Such deficits will produce deficits in the child's learning ability of two types. First, the child will not learn BBRs that are basic to learning more advanced repertoires. A child, for example, who has no or poor language BBRs will not have the wherewithal to learn to read. Second, deficit or inappropriate learning conditions can result in deficits in the pro-learning repertoire, or in acquiring the anti-learning repertoire, both of which will handicap the child in all learning tasks.

Since the deficits in the BBRs that compose mental retardation may result from a biological condition or from poor learning conditions, it is not possible to infer from the deficit behavior and poor learning ability themselves just what the cause is. That realization is fundamental, and it has fundamental implications for working with children who have deficits.

Childhood Autism

The *DSM-IV* presents a classification of Pervasive Developmental Disorders, which includes Autistic Disorder.

DSM-IV Description and the BBRs

The *DSM-IV* criteria of autistic disorder involve disturbances in social interaction, intellective functioning, and in activities and interests. In the first category the child shows lack of awareness of others' feelings, no pleasure in the comfort of others, no or impaired imitation, no or abnormal social play, and gross impairment in making friends. In the second category, the child does not communicate verbally or non-verbally, does not display imaginative ability, such as in taking roles or appreciating stories, speech is absent or disturbed, and even if there is speech, conversation is not sustained. In the third category the child has stereotyped body movements, is preoccupied with parts of objects, is upset by trivial environmental changes, and has a narrow range of interests and preoccupation with only one (American Psychiatric Association, 1994, pp. 70–71). These are descriptions of devastating deficit and inappropriate characteristics.

The PB Etiology Position

The *DSM III-R* suggests that a wide range of pre-, peri-, and post-natal conditions can cause "brain dysfunction and are thought to predispose to the development of Pervasive Developmental Disorders [that is, autistic disorder]" (American Psychiatric Association, 1987, p. 37). The *DSM III-R* also says there is no support for the view that autistic disorder can be caused by "parental personality and child-rearing practices" (p. 37). The *DSM-IV* does not include these statements. This change is interesting; the radical behaviorism approach to autism essentially took the position that autism had a biological etiology (Lovaas, 1966) and has not set forth a theory that autism is learned. Nevertheless, Lovaas (see 1977) went on to apply to the treatment of autistic children some of the same types of language training procedures developed in PB (see Staats, 1963a, 1968a, 1971a), showing the positive impact of training on the autistic child.

The PB view has always been quite the opposite of the biological position. The PB view recognizes that it is possible that biological conditions could limit the child's ability to profit from environmental experiences and thereby produce deficits in the BBRs. Whether or not that is the case, however, must be shown directly, not accepted on the basis of assumption, or on the basis of the type of "circumstantial" evidence that has been employed in twin studies of intelligence. *The PB theory is that, whatever behavior the autistic child displays, it is learned.* If there are biological conditions that impede or distort learning then just what is involved must be shown. The fact is there is no hard evidence of the biological causes of autism. And, the symptomatology of autism could be produced very straightforwardly by learning conditions inadvertently introduced by parents in homes that are otherwise quite normal.

The PB Theory of Autism

In the PB view the definition of autism in the *DSM-IV* is considered to consist of descriptions of the typical behaviors displayed by such children, organized into commonsense categories. Thus, lack of communication skills, imaginal skills, speech, conversation skills, friends, playing, and so on, all involve deficits in the child's language-cognitive BBR. All of these activities, even social activities, demand the child have acquired the various aspects of language. The child cannot have play interactions with other children, for example, without being able to respond to speech and to produce speech in return. So the autistic child, without language, will have deficits in the learning that comes from peer interaction. This is also true of acquiring interests in different activities. Without language, the child can only use (be interested in) objects on the basis of their primary characteristics. A toy car, for example, in terms of its basic properties is only an object—to mouth, to throw, or to pound. However, if the child can respond to such directions as "Let's play racing cars and see which one rolls down this board faster," then the car can be used, additionally, in a manner that is social and playful. If the child has the words for cars and what they do and what they are used for then the toy car can be used in an "imaginal" way. These types of activities are beyond the autistic child who has not learned normal language repertoires.

Other descriptions of the autistic child involve deficits in the development of the emotional-motivational BBR. Thus, the lack of emotional response to comforting and affection—so different from the usual child—is a frequent characteristic of autism, supposedly due to the child's biological abnormality. The PB view is that such symptoms simply indicate the child's learning circumstances have not produced a positive emotional response to being comforted and receiving affection. The fact that the child atypically does not make eye contact with the parent, does not approach the parent affectionately and seek the parent, calls for analysis in terms of the child's learning. The same also applies to the sensory-motor BBR. The autistic child typically has not developed repertoires in this area as well. Playing with toys and with other children demands sensory-motor skills. A child deficit in those skills will not engage in those activities. The autistic child typically will also have learned inappropriate sensory-motor repertoires such as repetitive movements, head-banging, and other forms of self-damage. Studies have shown that, when appropriate conditions are imposed, such behaviors can be removed by extinction (non-reinforcement) (see Wolf, Risely, & Mees, 1964).

"The most severely incapacitated are those who have widespread deficits in those basic behavioral repertoires ordinarily acquired early in life. . . . The autistic child . . . also . . . has learned bizarre and maladjustive repertoires of behavior that further prevent him from learning the necessary repertorial skills" (Staats, 1971a, p. 314). What is being said is that all of the symptoms by which autism is described involve either deficits in behavior or inappropriate behaviors. And, in each case, only the conditions of learning for the child may be the cause, without any biological causation. The

PB analysis of autism has been presented in various places, in the context of describing both normal and abnormal basic behavioral repertoires. Important in the etiology of autism is the cumulative-hierarchical process. For example, deficit learning conditions produce repertoire deficits that then produce social treatment that is deficit and inappropriate, in an interactional way. Because the child has deficits the parents try to press the child to learn and that results in the child acquiring negative emotional conditioning (anxiety) to learning situations and to the parent. This then provides the basis for further undesirable learning.

> With younger children the behaviors that are learned because they remove the child from anxiety-producing learning situations can vary widely. The child may "escape" the learning situation by insisting to the parent that he be allowed to perform the task himself, . . . even before the parent has finished the instructions. He may run to another activity, or begin another activity. The child may refuse to look at the relevant stimuli, or he may make other irrelevant responses.

> The types of behaviors the child will learn will depend upon which of them are successful in getting him out of the situation. These can range from the mild behaviors just described to those that are bizarre enough to be considered "crazy." The author recently encountered a case where the child would become visibly upset whenever the situation took on the appearance of formal training. He would then become hyperactive and move about with increasing rapidity and frenzy as the parent attempted more strongly to bring him into the learning situation. He would not respond to verbal stimuli. He would not attend. This would continue until the attempted learning situation was abandoned. He thus had been learning hyperactive frenzies because through this behavior he avoided the learning situations in which he ordinarily received punishment [the parent's impatience and disappointment], not reward. . . . [We will then] see a child who so successfully avoids situations that he suffers grievous deficits in the acquisition of his basic behavioral repertoires. These deficits will make learning even more trying for the child . . . [yielding] further punishment in learning situations. . . . [A] vicious cycle can be developed that hinders normal learning and . . . produces abnormal learning. . . . When such cycles are continued over a period of years they will result in . . . children we term emotionally disturbed, autistic. . . . [This] may include (1) self-destructive responses such as knocking one's head against the wall, biting oneself, and so on, (2) hyperactivity, (3) crazy behaviors such as monotonous rocking, weird gestures and facial expressions, uttering crazy noises, and so on. (Staats, 1971a, pp. 244–245)

The parent–child interaction can come to elicit primarily negative emotional responses in both, and escape from the interaction can in each case be a reinforcer. The PB theory of autism, thus, is that the interaction of parent and child does not provide learning conditions by which the child acquires normal BBRs. Rather, the child begins to acquire undesirable repertoires. And the cumulative-hierarchical learning of the child progressively develops along both paths. Very central is the extensive development of the anti-learning repertoire, including undesirable behaviors of all kinds that protect the child from the learning situations that have made the child uncomfortable. Evidence in support of the PB conception of autism is provided by research showing that autistic children can be trained in the normal BBRs (see Lovaas, 1977; Wolf, Risely, & Mees, 1964) that PB has analyzed and dealt with (Staats, 1963a, 1968a, 1971a). In the PB analysis *if these repertoires can be taught to children after they have become autistic, which means they have the anti-learning repertoires that make learning more difficult, then these children could have learned those normal BBRs at the beginning.* This is the position other works are now beginning to support (Merzenich et al., 1996). This suggests there is nothing biologically wrong with the children with respect to their potential for normal learning. The same is true of the "idiot-savant" phenomenon, where an autistic child who has pervasive deficits nevertheless has some special skill in music, art, number operations, and such. This is generally taken to mean that such children have generally defective brains but with one "bright" spot. There is no evidence to back this up. In the PB view special skill in one area means the child has the wherewithal to have learned skills to the same level in other areas.

ADULT DISORDERS

Several PB theories of the childhood disorders have been summarized to characterize the PB abnormal psychology. The following sections will do the same for several adult disorders.

Depression

Depression is one of the most common behavior disorders, occurring more with women than men, and frequently accompanying old age. Depression constitutes a widespread problem.

DSM-IV Definition

DSM-IV description of Major Depressive Episode includes such symptoms as dysphoric mood (depression) and loss of interest and pleasure in all or almost all usual activities and pastimes. The disturbance is salient and persisting—occurring "for most of the day, nearly every day, for at least 2 consecutive weeks. . . . during which there is either depressed mood or the loss of interest or pleasure in nearly all activities"—and involve[s] at

least four additional symptoms from a list including "changes in appetite
or weight, sleep, and psychomotor activity, decreased energy, feelings of
worthlessness or guilt, difficulty thinking, concentrating, or making decisions, or recurrent thoughts of death or suicidal ideation, plans, or attempts"
(American Psychiatric Association, 1994, p. 320).

Behaviorizing-Psychologizing the Definition of Depression

Depression was the second behavior disorder to be elaborated into a full
theory in PB (see Staats & Heiby, 1985). In treating this theory I will suggest, first, that the dysphoric mood described in the definition constitutes
a negative emotional state in PB. The emotional state is experienced for
"most of the day, every day," indicating that much more than ephemeral
emotional responses are involved. The negative emotional state is a function of the individual's life situation and emotional-motivational BBR, as
shown in Figure 7.3.

Placing depression disorder in the PB framework theory in this manner
has various implications. It can be expected, for example, that the negative
emotional state will induce other negative behaviors of a language-cognitive as well as a sensory-motor type. In the language-cognitive category are
the recurrent thoughts of death and suicide. What is described as feelings
of worthlessness and guilt, and it might be added of inadequacy, wrongdo-
ing, and the like, really refer to thoughts of (language behavior with respect
to) such things. This is true also of worry, self-blame, self-pity, and negative
appraisal of the future. Such verbal-behavior negatively impacts on others.

Other symptoms of depression refer to the characteristics of the emotional state itself. Thus, depressed individuals typically experience little or
no pleasure in usual activities, for example, in eating, and in sexual activity.
The PB view, following the algebraic sum principle, is that a strong negative emotional state subtracts from experiencing the positive emotional

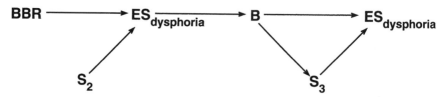

FIGURE 7.3   This model depicts the PB concept of the vicious cycle of depression
(and other mood disorders). Because of the individual's personality repertoires
(BBR) and the life situation (S_2), the individual experiences the negative emotional
state (ES) of dysphoria. The dysphoria in turn affects the individual's behavior in
undesirable ways. This behavior then affects the individual's social environment
(S_3) in negative ways; in this continuing development, that social environment further impacts on the individual to deepen the dysphoria.

responses usually elicited by food and sexual stimuli. The negative emotional state also lowers the extent to which stimuli will serve as positive reinforcers or incentive stimuli for the individual. For example, since food stimuli and sex stimuli no longer elicit such a positive emotional response, they will not strengthen food- and sex-securing behaviors. The depressed person, thus, displays less eating behavior (loss of appetite) which can result in weight loss. This is true also of sexual behavior, which diminishes in frequency. The emotional effects on behavior also involve the incentive function of stimuli. Positive emotional stimuli elicit approach behaviors; anything that diminishes that emotion will lessen their incentive strength. When the individual is depressed the positive emotional response to all stimuli is decreased, resulting in the typical decrease in activity and "energy." For example, the individual will have an attenuated emotional response to the announcement of a movie, and thus be less likely to go.

The negative emotional state will, on the other hand, *add* to stimuli that elicit negative emotional responses. The individual who is depressed, thus, will cry more easily than usual in response to bad news, or any sad event, and become annoyed or irritable more easily. Any stimulus that elicits a negative emotional response will be enhanced by the negative emotional state of the individual. This includes the enhancement of pain, as a new PB theory of pain indicates (Staats, Hekmat, & Staats, in press). The individual, as a consequence of the negative emotional state, is also likely to display sensory-motor characteristics of dejection.

In actuality these events interact. Let us say the negative emotional state begins because of some environmental loss that entails a number of negative emotional stimuli. The emotional state, in turn, affects emotional responding to life's other stimuli and, hence, the incentive and reinforcing value of those stimuli. And the emotional state affects the things the individual says to herself—the self-blame, the worry, the negative thinking. But these are powerful and continuing events that themselves elicit negative emotions that contribute to the negative algebraic sum of the negative emotional state. In further interaction the depressed behavior of the subject—the negative language behavior, the lack of participation in activities, the dejected motor behavior, and such—have an effect on the social environment, which then acts back on the individual. The spouse, for example, disaffected by the depressed person's negative talk, inactivity, dejection, and irritability, may be alienated and complain, threaten reprisals, and generally act negatively, all of which deepen the person's depression. This is schematized in Figure 7.3.

The Current Environment in the PB Theory of Depression

Analyses of depression have frequently considered environmental misfortunes such as death of a loved one, losing a job, moving away from family and friends, a failed marriage or rejection by a loved person, retirement, and old age. Some environmental events seem anomalous—like attaining a major life objective, receiving a promotion, or the birth of a child. But attaining something, in effect, can remove a life goal, and a promotion or a child may bring threatening responsibility. In PB terms "The environment in which the individual finds himself or herself may be deficient [involving losses]. . . [or] inappropriate—such as occurs when . . . a new boss . . . who dislikes the individual . . . makes unreasonable demands, . . . withholds usual rewards and recognition, and . . . creates special problems for the individual" (Staats & Heiby, 1985, p. 292).

Each misfortune actually consists of a large number of individual stimuli. The individual who loses a job, for example, does not just suffer one negative emotional stimulus. Many negative stimulus circumstances result, such as having to spend life savings, to resist buying needed or desired things, to withdraw from participation in recreations, and the like, all of which will elicit a negative emotional response. There are also a host of social stimuli that result from having lost status as an employed, worthwhile, contributing, successful member of society. These are stimuli that can elicit numerous, continuous, and strong negative emotional responses. Such negative emotional responses begin the continuing emotional state, dysphoria, that defines depression.

One of the things that has been confusing is that, although a good percentage of patients will have experienced a discrete, apparent misfortune before becoming depressed, many will not. Reactive depressions that involve a misfortune can more easily be seen to have a demonstrable cause. Let me suggest, however, that a person's life may involve many stimuli that elicit a negative emotional response even without the occurrence of some specific, dramatic loss. The individual may have a poor or non-existent family life, a non-fulfilling job, few friends and enjoyable activities, and so on. In such a case there may be no dramatic loss that precipitates depression. The precipitating event may occur within, such as the verbal projection this scenario is not going to improve. And, even when external circumstances appear very good, we cannot know what is occurring in the unobservable intimacies of the individual's life, as in marriage, in the discrepancy between a life-dream and reality, in the response to aging, and many others. It is easy to assume in such "unjustifiable" cases as these that the cause must be some biological condition, but the error is in our ability to analyze and apprise ourselves of the causal events.

The environmental and behavioral conditions of depressed people need to be studied systematically, so that we can have better knowledge of the variety of circumstances that can be involved. In the PB view the current life environment interacts with the individual's BBRs to produce dysphoria and depressed behavior, which further affect the environment.

Understanding the disorder calls for knowledge of these several sources of causation.

The Basic Behavioral Repertoires in the PB Theory of Depression

Not all individuals who experience a great loss in life become depressed. Their mourning does not begin the complex interactions that bring a persisting state with disabling symptoms. In the PB view such individual differences are due to variation in the BBRs. One individual, for example, may learn a very rich positive emotional-motivational repertoire, with positive emotional responses to many people, recreative stimuli, work stimuli, sexual stimuli, family stimuli, social stimuli (friends, relatives), religious stimuli, intellectual stimuli, political stimuli, as well as material things of various kinds. On the other hand, another individual may have learned a much more restricted, sparse positive emotional-motivational BBR. There may also be differences in individuals in the extent to which the *negative* emotional-motivational repertoire is learned. An individual may learn a negative emotional response—fear, anxiety, annoyance, hate, dislike—to many things.

The same is true of the sensory-motor repertoire. Some people have learned a variety of sensory-motor skills, in areas like playing tennis, repairing cars, sewing, cooking, playing an instrument, painting, playing with children, gardening, and love-making, among others. Other individuals will have learned a narrower range of sensory motor skills. Some sensory-motor skills also may affect the individual's physiology in various ways that may be relevant for depression, for example, recreational exercise may help determine the individual's weight and health, as well as physiologically (biochemically) affect the individual's emotion elicitation.

The same is true of the language-cognitive repertoire. One individual may have learned negative language-cognitive characteristics, such as generally labeling events, including those yet to happen, in a negative way. This individual may verbally criticize herself and generally describe herself in what we would call a negative self-concept. As another individual difference variable, some people are very "introspective." That is, they engage in a lot of self-language, whereas others may respond more to external stimulation, such as interacting with others, working on tasks, reading, and listening to television. Moreover, individuals who are introspective may vary in their perseveration and the depth with which they treat a topic. Some individuals who experience something positive or negative will examine the experience in detail, analyzing what happened, thinking of related issues, implications, and the possibilities of further development of the situation involved. Others will do so much less. These various differences will affect the positive and negative emotional responses people experience and, hence, their emotional states.

Depression Vulnerability.   These BBR differences are centrally important
with respect to how the individual will respond to a negative environmental development. Not everyone who loses a job, a loved one, one's health, or
whatever, becomes depressed. Some people, because of the nature of their
BBRs, are more vulnerable to depression than are others (see Carrillo, Rojo,
& Staats, in press). As in the above example, a person who describes herself in negative emotional terms will be more vulnerable to depression than
a person who describes herself in positive emotional terms. As another
example, a person who ruminates excessively over things that happen will
be more vulnerable to depression, in contrast to a person who gives each
situation its due and then moves on. Thus, characteristics of the individual's language-cognitive repertoire will contribute to vulnerability.

   With respect to the emotional-motivational BBR, a person who has a very
richly developed emotional-motivational BBR, in which there are many
stimuli that elicit a positive emotional response, will be less vulnerable than
a person with a less developed BBR. Let us take the example of two mothers, each of whom has lost an only child. The mother who has a happy marriage, rich sex life, a fulfilling career, compatible relatives, close friends,
various enjoyed recreations and cultural pursuits will weather that loss
much better than a mother with an empty marriage, no sex life, no career,
incompatible relatives, no close friends, recreations, or cultural pursuits
(Staats & Heiby, 1985). Each of these categories is a potential source of
multiple positive emotional stimuli. When those sources are few in the
individual's environment, or when the individual has not learned a positive
emotional response to such stimuli (see Rose & Staats, 1988), there is not
much to counterbalance the scales when negative emotional stimuli are
encountered in life. The individual is then *vulnerable* to depression.

   The same is true of the sensory-motor repertoire, for sensory-motor
skills are one usual means of "acquiring" positive emotional experience.
The individual who has the sensory-motor skills of being a carpenter, a
musician, an athlete, a cook, or a lover can gain important positive emotional stimuli through their use. The individual who has multiple repertoires in different areas will not experience a great loss if performance of
one becomes impossible. An individual, for example, who has the sensory-
motor skills involved in being a good tennis player, surfer, musician, social-
izer, and painter will not feel as much loss with an achilles tendon injury—
that prevents playing tennis—as someone who has few other areas of
sensory-motor development. Again, the richness of the development of the
sensory-motor BBR will affect vulnerability to depression.

   In the above section a person was described who has a poor family, work,
recreative, and social life who progressively realizes that her dreams and
hopes will never be fulfilled. These "realizations" (self-language) push her
into a depression. The person who has rich BBRs that obtain a rich family,

work, recreative, and social life, in contrast, will not engage in that type of negative appraisal and thus will be less vulnerable to depression. When considered within the framework of PB theory, it can be seen that the topic of vulnerability to depression, and other behavior disorders, deserves systematic research, including test construction.

Depression and the PB Principle of Compounding

The principle of compounding is actually involved in the above examples, but needs to be stated explicitly. The theory states that, because of the interaction of the various determinants of depression, the individual can experience a more intense negative (or positive) emotional state than external environmental circumstances warrant. The individual, for example, may lose a job. That event brings many negative emotional stimuli, and consideration of the various negative results of that loss should elicit a negative emotional state.

If, in addition, however, the individual describes what has happened as an indication of personal worthlessness—instead of, say, an economic downturn—that self-description and its continued elaboration can intensify and continue the negative emotional responding, deepening the negative emotional state. And that, in turn, will have the effect of eliciting further negative self-descriptions, descriptions of others, descriptions of other circumstances. In the person with vulnerable BBRs, losing the job can precipitate a negative "view" of the self and the world, an ample supply of negative emotional response elicitation. Worse, the individual's language behaviors, as well as her other symptoms, which make her ineffective in various settings, will be responded to by others in a negative manner. This will result in additional negative emotional stimulation. The simple job loss has in these various ways been compounded, which means a deepening of the negative emotional state beyond that which the current life situation itself warrants. (Compounding is important, also, in understanding the manic counterpart of depression [see Staats, 1989], but this cannot be developed here.)

Part of the theory task, thus, is the analysis of the various sites of causation of depression and the manner in which they interact to produce an *exaggerated* condition of negativity. Understanding this phenomenon involves understanding the basic PB principle that behavior can play two roles. A behavior may be a dependent variable, induced by a stimulus, but also be an independent variable as well, that induces yet other behavioral symptoms. The behavioral-environmental-BBR interactions in depression are part of the disorder and must be understood (see Staats, 1963a, 1968a, 1975).

Biological Conditions and Depression

There are twin studies that suggest depression is inherited (Allen, 1976). There is also a belief that misfunctioning biological mechanisms are the cause of depression. For example, Schildkraut (1970) proposed that depression is caused by a deficiency in norepinephrine in the brain, and mania (inappropriate euphoria) is caused by an excess in this substance, which aids transmission of nervous impulses. There are various studies that support this hypothesis, for example, by showing that depressed people have an excess of norepinephrine (one of the catecholamines) in their urine (Kety, 1975), and by showing that treating manic patients with lithium carbonate reduces the mania as well as the level of norepinephrine available in the brain. PB analysis, however, advises caution in interpreting such studies. Increases in norepinephrine may *result* from the depression rather than *produce* it.

In the PB view, it is possible that there are brain characteristics, *independent of BBR/environmental events*, that cause depression. The PB position, as has been indicated, is that the emotional response occurs essentially in the brain (see Staats & Eifert, 1990). Biochemical processes could directly affect the functioning of the brain to produce a negative emotional state. We see such an effect, usually in the opposite direction, when most people consume alcohol. Typically the individual's mood (emotional state) becomes happier. We can see the same effect in drug studies, where patients report being happier when administered antidepressant drugs. In PB terms the drug attenuates the negative emotional state of depression. And, as expected in PB, change in the negative emotional state will change behavior; with drug treatment "Pessimistic worry about future problems . . . showed the greatest change" (see Bower, 1994, p. 359). There is a current controversy concerning whether or not antidepressant drugs change personality (Bower, 1994). Psychological behaviorism provides a framework for resolving that controversy by specific analysis of what is involved.

It should be emphasized, however, that alcohol or drugs raise or lower (as in drug treatment of manic disorder) the individual's emotional state; however, this *does not mean that the individual's brain was malfunctioning beforehand*. Such results only demonstrate that chemicals can indeed directly affect the emotional mechanisms in the brain. Let me also make another observation in this respect. Maas, Fawcett, and Dekirmenjian (1972) showed that the reduced levels of catecholamines in depressed subjects return to normal when they are treated with antidepressant drugs. Such a finding, again, does not show that the depression began when the subjects' brain in and of itself became deficient in the catecholamines. The deficiency could have occurred because of environmental/BBR events that produced a negative emotional state.

Let me elaborate. The emotion mechanisms in the brain have been constructed by evolution so their function is to respond to environmental events. The PB hypothesis is that, when the individual with certain BBRs faces a life situation that elicits a negative emotional state, *this occurs by means of changing the physiology of the brain.* Generally, it is the individual's BBRs and life situation that determine the physiological state, rather than the reverse. Research needs to be conducted to test this theory. It is important to realize that whether the physiological state in the brain is caused behaviorally or by the brain independently, correcting that state will correct the depression. For that reason, studies that use drugs to change emotional states do not isolate just which—biological or behavioral—causation was involved in the first place. *An essential point is that pharmacological studies of this type do not provide evidence for the biological causation theory of depression.*

Again, other than the PB position, we have not had a theory framework in which biological and behavioral causation are interrelated. We need the unification of neurobiology and psychological behaviorism, and unified research efforts.

Heuristic Characteristics of the Theory of Depression

In describing the theory of depression examples have been given of research implications. One further example will be described to indicate something about the biological–behavioral interaction contained in the PB approach. The example refers to a recent study that found that the success of treatment of depression with antidepressant drugs is related to the individual's personality. The subjects under treatment suffered from major depression, and about half also received diagnoses of personality disorder (PD). Two-thirds of these patients had two or more such diagnoses. Patients diagnosed with no personality disorder did best four months after treatment started, those with one such diagnosis did less well, those with more than one such diagnosis did less well, and those with a diagnosis that included paranoid, schizoid, or schizotypal disorders did the poorest of all. Such results traditionally feed into a biological theory of depression, the relationship of personality disorders to depression enhancing the general suggestion there is some brain defect involved.

In contrast, the PB analysis is that the patients without a personality disorder are more likely to be suffering a depression because of environmentally caused problems. That is why these patients show more remissions; for the life problems pass, or the individual may adjust to them. Moreover, part of the depression in such cases results from the *compounding principle.* When the antidepressant drugs cut off the depression, the individual's unrealistic worries, guilts, and self-recriminations diminish and the individual behaves more positively. As a consequence, others treat the individual better, so a positive cycle is produced that reverses the vicious cycle involved in the depression.

The circumstance with those with personality disorders is not so positive. The behavior (BBR) that is part of their disorder is likely to be generating problems that are the primary cause of the depression. Moreover, as the number of those diagnoses (paranoid, schizoid, and schizotypal) increases, the disturbed behavior is more widespread, and there are thus more negative current life circumstances. These conditions produce the depression. Moreover, those with personality disorders have fewer behavioral resources for adjusting to environmental problems. Personality disorders will ordinarily continue. Even though the antidepressant medication reduces the negative emotional state, the individual with the personality disorder will continue to behave in the same disordered way, thus continuing the negative current life situation. This study should not support a belief in biological determination of depression. The PB theory of abnormal behavior provides a behavioral understanding of the findings.

Moreover, there are a host of empirical questions suggested by this analysis. For example, one line of research would investigate the extent to which the patients without personality disorders, in comparison to those with such disorders, are reacting to the occurrence of new life problems. Another study, which presents technical problems, would concern the extent to which the differential effects are the result of the reduction in compounding produced in patients without personality disorders. Another line of research would seek to establish the extent to which the depression of patients with personality disorder diagnoses is caused by the behavior of the patients themselves. This line of research would investigate this effect in relationship to the different diagnoses. This, of course, is a type of research that is important with respect to various disorders, not just depression.

A major point here is that we need to make PB analyses of the manner in which the behavior of patients with different types of disorders contributes to the causes of their disorders, as well as how that behavior is determined by BBR deficits and inappropriacies. In depression, for example, such study is necessary before interpreting just what the role is of drugs, for the drug-induced alleviation of the negative emotional state can set in motion behavioral processes that are a large part of the treatment effect.

The Anxiety Disorders

The anxiety disorders are generally considered as a class, as indicated in the following succinct description.

DSM-III-R Definition

The characteristic features of this group of disorders are symptoms of anxiety and avoidance behavior. In Panic Disorder and Generalized Anxiety Disorder, anxiety is usually the predominant symptom, and avoidance behavior is almost always present in Panic Disorder with Agoraphobia [phobia for being out of doors]. In Phobic Disorders anxiety is experienced if the person confronts the dreaded object or situation. In Obsessive Compulsive Disorder anxiety is experienced if the person attempts to resist the obsessions or compulsions. Avoidance behavior is almost always present in Phobic Disorders, and frequently present in Obsessive Compulsive Disorder. (American Psychiatric Association, 1987, p. 235)

Phobias occur to such things (stimuli) as being on an elevator or airplane, seeing a particular animal (dogs, insects, snakes), or being called upon to speak in public. Panic disorder involves an intense, unexpected, repeated fear or discomfort with physiologic concomitants such as shortness of breath, dizziness, palpitations, trembling, and sweating. Obsessive–compulsive disorder is divided. As *DSM-IV* indicates, obsessions are considered as "recurrent and persistent thoughts, impulses, or images that are experienced . . . as intrusive and inappropriate and that cause marked anxiety or distress . . . [and that] the person attempts to ignore or suppress . . . or to neutralize with other thought or action" (American Psychiatric Association, 1994, pp. 422–423). Compulsions are defined as "repetitive behaviors (e.g., handwashing, ordering, checking) or mental acts (e.g., praying, counting, repeating words silently) that the person feels driven to perform . . . [that] are aimed at preventing some dreaded event or situation" (American Psychiatric Association, 1994, p. 423). Generalized anxiety disorder involves unrealistic or excessive anxiety and worry about two or more areas of life, such as one's children's safety or one's job or health, for six months or longer, most days, with physiological signs of negative emotion.

The PB Emotional State and the Anxiety Disorders

In introducing the concept of the emotional state in the preceding chapter, it was stated there are only two types of emotional response—positive and negative. The different negative emotions commonly referred to—such as anger, fear, hate—are the same with respect to the emotional response itself. The distinctions among such emotions result from differences in the situational stimuli that are involved and in the behavior made to those stimuli. Thus, although a hated person and a feared person both elicit a negative emotional response, there are stimulus differences that elicit different behaviors.

The same thing is true of the emotional state. It can vary in intensity. And it can vary in constancy. And it can vary in direction—positive, negative, or neutral. And the emotional state may be produced by stimuli that have different characteristics. For example, the stimuli may be explicit, as with the loss of a loved one. In contrast, the negative emotional responses elicited by one's own life situation or one's behavior may not be so explicit. Moreover, the negative emotional stimuli may be actual or portrayed in language (as in worry) and thus be "potential" or "threatening." For example, a downturn in the economy, an increased mortgage on a new house, an impending restructuring of the individual's employing company, and children who will soon need college tuitions are threatening events. It may turn out, however, that the individual retains her job, continues to have an income, does not have to pay for her childrens' college tuition. Nevertheless, the negative emotional responses can be experienced beforehand through language "anticipations" that produce an anxiety state (Staats, 1963a).

And different circumstances can produce the negative emotional state; for example, it may result from losses of positive emotional stimuli, or the presentation of negative emotional stimuli. Since the emotional state is produced by multiple stimuli, there can be various combinations by which a negative state of a certain intensity can be reached. In one case moderate negative emotional stimuli and the paucity of positive emotional stimuli can produce a negative emotional state. In another case, the same level can be attained where the negative emotional responses are intense, but are counterbalanced to a some extent by strong positive emotional responses elicited by life circumstances. There may be differences in the effects of these states, even though their intensities are equal.

Frequently in life there are positive emotional stimuli mixed with negative emotional stimuli, actual and potential, where the outcome could be positive or negative. Take a career woman with a promotion pending, a new love and relationship that could go either way, the responsibility for the company party, a large project that may succeed or fail and add or subtract from her promotion chances, an upcoming city tennis tournament that will determine her state ranking, and the problem of resisting her parents' request that she move back in with them without alienating them. Worry about losing such strong positive emotional stimuli, and receiving the negative, can both contribute to an anxiety state. Such life stimuli, all calling for time and effort, may also elicit excessive activity, and too little sleep, and thereby add to the negative emotional responses. Moreover, the negative emotional stimuli—such as work deadlines and competitions, social demands, and parental demands—will elicit negative emotional responses that contribute directly to a negative emotional state. An emotional state produced by such circumstances, where activity remains high, will be labeled as anxiety (or stress). This anxious individual experiences an emotional state that is negative and includes pressure and tension along with sustained activity, which is different than the experience of depression.

Differing emotional states can result from the various arousing stimuli that can occur. We need additional evidence on the emotional states that people can experience. One implication would be to use the PB theory with which to construct an instrument to survey differences in the experience of people with disorders involving negative emotional states. And comparisons should also be made in the physiological symptoms that are displayed—for example, by depressed, phobic, GAD, panic disorder, and obsessive–compulsive patients (as well as those suffering from stress).

The PB theory is that the emotional state is a function of both the individual's BBRs and current life situation. Only some of the individuals subjected to the same pressurized life situation will experience an anxiety state. But there are also differences in the nature of the complex life situations faced.

Personality (the BBRs) and the Anxiety Disorders

This topic has been dealt with more deeply in the PB theory of the anxiety disorders (Staats, 1989), but the approach can be illustrated here.

The Emotional-Motivational BBR. The emotional-motivational BBR is defined by all of the stimuli that would elicit either a positive or negative emotional response in the individual. But there are individual differences in the balance that is learned. Thus, some individuals have an emotional-motivational BBR that tilts them in the negative direction and others in a positive direction. Let me illustrate, with a mother who has a negative emotional response to many potential things such as dogs, being alone, contagious germs, illness, various failures, being different than others, not keeping up appearances, economic conditions, international tensions, parental censure, sibling competition, loss of sexual attractiveness and performance, loss of husband or his affection, infidelity, loss of friendships, planning trips and social affairs, as well as the uncertainties of children's health and school and social success, and on and on. The mother is concerned that her young child may get chilled, play with the rough boy down the street, eat junk food, get too tired, play too hard, be accosted by strangers, touch contaminated things, not behave properly in the presence of her husband's boss, and on and on.

A mother with such an emotional-motivational repertoire is likely to provide conditioning experience to her children that will produce the same type of emotional-motivational learning. The child need not experience anything unusual—raised with an "anxious" parent the child will learn that the world contains many "fearful" stimuli. Other things being equal, an individual raised that way will experience more negative emotional responses and states than an individual raised without that conditioning. And, PB theory states the "anxious" individual will be vulnerable to acquiring an anxiety disorder. Research of a prospective-longitudinal and psychometric nature should be conducted in this context. This would involve constructing a test to measure children's negative emotional-motivational repertoire. Children then measured should be followed, to ascertain who develops an anxiety disorder, as a means of studying the contribution to vulnerability of having a negative emotional-motivational BBR.

The Language-Cognitive Repertoire. In the above example, much of the child's conditioning will be conducted through language. The mother who cautions the child about all the things she has a negative emotional response to will be conditioning the child to have a negative emotional response also to those things. Through language conditioning the child can become conditioned widely and easily, and imperceptibly. The mother who says things like, "I hope you pass the test," "I wonder whether enough of your friends will come to the party," "Dad is really late, I hope he didn't get in an accident," "The flu is going around so don't play touching games," is training her child to negative emotional responses, albeit in a way that will not be noticed.

Moreover, in this process the child will learn also word sequences (modes of thought) that are of a similar nature. For example, let us say that two students face an important test and one describes how little time she has to prepare, how she does not have the right background, how she does not learn or retain material in this field, how tough her competition is, how anxious she becomes in test situations, and how uncertain her performance is likely to be. Let us say the other student describes the same things in positive terms, and a third student does neither, simply going about the business of preparing for the examination. The upcoming test will elicit more anxiety in the first student, and much less in the second two. The important thing here is that these individual differences in language behavior are important in the development of the anxiety disorders. A person who has such a "negative" language-cognitive repertoire, and who employs it widely in response to life events, will experience a great deal of negative emotionality that may contribute to a continuous anxiety state, a basis for one of the anxiety disorders, when the actual events of her life are no different than they are for others who do not display negative language and do not suffer an anxiety disorder.

> There are wide differences between people in their language-cognitive repertoires . . . [as] involved when we describe someone as (1) overly conscientious, feeling anxiety unless they do things just right; (2) negative in outlook, especially about themselves; (3) a worrier who frequently anticipates negative occurrences; (4) believing that what they think is what will happen . . . . [These are] descriptive of people with anxiety disorders. . . . It is the present view that what we call vulnerability to development of an anxiety disorder involves the individual's personality repertoires, because these repertoires can set the individual up for development of a disorder. It should be possible to study such things prospectively. Thus, it should be the case that if we isolated a group of subjects who displayed a strong tendency to describe events—including pending events—in terms that elicit negative emotional responses, we would have a group that would display a greater frequency of development of an anxiety disorder than would a group of individuals who describe things neutrally or positively. We need such prospective research. But we must first define the language-cognitive repertoires that make the individual vulnerable to the development of clinical psychopathology. (Staats, 1989, Chap. 5, p. 60)

A supportive PB account of worrying further develops the importance of the language-cognitive BBR in the development of an anxiety disorder.

> Worry may be construed as distressing and pervasive thoughts, self-verbalizations, and rumination that are crystallized on domains of prime significance to the worriers. These domains include health, illness, family, financial, academic, environmental, religious, vocational, interpersonal situations, future catastrophes, and personal control-related issues . . . . Worrisome individuals tend to experience more trait anxiety, state anxiety, social anxiety, self-blame, low thrill seeking, low boredom susceptibility, depression, self-esteem problems, rumination, obsessional symptoms, unpleasant thoughts, public self-consciousness, negative daydreaming, cognitive intrusion, sleep problems, avoidance problems, wishful thinking, attention focusing problems, distractibility, hypervigilance, and health concerns . . . .
>
> Excessive worry is considered the prime symptom of generalized anxiety disorder . . . . The majority of anxiety disorder patients spend 50% or more of a day worrying. (Hekmat, Edelstein, & Cook, 1994, p. 4)

Many contemporary behavior therapy descriptions use a general cognitive–behavioral theory-language. Worry is thus treated as an unanalyzed cognitive process. These clinical descriptions support the PB position; but PB provides the principles and concepts by which to treat what worry is and how people learn a "worrying" repertoire (part of the language-cognitive BBR) that produces anxiety.

The Sensory-Motor Repertoire and the Escape-Avoidance BBR. The experience the anxious mother provides the child not only produces negative emotional stimuli, but it also trains the child to be vigilant of the environment with respect to possibly harmful stimuli. Such vigilance may be considered a sensory-motor characteristic of an anxious person.

In addition, although glossed over in the *DSM* definitions, avoidance plays a prominent role, especially in some of the anxiety disorders. For example, escape behavior is central in obsessive–compulsive disorder (OCD). The individual may step on every line on the cement pavement, return again and again to check whether the door is locked, repeatedly wash hands or take showers, or avoid touching door handles by putting on gloves or using a handkerchief as a buffer. These behaviors provide escape from the negative emotional response that would be experienced if the behaviors did not occur. The phobic person, also, is characterized by escape-avoidance behavior with respect to the feared objects. The person with PTSD generally avoids situations that elicit anxiety. In the PB theory there is a sensory-motor personality characteristic that may be called the "escape and avoidance" BBR, which includes language-cognitive escape-avoidance behavior.

Simple phobics characteristically avoid representations of their phobic object or situation. Sometimes these representations may range far and wide across a number of generalization gradients, including images, thoughts, and objects that seem only remotely related to the original phobic object. By all reports . . . the same can be said for PTSD. (Barlow, 1988, p. 523)

Barlow does not analyze what representations are, how they are learned, and how they operate to produce anxiety. Moreover, the behaviorism he employs does not provide such analyses, nor the foundation principles and concepts necessary. Skinner's (1975) position does not provide a basic theory for understanding how language (thoughts and images) can produce anxiety, or how anxiety can affect behavior. Psychological behaviorism's basic theory of language provides the necessary principles and concepts.

For example, let us refer to Barlow's description and ask what is happening behaviorially. What are the "representations" that are avoided? In the PB framework representations are constituted of language behavior; for example, worry includes saying implicitly words that elicit negative emotional responses. And avoidance of negative-emotional language behavior constitutes a type of escape-avoidance behavior. The individual may thus occupy herself with alternate language behaviors to blot out the feared responses—as in praying or counting silently. Language-cognitive escape-avoidance behaviors will be illustrated further in the context of the disorders described.

Generalized Anxiety: Basic in the Anxiety Disorders

The PB view (Staats, 1989; Sternberger & Burns, 1992) is that generalized anxiety disorder (GAD) represents the basic anxiety disorder—that all cases of clinically relevant anxiety disorders involve a person who generally experiences anxiety to a greater extent than is usual. The person diagnosed solely with the generalized anxiety disorder may not have developed specific phobias, panic disorder symptoms, obsessive–compulsive behaviors, or the additional things involved in PTSD. Thus, the other disorders involve elements in addition to those of GAD.

Phobic Disorder

The general anxiety disorder (GAD) may not reach clinical proportions with the person diagnosed as phobic, but this person has a more than usual level of anxiety. Such a person is vulnerable to developing stronger than usual negative emotions to specific things. For example, the individual may be uneasy about flying, in which case, reading about air crashes can provide additional negative language conditioning of emotional responses. The individual may image crashes, worry about what would happen to children, spouse, and career if killed in a crash, and such, all of which will produce additional conditioning. Once this occurs to the level that the individual avoids flying, the phobia becomes more intractable. Additional negative emotional responses are elicited by others pressing one to fly, by being thought of as odd, and such. And the individual's avoidance behavior prevents the individual becoming accustomed (extinguishing negative emotions and learning positive emotions) to flying.

Panic Disorder

The person who develops panic attacks is an anxious person also. The panic attack seems to occur without stimulus elicitation, because the stimuli are largely self-produced and not obvious. To illustrate this, let us use the case of nocturnal panic states. The anxious individual awakens from sleep experiencing a negative emotional response with physiological stimuli (such as a pounding heart and rapid breathing), perhaps a concomitant of dreaming. But what occurs then is that the physiological stimuli themselves elicit a fear response. Let us say the individual worries, "God, am I going to have a stroke?" This maintains and increases the negative emotional responding and the physiological stimuli. This then leads to further ominous descriptions. This compounding can quickly build to the panic state. We can see this in clinical descriptions, for example, "a patient may become alarmed by a decreasing heart rate that occurs during relaxation—a cue to which the panic-prone patient is very sensitive, and which may therefore trigger a panic attack. . . . Similarly, a sleeping individual may be oblivious to his or her environment, but may remain attuned to personally significant stimuli" (Barlow, 1988, p. 86). Among panic-disorder individuals the "symptoms reported with the greatest frequency were strong, rapid, or irregular heartbeat; shortness of breath; hot and cold flashes; choking or smothering sensations; trembling; and fear of dying" (Barlow, 1988, p. 87).

Besides the general anxiety these individuals also have specific fears concerning health, are vigilant concerning body sensations and states, and have learned a negative emotional language-cognitive BBR concerning such matters. The occurrence of physiological sensations then triggers the compounding interaction of these various repertoires. Such attacks increase the individual's fear responses generally to health, the individual's self-concept becomes more negative, and the individual becomes a more anxious person, in a vicious cycle development.

Obsessive–Compulsive Disorder

With these descriptions in hand it is possible to deal with obsessive–compulsive disorder (OCD). To begin, in the PB view the terms obsession and compulsion are not clearly used. Let us ask first, thus, what is it that allows us to differentiate obsessions and compulsions and to see their commonalities as well? To begin the clarification, the obsession occurs and the individual struggles to replace it. However, the compulsion occurs before the feared event, thus postponing that event. There is an analogy to be found in animal studies. A negative reinforcer can be applied in different ways to affect learning. Let us say that two animals separately receive experience in which the floor of an operant apparatus is electrified to deliver a sustained shock until a bar is pressed. In one case, let us say, the shock is turned on again after a systematically varied period, until the animal again presses the bar and this is repeated. The animal will be conditioned to press the bar. In the other case, however, let us say the animal learns to press the bar this way, but with an additional contingency. Every time the animal presses the bar this has the effect of lengthening the period slated before the next delivery of shock. Under the first, *escape,* condition, the animal will learn to press the bar as soon as the shock comes on. That is like the obsession. The shock is the feared cognition. In the second, *avoidance,* condition, the animal will learn frequently and continuously to press the bar so that the shock is not experienced. This is like a compulsion.

When analyzing the behaviors involved other aspects are clarified. Actually, both obsessions and compulsions involve feared stimuli, and in both cases those stimuli are self-produced. The individual who is compulsive originally had an image of an unlocked house, or a thought of contamination, as examples. To exemplify an obsession, let us take a mother who has a repetitive image of doing harm to her children. There is no difference, in principle, with respect to the type of stimulus. Obsessive stimuli and compulsive stimuli elicit a negative emotional response.

Typically, however, there is a difference on the escape response end. With obsessions the *escape* behavior is of a language-cognitive type. The mother with an image of throwing her infant out of a window struggles to replace that image with one of caring for the infant or some other response that removes the negative emotional image. However, the *avoidance* behavior in the compulsion is of the sensory-motor variety. The individual originally afraid of the unlocked house returns to the house; the individual who is afraid of disease and dirt must wash her hands.

The behaviors involved in compulsions and obsessions are exhausting, and self-demeaning in their "craziness," bringing on additional negative emotions and increasing the anxiety state. They are non-effective, for they do not get at correcting the problem, which is that of the generalized anxiety the person suffers from her BBRs and life situation. "If one evaluates a patient with unbearably severe generalized anxiety, recurrent panic attacks, debilitating avoidance, and major depression all occurring simultaneously, the diagnosis is probably OCD. For OCD is the devastating culmination of the most intense manifestations of emotional disorders" (Barlow, 1988, p. 598).

In the present conception, what this means is that the OCD patient has learned the inappropriately negative emotional-motivational BBR, the negative emotion-producing language-cognitive BBR, and the escape-and-avoidance BBR in full measure. In addition, the OCD patient has developed all the symptomatology that can result from such BBRs—the phobias, GAD, and panic attacks. Centrally, what is involved is a cumulative-hierarchical learning process where the individual learns ways of avoiding phobic objects. But these behaviors in their unreality and ineffectiveness simply produce more negative emotional stimulation, that is, a heightened general anxiety state. That development then yields panic disorders, which increase the individual's fear of what is happening and her inability to cope. Effects on the social environment—loss of status and confidence in the disordered individual—bring increased anxiety. Fearful thoughts begin and the patient struggles desperately to escape and avoid them, and thereby also to regain her control and confidence in herself. What is involved is a cumulative-hierarchical learning process.

With respect to OCD it is interesting in this context to note that groups have developed general and stylized language-cognitive behaviors for avoiding anxiety-producing stimuli. For example, meditation devices, like the repetition of a mantra, can function as a type of escape mechanism, preventing the individual from verbal and imaginal responses that would elicit negative emotional responses. The individual can remove anxiety-producing sexual, violence, or failure images by this means. Various religious rituals have that same function, such as prayer that may be practiced to a furious intensity in order to avoid thinking about other, sinful things. Thus, the avoidance is accomplished by having other behaviors occur that are incompatible and that prevent the negative cognitions from occurring. The added "appeal" of such avoidance behaviors is that they are "group validated," not "crazy," and thus do not themselves elicit anxiety. Are there general "skills" involved in being an avoider of anxiety-producing cognitions? Do those with anxiety disorders have richly developed escape-avoidance BBRs including language repertoires? Are such repertoires "causes" in the anxiety disorders? Psychological behaviorism answers yes, but the questions call for research.

Post-Traumatic Stress Disorder (PTSD)

With this disorder there is a specific experience that seems to precipitate the disorder, such as a dreadful war experience, or sexual or violent assault. In PTSD the individual may experience various symptoms, such as disturbed sleep, reliving the experience, phobic responses to stimuli like those in the original experience, as well as general life disturbance (such as job, marital, and social instability).

Ordinarily the focus of interest with respect to PTSD is the traumatic experience. In the PB view, however, longstanding PTSD cases constitute a complex disorder involving deficit BBRs and inappropriate BBRs (such as generalized anxiety and a well-developed escape-avoidance BBR) and a cumulative-hierarchical learning development. Thus, a war veteran with such problems may return and exhibit problems in work and family relations. For example, the individual may experience anxiety in work situations that are challenging, and engage in various avoidance behaviors to those work situations. The failure that results may then be blamed on the original trauma. The blaming is a form of escape from anxiety. Experiencing anxiety to work situations is a general problem that will impact centrally on the individual if he is reduced to seeking unchallenging jobs that elicit a negative emotional response for that reason. When the individual's life failures elicit a negative emotional state, drinking, which reduces that state, may then enter as an additional problem. These various escape-avoidance behaviors that do not deal with the problem and that thus exacerbate life's problems are central in chronic PTSD. It should be remembered that most people who experience traumatic events do not develop PTSD, so the trauma alone is not the cause. A more complete analysis of this disorder is presented in PB (see Staats, 1989).

The Current Life Situation and Stress

It has been recognized generally that environmental losses are involved in many cases of depression. And the life situation is important in the consideration of the anxiety disorders. For example, in the case of PTSD, environmental events loom as an important cause, but current life events should be more the focus of attention than they are. In general, how various life situations (sometimes self-caused) can produce an anxiety state in the individual need to be systematically considered and studied.

Interestingly there is another problem area in psychology that has been concerned with anxiety- or dysphoria-producing environmental circumstances. Called *stress* or *stress management,* the tradition of the field is separate from the study of depression and the anxiety disorders in abnormal psychology. More than with depression and the anxiety disorders, the study of stress arose within a conceptual framework concerned with how certain environmental situations can produce medical problems—such as hypertension. It is typical of psychology that these very closely related types of phenomena—depression, anxiety disorders, and stress-psychosomatic problems—are generally studied and considered separately.

The incongruity of this separation can be seen from the fact that the same types of environmental events are considered in the three areas. As an example, let us take the Social Readjustment Rating Scale (Holmes & Rahe, 1967), which was composed to measure the stress—amount of readjustment—that life events cause. The most stressful events included are death of spouse, divorce, marital separation, death of a close family member, personal injury or illness, marriage, being fired at work, marital reconciliation, retirement, change in the health of a family member, pregnancy, sex difficulties, gain of a new family member, business readjustment, change in financial state, death of a close friend, change to a different line of work, change in number of arguments with spouse, mortgage of $10,000 or more, foreclosure of a mortgage or loan, change in responsibilities at home. Others listed are trouble with in-laws, wife begins or stops work, beginning or ending of school, trouble with boss, change in residence, schools, or social activities. The important point is that most of those events can also be inducers of *depression* and *anxiety.*

The PB position is that the different problem areas should be studied in an interrelated manner. There are various stressing environmental events. The field of stress needs to study them, along with the physiological symptoms that result from them. But they need also to be studied in a broader context. Are stressful environmental events different for depressed people, psychosomatic people, and for those with an anxiety disorder? For example, there are cataclysmic events—like the death of a loved one—and there are longstanding, day-to-day events—like a pressurized, anxiety-producing, threatening work situation. Does the first type of event tend to elicit depression and the second either an anxiety disorder or psychosomatic illness? Are environmental events different for those with different anxiety disorders? Or are the differences with respect to disorder primarily a function of the individuals' personality (BBRs)? These questions call for systematic consideration and study.

UNIFIED PB ANALYSIS AND DSM CLASSIFICATION

The traditional taxonomies of the behavior disorders began with the idea that there are discrete *mental diseases* with symptomatologies that lend themselves to classification, as indicated in the *DSM* series title. Freud's psychoanalytic theory was the basis for attempts to construct a general, unified theory of abnormal behavior (see, for example, Cameron, 1963; Fenichel, 1945). For a time this approach had a general influence, which has diminished in the past few decades. Moreover, the concept of mental disease has not been supported by evidence. With the weakening of such conceptual foundations, the field has become more descriptive, less conceptual and explanatory, lacking interest in analyzing the various disorders within a unified theory. This trend is continued in *DSM-IV.* The grouping of disorders into classes is done on the basis of symptom commonality. The assumed but undeveloped explanatory conception is biologically oriented, with a recognition that the environment can play a role in at least some disorders.

But having an explicit, unified set of principles and concepts that is explanatory is an obvious advantage in understanding phenomena in any science. Analyzing a wide range of behavior disorders within such a unified set of principles and concepts is central in the PB theory of abnormal behavior. One advantage is that of indicating the relationship among the various disorders. As an example, let us take the *DSM-IV* developmental disorders, including the subclassifications of mental retardation, pervasive developmental disorders (autism), and the specific learning disorders (such as reading, writing, and arithmetic disorder). The *DSM-IV* is only descriptive; as a consequence the several disorders appear to be independent and unrelated, with a suggestion of separate brain defects.

Within PB's explanatory theory, however, the relationships of the several disorders can be seen. Centrally, the basic framework is that child development involves the cumulative-hierarchical learning of the BBRs (personality). The various behavior disorders involve problems in that cumulative-hierarchical learning. Where and when the problems arise in that learning is important. In terms of time, for example, the circumstances are very similar for mental retardation and autism. The problems of learning begin early and for this reason are more pervasive. Nevertheless, in *DSM-IV*, Mental Retardation constitutes a different classification category than the Pervasive Develop-mental Disorders such as Autistic Disorder. The fact is, there is important overlap in terms of the central deficits that occur in the two disorders. For example, in severe cases in both, the learning process begins to go awry in the first years in such central areas as language development (learning). Language constitutes a very central BBR for the child's later learning. The deficit in language development brings to a halt much of the child's general cumulative-hierarchical learning, setting the stage for developing further problems of learning in both disorders.

Thus, the deficits may be similar with respect to the language-cognitive and sensory-motor BBRs. What is the difference between the mentally retarded and the autistic child? These children differ in such things as learning of the emotional-motivational repertoire. The mentally retarded child may have language-cognitive deficits that are as severe as those of the autistic child, but nevertheless may learn a positive emotional response to the parents, along with sensory-motor behaviors of seeking and giving affection. That difference can help establish the differential diagnosis, as in the lack of approach behaviors to parents displayed by the autistic child but not the retarded child. The two disorders also differ greatly in their anti-learning repertoires. The retarded child can escape learning situations by "acting dumb." The autistic child can learn bizarre behaviors to escape from the training periods the well-intentioned parent attempts to give the child. On the other hand, bizarre troublesome behavior, when there is pressure to learn, leads to unpleasant parent–child interactions. For example, when extremely inappropriate behaviors require physical restraint these encounters produce mutually unpleasant experiences. Love is learned, and when the learning experiences are deficit on the positive side and full on the negative side, the balance can be negative. Although a mentally retarded and an autistic child have the same IQ (language-cognitive BBR development) deficits, they typically differ in their emotional-motivational repertoires (to parents and hence others), and in their anti-learning sensory-motor repertoires. The *unified* analysis helps in understanding both disorders, as well as their relationship to each other.

Specific developmental disorders, like reading, writing, and arithmetic disorders, in contrast to the other two disorders, occur at a *later* point in the child's development. The child prior to the development of the disorder may have acquired normal language-cognitive, sensory-motor, and emotional-motivational BBRs. The child's abnormal development may not begin to occur until the child enters school. Starting at a later time in the cumulative-hierarchical learning process the effects on the BBRs are less severe and general than in mental retardation or autism. However, the cumulative-hierarchical learning of language-cognitive academic BBRs may be specifically or generally stopped or hindered at the point the disorder appears. And that may set the cumulative-hierarchical-learning foundation for the other abnormal developments, such as school phobia and child, adolescent, and finally adult antisocial behavior disorder. The important point here is that the learning disorders are to be considered in a related manner to each other and to mental retardation and autism, within the same set of principles and concepts.

The PB theory also provides a means of relating depression, stress-related problems, and the anxiety disorders, including an ordering of the severity of the latter. The same principles apply, and there is overlap in causative variables, the involvement of the three BBRs, and the role of the negative emotional state. There are also differences among the different disorders, especially in the escape-avoidance behaviors that have been learned as a means of reducing immediately experienced negative emotion. It can be expected that important heuristic developments will arise from consideration of the behavior disorders within a general unified theory.

CONCLUSION

The knowledge of abnormal psychology—the observations of the behavior of clinical patients—has been organized into taxonomies of the behavior disorders. These naturalistic observations have not been established via experimental analysis of behavior technology, or even other behavioral methods, and are not accepted in radical behaviorism. In PB the knowledge of the traditional field of abnormal psychology is considered valuable. The PB methodological philosophy, however, holds that the naturalistic observations made in abnormal psychology can only be made *behaviorally* valuable by means of multilevel theory construction, elaborating concepts and principles from the basic laboratory principles in a step-by-step manner until a theory is created that can make the naturalistic observations understandable in objective, empirical, heuristic terms. This chapter shows how a theory of abnormal behavior, and theories of the individual behavior disorders, can be linked to and derived from the multilevel theory-construction program of PB, validating its concepts and principles.

Central in this development is the theory of abnormal behavior presented at the beginning of the chapter. First, as Figure 7.1 indicates, the field of abnormal psychology must systematically research the learning that produces abnormal behavior. But, although it is generally acknowledged that learning plays a role in various behavior disorders, there has been no study of such learning. To know how learning operates demands that it be observed, in a detailed manner, over the cumulative-hierarchical periods involved, which means long years. Such research would be difficult and costly, but until we conduct that study we cannot know the importance learning has in the production of the behavior disorders. That this is not understood is very revealing.

Moreover, according to the PB abnormal psychology, the theory of personality plays the crucial role. For a theory of abnormal behavior must rest on stipulating the BBRs (personality) that typically are the proximal causes of the behavior disorders. The descriptions of abnormal behavior (as in *DSM-IV*) yield some knowledge of the BBRs. But it should be remembered that those descriptions are of behavior. While those behaviors are in the individual's BBRs, they are but a sample; other aspects of the abnormal BBRs will not be revealed by observing behavior. Take reading disorder, as an example, where the *DSM-IV* focuses on the absence of reading. That description, however, does not indicate what the reading BBR is—hence what the disorder involves, the learning problems that produce the disorder, or how to treat the disorder. Reading disorder is a personality disorder, and a theory of that disorder demands a personality theory that specifies the reading BBR—and how it is or is not learned. More generally, abnormal psychology must have access to a personality theory that stipulates the normal personality repertoires. The abnormal psychology then must work out what has gone wrong that has produced abnormal personality repertoires. This position, again, calls for new directions of research development.

The PB position also calls for new consideration of the abnormal behaviors that are important in classifying the disorders and in diagnosing individuals. In addition to pure description, we need systematic study of the *effects* of abnormal behaviors in the *explanation* of the disorders. For the PB theory of personality is an interactional theory—it recognizes that abnormal behavior produces conditions that have causative effects. Sometimes the behavior has effects on others that exacerbate the problem—as in the case of the behavior of the depressed person that produces criticisms in family members that have the effect of deepening the person's depression. Sometimes the behavior has effects on the person herself—as in compounding where the depressed person's self-condemnatory language behavior elicits negative emotional responses that add to the person's negative emotional state. We need general and systematic research to study how abnormal behavior has a causative effect in the behavior disorders.

And, finally, we need study of the current life situations that exert causative effects in the production and maintenance of behavior disorders. This need has been recognized—as in the study of stress—but we need systematic and profound study.

There has not been a general and unified theory of abnormal behavior since the psychoanalytic attempt (see Cameron, 1947; Fenichel, 1945). The PB analysis of abnormal behavior and the behavior disorders produces a unified theory. It is suggested that this theory should be used and further developed as the framework for specialized theories of the behavior disorders that have not yet been treated, or those only dealt with incipiently. Moreover, the theory suggests various new directions for empirical development.

CHAPTER 8

Psychological Behavior
Therapy/Analysis

Treatment methods are derived from mother conceptions regarding human behavior. For example, for those who believe abnormal behavior is caused by demonic possession, treatment involves exhorcizing the demon. In the psychoanalysis conception abnormal behavior occurs because of unconscious personality conflicts resulting from childhood experiences. Psychoanalytic treatment thus aims to uncover and resolve the individual's childhood experiences and unconscious conflicts. Rogers (1951) inferred that individuals have a "life force" that strives for growth and self-actualization; with behavior problems occurring when the life force is restricted by social pressure and the individual ceases to know herself. Treatment, thus, attempts to produce a warm, accepting therapy atmosphere, where the individual is safe to express anything and can come to know herself and behave according to her true nature. The unified, multilevel PB theory also involves, and provides for, a conception of psychological behavior thrapy.

THE BEHAVIOR THERAPY CONCEPTION

Our behavior therapy also grew out of a conception, whose history and growth is complex and not well understood. It has come to be generally believed that Skinner's radical behaviorism provided the basic foundation for behavior therapy, behavior modification, behavioral assessment, and applied behavior analysis. That is not the case. In actuality, the various first- and second-generation behaviorisms together provided the basic conception that was responsible. And that conception was rather simple, namely, that abnormal (or problematic) behavior is behavior and can be treated by use of

304

conditioning principles. That simple conception, common to each of the behaviorisms, has the same directives for treatment regardless of the behaviorism used.

Actually, the first applications of the conditioning principles to problems of behavior did not begin in Skinner's radical behaviorism. Systematic work at several different places got the behavior therapy conception under way. One source was in Great Britain (see Eysenck, 1960a). It employed a general conditioning perspective. Another was the program conducted by Joseph Wolpe (1958), influenced by Hull's (1943) theory. Another of the several foundations was stimulated by PB analyses and formal and informal research (Staats, 1956, 1957a; Staats, Staats, Schutz, & Wolf, 1962). These developments fed into radical behaviorism (see Ayllon & Michael, 1959; Wolf, Risely, & Mees, 1964), producing a combination that was a central foundation of behavior modification and behavior analysis.

It is the case, however, that the fields of behavior therapy and behavior modification later came to be conducted, in good part, by behavioral psychologists who were trained in Skinner's principles and in his methodological philosophy. They thus considered themselves to be working within this theory and, in fact, their work was influenced by the characteristics of the approach, as will be indicated. Radical behaviorism has come to be the basic behaviorism that is most generally employed, so the approach has and does cast a very large and influential shadow on the general field of behavior therapy and related endeavors. Various characteristics of behavior therapy are a result of the radical behaviorism influence, including characteristics that are not recognized.

Let me explain. Skinner's radical behaviorism was developed in the context of animal behavior research that pertained 65 years ago. It does not have the basic nature of a behaviorism developed in the modern context. For that reason radical behaviorism is not a good foundation for behavior therapy. Trying to use it in that manner has left the field of behavior therapy rudderless in various ways. Because this behaviorism does not have characteristics by which to develop needed elements for the subject matter, it has been necessary to seek answers from other approaches. For example, since radical behaviorism did not accept or justify the use of verbal psychotherapy methods, or provide guides for doing so, behavior therapists (including radical behaviorists) first rejected psychotherapy. Later guides were sought in cognitive psychology. Because this problem pertains to various areas, behavior therapy has been forced to include disparate and unrelated materials. Today the field is unsure of its identity, its philosophy, its methodology, its theory, and its subject matter. While our field has brought science to clinical psychology, producing a plethora of research accomplishments, valuable therapy methods and assessment instruments, behavior therapy is at the present time, eclectic and mixed up (Staats, 1995).

The purview and program of development for behavior therapy must be derived from a mother conception. A primary weakness of radical behaviorism is that it cannot provide that purview and program. The fact is it never has—behavior analysis actually had to give up the restrictiveness of experimental analysis of behavior in order to use the simple framework provided by our early behavior therapy methods. *Radical behaviorism is a two-level theory.* Its basic level—where its systematic development is focused— is that of animal behavior. Its other level is human behavior. But Skinner considered this development a philosophy. He never developed this level systematically like the basic level; and he provided almost no empirical or theory guide for doing so. Skinner's radical behaviorism (1948, 1953, 1957, 1975) never included human research, let alone clinical research. It contains almost no analyses of learning in the naturalistic situation—parent to child, for example. There are no behavior analyses of abnormal behavior in Skinner's works, of behavior disorders, of treatment methods, of behavioral assessment, and so on. Radical behaviorism, as a two-level theory, does not ask that behavior therapy develop itself within the other fields of psychology, using materials from those fields in doing so. As a guide, radical behaviorism provides a program for isolation (Fraley & Vargas, 1986; Skinner, 1988).

Psychological behaviorism, in addition to employing basic animal learning-behavior principles, was also developed in the human research context. This development enabled it to contribute to the foundations of modern behavior therapy and generally to address human behavior. In its 40-plus years of development it has provided a conception with a program and a purview for conducting and expanding behavior therapy. The purpose of this chapter is to indicate how psychological behavior therapy (PBT) can now provide a foundation for the present and future development of the field of behavior therapy. It will be proposed that behavior therapy needs a behaviorism foundation that establishes the basis for relating in a mutually heuristic manner to the other fields of psychology—from basic animal learning, through human learning, social psychology, child development, personality, personality measurement, and abnormal psychology. That means a multilevel theory framework is needed, as will be illustrated.

THE BASIC LEARNING/BEHAVIOR LEVEL

The basic level of PB studies the elementary principles of conditioning (the primary level of study of the second-generation behaviorisms). Both the principles of classical conditioning and of reinforcement can be applied to the analysis of a human behavior for the purpose of changing that behavior. Much of the published work of behavior therapy involves this level of study, and this level remains important to behavior therapy.

Studies with Adults

Behavior therapy began with such studies and analyses. For example, Walton (1960) reported a patient who scratched her neck compulsively, creating a skin problem. His analysis was that the behavior was supported by social attention, and the method of treatment consisted of extinction. Raymond (1960), as another example of a British behavior therapy study, paired pictures of baby carriages with a negative unconditioned stimulus and thereby successfully treated a patient's fetish for baby carriages. As has been indicated, PB analyzed the opposite speech of a schizophrenic patient as a behavior, produced by the reinforcement of hospital staff, that could be treated by extinction and by reinforcement of normal speech (Staats, 1957a). Jack Michael—who had been exposed to this analysis and a previous informal PB use of reinforcement to treat a problem of behavior—then worked with his student Teodoro Ayllon (Ayllon & Michael, 1959) in a study that verified the PB behavior modification principles, in the hospital setting, with various symptom behaviors of psychotics. Eysenck's (1960a) collection of behavior therapy works did not include any of the American studies that had begun, because they were dispersed and unknown, but during a visit to England in 1961 I had a chance to initiate the connection.

In my first PB account of abnormal behavior and treatment (see Staats, 1963a, chap. 11) I employed the few behavioral studies then available. The position went past these studies systematically to indicate in specific analyses that the gamut of abnormal behaviors were learned—schizophrenia, physical (and sensory) disabilities and the problems involved, compulsive disorder, delusional behavior, phobic disorder, psychosomatic illnesses, paraphilias, alcoholism, criminality, and juvenile delinquency (in addition to the childhood disorders). The PB theory said that conditioning principles could generally be applied to the analysis and treatment of behavior disorders. This account constituted a blueprint for the new applied behavioral field, a blueprint that was not available in radical behaviorism or social learning theory. Included in this was the projection of a new field of "learning psychotherapy" (Staats, 1963a, pp. 506–511), as I first called it.

> [A]djustment to life in our society demands extremely complex behaviors. The individual must acquire intricate language behaviors, complicated social behaviors, work skills, and so on, in order to gain the reinforcers available in our society. Moreover, these behaviors must be under complex stimulus control, and the consequences of these behaviors must have customary reinforcing value for the individual if his adjustive behavior is to be acquired and main-

tained. Otherwise, competing and perhaps inappropriate behaviors may replace the adjustive behavior.

. . . [A]n analysis of complex human behavior in terms of learning principles leads readily to the view that behavioral difficulties may best be explained and manipulated through the application of the laws and procedures of learning. . . . Eventually, from such a rationale, *programs* of treatment . . . might be devised for dealing with behavior disorders. Thus, if a person exhibited a deficit in social behaviors, a gradual program for training such behaviors might seem appropriate. A program for establishing work skills and general work habits might be another. In many cases the development of, or change in, the functional language might be indicated, and so on. The problems of behavioral disorders when described in learning terms seem to involve many areas of training, and the types of learning programs that would seem necessary to solve those problems might eventually be large in number. . . . (Staats, 1963a, pp. 506–508)

We can see in this one PB excerpt the basis for an interest in training social skills and assertiveness, work skills, and for considering self-reinforcement problems, all of which later became focuses of interest in the new behavior therapy development. The analysis, importantly, helped introduce the necessity of therapy to produce adjustive types of behavior. Available studies concentrated on reducing abnormal behavior symptoms (see Allyon & Michael, 1959; Eysenck, 1960a; Raymond, 1960; Walton, 1960). PB's call for a behavioral clinical psychology helped stimulate the many works that did indeed establish that field.

The next year a PB collection was published (Staats, 1964) that presented a range of studies applying conditioning principles to the study of human behavior. One part, entitled "Behavioral Treatment," presented the original studies that I felt showed clearly the functioning of behavior principles and could be used as models. This included the work of Ayllon and Michael (1959) and Ayllon and Haughton (1962), showing how symptomatic behaviors of schizophrenics could be decreased or produced through reinforcement principles, a study showing that speech could be reinstated in two mute schizophrenics through reinforcement (Isaacs, Thomas, & Goldiamond, 1960), and a study showing that crying at bedtime could be decreased using extinction (Williams, 1959).

The 1963 and 1964 PB books were followed by more specialized behavioral collections of studies aimed specifically at the clinical field. Thus, Ulman and Krasner (1965) not only added additional studies for the growing behavioral audience to peruse, but also dubbed the emerging field "behavior modification." Their book consisted largely of case studies involving one subject, treating problem behaviors that had inadvertently been reinforced and needed to be extinguished, weakened by punishment, or replaced by normal behaviors that were made stronger by reinforcement, principles advanced in the first PB analysis (Staats, 1957a). Not all of the studies were clear in their analysis of the problem behavior (as was true also of Wolpe, 1958) or in the procedures that were employed, but they dealt with a variety of cases, such as those already described, plus anorexia (Bachrach, Erwin, & Mohr, 1965), hysterical blindness (Brady & Lind, 1961), and tics (Barrett, 1962), as well as a number that dealt with problem behaviors in children. Krasner and Ullmann also organized a series of talks, at the Palo Alto Veterans Administration Hospital, where the nucleus of the new American "behavior modifiers" described their programs of work. These papers were published as chapters of another behavior modification book (Krasner & Ullmann, 1965).

My talk in the 1963 Krasner-Ullmann series described the behavior modification work I had done since 1957 as well as the token reinforcer system I had developed for children. The system had been disseminated to Jack Michael in 1958 and to Teodoro Ayllon in 1961 with the suggestion that he use it in training functional behaviors in psychotics. Ayllon and Azrin (1968) at Anna State Hospital, introduced a token reinforcer system (token economy) and demonstrated that patient behaviors—such as self-care and daily routine endeavors—could be maintained by such reinforcement. Atthowe and Krasner (1968) also set up a token economy in a psychiatric ward and studied the effects on such behavior. These were critical studies in extending behavior principles to adults. In this period the field of behavior modification exploded into many studies. Conditioning principles, sometimes with token systems, were applied to stuttering and fluency (Lanyon & Barocas, 1975), dropping out of treatment (Baekeland & Lundwall, 1975), neurotic depression (Hersen, Eisler, Alford, & Agras, 1973), fluid overload in a hemodialysis patient (Barnes, (1976), stopping smoking (Elliot & Tighe, 1968), drug abuse (Boudin, 1972), social skills training (McFall & Twenty-man, 1973), antilitter procedures (Chapman & Risley, 1974), job-finding (Jones & Azrin, 1973), elimination of vomiting (Azrin & Wesolowski, 1975), teacher attending behavior (Cooper, Thomson, & Baer, 1970), chronic cough (Alexander, Chai, Creer, Micklich, Renne, & Cardoso, 1973), delusional and hallucinatory speech (Davis, Wallace, Liberman, & Finch, 1976), spasmodic and congestive dysmenorrhea (Chesney & Tasto, 1975), fecal incontinence (Engel, Nikoomanesh, & Shuster, 1974), increasing heterosexual responsiveness (Barlow & Agras, 1973), and many others. From the early direct use of conditioning principles and procedures various techniques were elaborated including methods of practicing skills, videotapes, watching models, contingency contracts, demonstrations, and so on. And improved methods were introduced for study of functional behaviors with single subjects in the naturalistic situation, such as AB and ABA experimental designs and time sampling.

Today behavior therapy includes many practitioners and many researchers and is an established field with many hundreds of works, case studies, experiments, research methodologies, clinical procedures, behavioral assessment instruments, therapies, and theories—with more produced each month. A modern textbook in behavior therapy includes chapters in obesity and eating disorders (Craighead & Kirkley, 1994), sexual dysfunctioning (LoPiccolo, 1994), pain and stress management (Keefe & Beckham, 1994), addictive behaviors (Larimer & Marlatt, 1994), treatment of schizophrenia (Bellack & Mueser, 1994), and social skills training (Dow, 1994). There were various sources that began this tradition; and it is significant that PB is one of them. There is clear continuity of tradition, but it has been greatly elaborated by many behavioral psychologists contributing many new elements.

Studies with Children

Behavior modification work with children is widely considered also to have derived from Skinner's work. Actually, there is almost no mention in his works (Skinner, 1948, 1953, 1957) of analyses of children's learning. The early work with children that derived from Skinner's behaviorism dealt with laboratory samples of simple behaviors using the method of experimental analysis of behavior that was projected as the only method (Azrin & Lindsley, 1956; Bijou, 1955, 1957; Gewirtz & Baer, 1958).

In both respects PB was significantly different. I was convinced from my analyses and works that conditioning principles applied not only to adult behavior but also to child learning. For example, in 1956 I made a reinforcement analysis of the problem of getting a child to use a prosthetic arm, which an occupational therapist employed successfully. This was supportive, but involved simple behavior. I concluded that, to really demonstrate the value of conditioning principles, it was necessary to demonstrate how complex functional human behavior and problems of human behavior could be treated using those principles. I thus considered various problems that could be dealt with in this framework. I had already entered a major study of language, and previously had worked with children with reading problems. Reading was complex and problems of reading were very serious. So this became a PB focus of study.

The basic conception was that some young children do not learn to read because they are not adequately prepared by previous learning and because of inadequate reinforcement for working at the task. By 1958, when other behavioral works were just beginning to study only simple behaviors, I and my associates[1] had already completed a study on reading in a public school, in which adolescent children participated over a period of several months. That study served as the foundation for securing a U.S. Office of Education research grant for the study of reading and problems

---

[1] Judson Finley, Karl Minke, Richard Schutz, and Carolyn Staats.

of reading. This PB program of research had an influence on the development of child behavior therapy, in several different areas.

Developmental Disorders. The 1958 study—disseminated but not published—done with adolescent dyslexic children in a public school, showed that these children, who had been "problem learners," became conscientious students when my token reinforcer system was used in conjunction with reading materials that I designed according to behavior principles. Each reading response was reinforced by tokens, backed up by material reinforcers the subjects selected (sporting equipment, clothing, tickets to movies, whatever). The study provided powerful support for the efficacy of the token-reinforcer system as a general tool. A subsequent study with four-year-olds involved learning to read single words, followed by learning to read the words in sentences, followed by these elements appearing in short stories (see Staats, Staats, Schutz, & Wolf, 1962). Reinforcement was presented sometimes (A) and not presented other times (B) to yield an AB design with some subjects and an ABA design with others. It was clearly shown that reinforcement was crucial. Even preschoolers could learn well if reinforced. Various studies were conducted in this program (see also Collette-Harris & Minke, 1978; Ryback & Staats, 1970; Staats & Butterfield, 1965; Staats, Finley, Minke, & Wolf, 1964; Staats, Minke, & Butts, 1970), showing that reading learning problems can be prevented by the use of good learning conditions and can be treated through changing to those conditions. Children with severe learning problems increased in tested reading achievement, school attendance, and in grades as a result of the PB treatment, and classroom conduct problems decreased.

In the course of the research program these behavior therapy methods were applied to different types of children who had reading problems—culturally deprived, mentally retarded, dyslexic, conduct disordered, and emotionally disturbed children. Moreover, PB projected the need for extending the token-reinforcer methods and behavior analytic principles widely to "special populations of children" (Staats, 1963a, p. 456). I specifically said that "many children labeled as mental retardates or autistic children are only victims of poor training conditions" (Staats, 1963a, p. 456) and that "[t]he present methods would seem to be useful in the study of the acquisition of complex behavioral repertoires of immediate significance to human adjustment . . . e.g., remedial reading programs, the training of autistic children, . . . deaf children, mutes, etc." (Staats, Finley, Minke, & Wolf, 1964, pp. 146–147). I also said that these methods could be used by various professionals—teachers, social workers, child psychologists, and clinicians—as well as subprofessionals. In addition to reading, the research program included number concepts, arithmetic, and writing, and the need for further work in these areas was also projected. Figure 8.1

312 *Behavior and Personality*

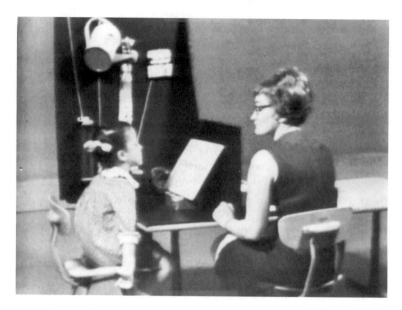

FIGURE 8.1 The PB child learning apparatus. A graduate student using one of the procedures in training a culturally deprived four-year-old child to read the numbers. The numbers (1 to 10) are on the large card, the trainer is randomly naming the numbers and the child responds by pointing to the appropriate number and repeating its name. The tokens (marbles) are delivered via a chute in the apparatus into the box that is behind the card. The tokens are placed by the child into one of the containers beneath the particular toy she wishes to work for. The card also partially obscures a window in the apparatus within which smaller cards with typed letters, words, or numbers can be shown for training in reading, number discriminations, counting, and such.

shows a four-year-old child involved in learning to read, using the PB token-reinforcer methodology and apparatus (see Staats, 1963a, 1968a).

This theoretical-empirical-methodological development provided a blueprint for extending behavioral methods widely to the treatment of children's problems. No other behavioral or social learning theory work provided that blueprint. The PB studies were included in many behavior modification readings books (for example, Ashem & Poser, 1973; Becker, 1971; Graubard, 1969; Harris, 1972). They were recognized as beginning the child behavior modification area (O'Leary & Drabman, 1971), which led into the contemporary developmental disabilities area in the field of behavior analysis. This area was later elaborated by radical behaviorists (see Sulzer-Azeroff & Mayer, 1986), who used the behavioral methods of training in research in arithmetic, writing, spelling, written composition and oral communication, handwriting, and school attendance—and was considered to have sprung from radical behaviorism. But the PB developments of the 1950s and 1960s became one of the foundations of behavior analysis as well as behavior therapy. One area that was influenced is now called classroom management.

Classroom Management. Montrose Wolf, who had contributed as a graduate assistant from 1960–1962 in some of the PB studies with children, played a very influential role in combining the PB developments with radical behaviorism in a manner that led to continuing research development. Following his Ph.D. at Arizona State University, Wolf went to the University of Washington where he introduced the PB token reinforcer procedures to the work there dealing with programmed instruction applied to mental retardates (see Birnbrauer, Bijou, Wolf, & Kidder, 1965). This project had been obtaining "[l]ittle, if any, improvement in sustained studying behavior" but introduction of the PB token reinforcer system "did indeed establish and maintain higher rates of effective study and greater cooperation" (Bijou, Birnbrauer, Kidder, & Tague, 1966, p. 512). With respect to the teaching materials, "instruction in sight vocabulary [was] patterned after the work of Staats, Staats, Schutz, & Wolf (1962)" (Bijou, 1965, p. 73).

Having first introduced the reading training with public school children, the behavioral training methods and token reinforcer system of PB were projected for use "in various situations, such as settlement houses, homes for juvenile delinquents, prison training programs, parts of adult education, and so on" (Staats & Butterfield, 1965, p. 939). Wolf went on to the faculty of the radical behaviorism program at the University of Kansas, where his student, Elery Phillips (1968) had a group of juvenile delinquents live in his home organized around doing academic studying and other tasks under a token reinforcer system. Called Achievement Place, this work was extended into a long-term treatment facility (Wolf, Phillips, Fixen, Braukman, Kirigan, Willner, & Schumaker, 1976).

Others began to introduce reinforcement methods into classrooms. Wolf and his associates (Allen, Hart, Buell, Harris, & Wolf, 1964; Harris, Johnston, Kelley, & Wolf, 1964) modified children's behavior to solve problems in the nursery school setting. There were works to extend this (Bushell, Wrobel, & Michaelis, 1968) and a number of studies were done demonstrating how misbehavior in the classroom could be dealt with using reinforcement principles (see Fargo, Behrns, & Nolen, 1970). Wolf and his associates also helped introduce the token reinforcer system to the classroom as a means of improving academic behavior (MacKenzie, Clark, Wolf, Kothera, & Benson, 1968). Today there are many studies that have extended treatment methods that are built around the tradition of using PB token reinforcer methods in the classroom to increase academic achievement.

Direct instruction employs general case programming, antecedent arrangements within classrooms and within teacher–student interactions, and reinforcing

consequences, including teacher approval and point systems. . . . [This] has
been replicated across numerous content areas (e.g., reading, mathematics,
language, science, logic), across different populations (e.g., regular and special
education students, including those with severe handicaps) . . . and across age
levels (e.g., preschool through secondary-aged students) . . . [G]ains on academic tests and in classroom behavior have resulted. (Walker, Greenwood, &
Terry, 1994, p. 229)

This large field of behavior therapy embodies the early PB blueprint,
although now that tradition is widely thought to have derived from radical
behaviorism (see Walker, Greenwood, & Terry, 1994).

Behavior Problems and Behavior Management. The PB research program also concerned problem behaviors in children other than those of
academic achievement. For example, PB presented the first behavioral
analysis of eating problems (see Staats, 1963a, pp. 373–377). This initial
analysis was later supported in the work of Browning and Stover (1971) and
behavioral work on this problem still continues (Rickert, Sottolano,
Parrish, Rileyk, Hunt, & Pelco, 1988). The first full behavioral analysis of
what is involved in toilet skills, how the skills are learned and can be
trained, and how the learning can go awry, was made in PB (see Staats, 1963a,
pp. 377–379). This analysis, as with others, was based upon the author's
work with his own daughter's toilet training. Giles and Wolf (1966) established toilet training in several retarded subjects by similar reinforcement
procedures. Foxx and Azrin (1973) systematically studied this area and
produced a rapid toilet-training program that could also be used with
retarded children.

The general problem of socially controlling the child's behavior was analyzed in PB in terms of the manner in which the child learns not to do
things she wants to do and to do things she does not want to do (Staats,
1963a, pp. 384–386). Central in the account were how language stimuli
come to exert that control through reinforcement principles. The PB
account indicated that children who have not learned such social controls
are considered to exhibit the "behavior problems" of conduct disorder
(Staats, 1963a, pp. 479–483), adding that "[the] defective verbal control of
behavior plays a part in other forms of maladjustment" (p. 480).

This was part of the general PB position that problems of children's
behavior generally arise in the faulty application of reinforcement principles (Staats, 1963; Staats & Staats, 1962; Staats, Finley, Minke, & Wolf, 1962;
Staats, Staats, Schutz, & Wolf, 1962). Wolf and his associates enlarged the
context by treating other problems of children. For example, Harris, Johnston,
Kelley, and Wolf (1964) analyzed and corrected the teachers' inadvertent
reinforcement of a nursery-school child crawling in class, rather than stand-

ing erect. These studies suggested that additional problem cases be found and treated in the school setting. Patterson (1965) decreased the rate of inappropriate disruptive behavior in the classroom by giving token-reinforcers for intervals that were free of such problem behaviors. Following this period child behavior modification studies multiplied rapidly (see Ashem & Poser, 1973; Becker, 1971; Graubard, 1969; Harris, 1972). Studies of the use of reinforcement procedures for changing undesirable behaviors in children in various settings continue to constitute an important part of the field (Iwata, Pace, Kalser, Cowdery, & Cataldo, 1990; Kazdin, 1994; Rolider & Van Houten, 1985).

Parent Training (Management). As will be indicated additionally further on, detailed research using conditioning principles in child raising was begun with PB in 1960. That work and the formal behavior modification studies conducted in PB were the foundations for the general PB position I summarized in the chapter "Child Development and Training" (Staats, 1963a, pp. 366–411). This was the first detailed behavioral analysis of the development of the child's behavior and the manner in which the parent is involved in that development. Analyses were presented of how the parent trains the child in sensory-motor development, feeding (including the creation of feeding problems), toilet training and toilet problems, crying and problems of crying, independent and dependent behavior, social control and lack thereof, social reasoning (good and bad), sex behavior and problems of sex behavior, working behavior, language, and others. The PB account also dealt with the parents' use of punishment. Finally, after presenting these analyses, PB advanced the position that the parent, whether intending to or not, *is the trainer of the child*. There was no corresponding material in either radical behaviorism or social learning theory works of that time, and PB subsequently elaborated that position (Staats, 1968a, 1971a, 1975).

> [The] learning analysis of the acquisition of behavior leads to a focus upon the parent as a *trainer* . . . [who] manipulates many conditions of learning that will determine . . . the behaviors the child will acquire. . . . [T]he parent could be an active participant in arranging circumstances to most efficaciously produce an abundant, rich, adjustive behavioral repertoire. . . . Faced with a training task of such imposing responsibilities, it would seem that the parent would need an understanding of the principles of behavior by which children learn . . . an analysis . . . of the various specific training problems he faces . . . [and] how not to shape undesirable behaviors, or, when they have developed, how to decrease them benignly. (Staats, 1963a, pp. 412–413)

This account could only present a small part of what had been found in PB research that applied its learning principles and procedures to raising children. One general position was that the child who thereby learns a rich set of BBRs is advantaged when going to school, the child whose training produces sparse BBRs is disadvantaged. One goal was to demonstrate empirically that suitably trained adults, following well-worked-out training methods, could successfully conduct training that produces complex and important repertoires in the child. This was done in a series of studies, beginning by having graduate students with no special experience with children train four-year-olds in reading, arithmetic, and writing repertoires (Staats, Brewer, & Gross, 1970; Staats, Staats, Schutz, & Wolf, 1962; Staats, Minke, Finley, Wolf, & Brooks, 1964; Staats, Finley, Minke, & Wolf, 1964). Additional studies showed that the PB method of reading training could be successfully employed by volunteer housewives and other non-professional personnel (Staats & Butterfield, 1965; Staats, Minke, Goodwin, & Landeen, 1967; Staats, Minke, & Butts, 1970). At this time the general position in the fields of education and clinical psychology was that parents should not try to be their children's therapists and teachers. Ryback and Staats (1970), however, showed explicitly that when using specified and systematic materials and procedures average parents could successfully work with their reading-disordered children—even those this involves a complex repertoire, not just simple behaviors. One child had been diagnosed as mentally retarded, another to have emotional problems, another to have a learning disability with minimal cerebral dysfunction. In child training that varied from 35 hours to 65 hours, the parents used the PB materials and procedures to produce in their children increases of at least one grade level in reading skill on a standardized test. Thus, the PB concern with parents as trainers of their children began in 1960 with systematic work with the author's children. In lectures in 1963 I played an audiotape where I was using my token-reinforcer system to train my two-year-old daughter to read. This work was extended in formal studies with other children and other adults as trainers. The general aim of providing training to parents was specifically indicated (see Staats, 1963a).

> [T]he weakest link in the child's cognitive development and in our educational system . . . [is that w]e leave the training of the various aspects of the *basic behavioral repertoires* in the hands of individuals [parents] who have no special training with respect to what the child needs in his basic behavioral repertoire, or of the principles by which the repertoire is acquired, or indeed of methods to produce the learning. . . . [O]ne of the purposes of the [PB] analyses is to produce information yielding training procedures appropriate for utilization by parents (Staats, 1968a, pp. 467–468). It is suggested that the use of these materials can be expected to constitute preventive treatment of central problems of child behavior and child development. Moreover, the materials can be used as behavior modification methods by parents whose children have already developed problems of development. (Staats, 1971a, pp. viii–ix)

This development within PB was taken up by the burgeoning field of behavior modification. Although not with parents, Wolf showed that nursery-school staff could be taught how to use behavior principles in dealing with simple problem behaviors (see Harris, Johnston, Kelley, & Wolf, 1964; Hart, Allen, Buell, Harris, & Wolf, 1964.) Another step toward providing parents with training information was taken in a study by Hawkins, Peterson, Schweid, and Bijou (1966). The mother was signaled when to reinforce her four-year-old boy with attention and approval, and when to tell him to cease an undesirable behavior, as well as when to use a time-out procedure. Although the child had been uncontrollable, the parent-training program was effective in reducing undesirable behavior and increasing desirable behavior.

O'Leary, O'Leary, and Becker (1967) had someone trained in behavior modification work with two siblings to reduce their aggressive behaviors and increase their cooperative behavior. Then the maintenance of the improved interaction was turned over to the mother. Zeilberger, Sampen, and Sloane (1968) trained a mother in the home in how to use time-out for inappropriate behavior, to praise appropriate behaviors, and to ignore minor disruptive behaviors. The objectives that were attained were to decrease physical aggression and to increase following instructions in the four-year-old child. Andronico and Gueney (1967) also studied how parents could be used for therapeutic purposes with respect to the school situation.

Another program that fed into this development was that of Patterson, beginning with interest in the parents and the peers of delinquents as reinforcing agents for children (Patterson, 1959, 1963). The focus was on the relative reinforcement value of such people, and on how responsive the child is to the reinforcement value of others (see Patterson, 1965a), rather than on the manner in which parents train their children in important types of behavioral repertoires. However, his work later turned to a concern with problems of aggressive behavior and the child's experience in the coercive home (Patterson, 1976) and to the role of parent training in treating such problems (Patterson, 1985). Wahler and Foxx (1980) provided a family-treatment package for dealing with children with aggressive behavior.

The continuity between the early PB developments and contemporary behavior therapy can be seen in another example. PB's analysis of child behavior problems emphasized the importance of the child's language development, especially that of following instructions, an analysis based on how the child learns the verbal-motor repertoire. It was said the child learned such "compliance" by virtue of training involving reinforcement principles. "Ordinarily, a child receives many trials where in the presence of such verbal stimuli as 'Stop that please'; 'I'm sorry, I'm using this now'; 'I am already playing with this toy'; 'you will have to be quiet now'; 'leave that alone'; 'don't touch that'; 'that belongs to me'; he will not be reinforced for the on-going behavior" (Staats, 1963a, pp. 384–386).

Let us say that a child requests a piece of candy before dinner. . . . [Then] the
parent says, "No, you can't have candy before dinner," [but] the child . . . continues . . . to wheedle, to whine, and finally to cry. If the parent does not
reward this behavior . . . [the parent's words] will [come to] control "desisting" behavior. . . . [But] if the behavior is rewarded the parent will have trained
the child to respond in a very inappropriate way. (Staats, 1971a, pp. 75–76)

The continuity can be seen in the following description of an ongoing work.

When a parent issues an undesirable command to a child (e.g., "go to bed"),
the child is likely to respond by whining, protesting, and refusing to comply
with the command. Some parents "give in," or remove the command, in order
to stop the protesting. Unfortunately, they also unintentionally reinforce the
very behavior they are attempting to avoid. (Wierson & Forehand, 1994, p. 146)

These authors have provided a training program for parents by which to
teach them how to train their children in this very important area. Let me
mention a few others of the many studies showing that many parents need
to be trained in behavioral ways of training their children. Moran and
Whitman (1991) have presented evidence that parents can be trained in
how to train their autistic children as have Laski, Charlop, and Schreibman
(1988) and others. Moran and Whitman (1985) have also employed a play-
oriented parent-training program for mothers of retarded children. Sanders
and Glynn (1981) trained parents in behavioral management procedures.
The continuity from the PB beginnings is clear, although today many of
those who work in the area consider their work to have derived from the
radical behaviorism tradition.

Autism and Other Childhood Disorders

The early PB framework involved the straightforward application of behavior principles and was thus very compatible with radical behaviorism. This
has been illustrated in several lines of behavior modification that involved
PB/radical behaviorism combinations. The same applies to another line of
research. That is, Lovaas had an experimental research program at the
University of Washington, working on such topics as the interaction between
verbal and non-verbal behavior (Lovaas, 1961), the effect on food intake of
being conditioned to say food words (Lovaas, 1964), and the cue properties of words (Lovaas, 1964). He employed Skinner's experimental analysis
of behavior technology as applied to a simple laboratory response. The PB
program, however, beginning in 1958, involved working with individual
children in producing functional language development in the *naturalistic*
situation (see Staats, 1963a, 1968a, 1971a). This development stipulated
the principles and conditions that apply to normal language development
in the child. When Montrose Wolf went to the University of Washington,

one of his central works involved applications of the child behavior modification principles to treating real behaviors of an autistic child and included concerns with creating normal behaviors (Risely & Wolf, 1967; Wolf,
Risely, & Mees, 1964). Lovaas and his associates later began a long-term,
extensive study of autistic children, first to reduce undesirable behaviors
and then to produce desirable behaviors (Lovaas, Berberich, Perloff, &
Schaeffer, 1966; Lovaas, Freitag, Nelson, & Whalen, 1967). Skinner (1957)
said very little about how to train children in language repertoires, whereas PB presented principles, analyses, and empirical methods and findings
on this subject matter. PB dealt with the conditions of learning and indicated that its training procedures applied to autistic children (see Staats,
1963a, 1968a, 1971a). Although his program progressively began dealing
with how autistic children could be trained in language repertoires in the
manner dealt with in PB, Lovaas has considered his orientation to be that
of radical behaviorism. Lovaas' project has trained many behavior therapists in working with autistic children, has devised techniques for working
with such children, and has shown in detail how such children are capable
of learning that repairs deficits and moves them in the direction of normality (Lovaas, 1977). Various other behavior therapists have set up similar
programs to provide therapeutic training to autistic children (Schreibman,
1994) and this development constitutes one of the most impressive achievements of behavior therapy.

Sex Behavior and Sexual Problems. Psychological behaviorism made the
first behavioral analysis of the learning of sex behavior and how problems
can occur in that learning (Staats, 1963a, pp. 398–403). This analysis
described how the child learns her sex identity—considered behaviorally as
the stimuli that come to have sexual reinforcing value for the individual.
The problem of restraining sex behavior without creating problems of later
sexual activity were described, as well as a framework for preventing such
problems. The analysis recognized that, in addition to the learning with
respect to what will be sexually arousing, the individual must learn sex
behavior, and the individual must learn the behaviors that get the individual into sexual situations where the sex behaviors can be learned. "[V]ari-
ous types of social behaviors must be acquired if the individual is to
"obtain" the customary sex reinforcers [such as] dating, courting, recreational and sports skills with both sexes, work behaviors, and so on" (Staats,
1963a, p. 401).

A behavioral approach to sexual dysfunction later developed that remains
one of the field's active areas (see LoPiccolo, 1994). The area focuses on
dealing with problems after they have arisen. As valuable as this work is, the
field needs systematic behavioral study of how sexual "identities" and
"misidentities" and sexual dysfunctions are learned. Such studies would

serve as the basis for materials for parents to employ with their children. As will be further indicated, prevention is a focus of psychological behavior therapy. Finally, PB's early call for work in training social skills also involved the PB analysis that social skills are basic to sex adjustment. Social skills training and its study has become one of the mainstays of behavior therapy (Dow, 1994).

These various developments occurred within the general behavioristic framework that abnormal behavior is learned and can be changed through manipulating conditioning principles. This constitutes an application of the basic principles of animal learning-behavior. Such applications are important but they are not sufficient, as will be indicated.

THE HUMAN LEARNING/COGNITIVE LEVEL

The second-generation behaviorisms, including Skinner's, are two-level behaviorisms. But the basic level of conditioning principles does not suffice in dealing with the various interests of behavior therapy. PB takes the position that lack of recognition of the multilevels of theory has brought different approaches into conflict with one another. Behavior analysis, for example, rejects the cognitive behaviorism approach for being "mentalistic." What is really involved is that radical behaviorism does not have the concepts and principles by which to behaviorize "cognitive" analyses. And the cognitive behaviorists, who employ radical behaviorism in the behavioral part of their interests, also have the same inability to connect conditioning principles with their interests in "cognitive" phenomena. So they are eclectic, using behavioral and cognitive concepts, but not relating them. The multilevel approach of PB, however, provides the means by which to understand "cognitive" phenomena and methods of treatment within a consistent theory of concepts and principles that includes basic conditioning principles. This section will concern the relevance of the human learning/cognitive level of study for behavior therapy.

To begin, when the emerging field of behavior therapy adopted Skinner's basic statement of the conditioning principles, it came also to adopt other features of this behaviorism, such as emphasis on the experimental-analysis-of-behavior methodology. Through the 1960s, thus, behavior therapy was restricted almost entirely to two-level works that involved extending a conditioning principle to the treatment of an explicit behavior problem. Thus, the animal model of study was adopted as *the* method for dealing with human behavior. Verbal psychotherapy was beyond the pale. That, however, was never the PB position. PB, because it had a different theory of language than Skinner's (1957), always differed from radical behaviorism in this area. The PB position was first indicated in a section entitled "Verbal Learning Psychotherapy" (Staats, 1963a, pp. 509–511).

> Traditional treatment [involves] . . . the psychological practitioner and the patient interacting on a verbal level. . . . [I]t should be possible for psychotherapy, in any of the areas of behavioral maladjustment . . . , to take place on a verbal level. Deficit behaviors, inappropriate behaviors, stimulus control, the reinforcer system, should all be accessible to change through verbal means. . . . Through verbal psychotherapy, reasoning sequences appropriate to physical and social events could be established . . . [as well as] the extinction of avoidance or anxiety responses. . . . (Staats, 1963a, pp. 509–511)

The new behavior therapists/analysts in 1963 were caught up with establishing that behavior problems could be treated using conditioning principles. Psychological behaviorism, which already had a decade of human behavioral research, had advanced beyond that to include an interest in changing behavior through language. This was one of the differences that separated radical behaviorism and psychological behaviorism, and it was another decade before the field of behavior therapy came to accept that verbal psychotherapy should not be rejected.

The PB position was that its human learning principles—in addition to the basic conditioning principles—had direct applications to the treatment of human problems. Unlike radical behaviorism, one of PB's focal developments was study of the language repertoires, what they are, how they are learned, and how they *function* to affect the individual's experience, learning, and behavior. Psychological behaviorism treated how they functioned interpersonally, as in communication, and intrapersonally in such things as problem solving, originality, and creativity (see Staats, 1963a, 1968a). This advancing framework suggested that *how the language repertoires function intrapersonally concerns, in good part, the phenomena studied in cognitive psychology*, hence the title *Learning, Language and Cognition* in one PB work (Staats, 1968a). Finally, a specialized article introduced the terms "language behavior therapy" and its synonym "cognitive behavior therapy" (Staats, 1972). What was called language (cognitive) behavior therapy outlined the ways in which the individual's language repertoires could be employed to change the individual's behavior, in the traditional "talk" psychotherapy setting.

As an example, one of PB's developments at the human learning level of study is the method of language conditioning of emotion, whereby emotional words are paired with new stimuli and the latter thereby come to elicit an emotional response. Hekmat (1972, 1973, 1974; Hekmat & Vanian, 1971) began using the language conditioning method in the context of clinical treatment. With snake-phobic subjects the word "snake" was paired with positive emotional words. The result was the negative emotional response of the subject to the word snake, and to snakes themselves, was attenuated, and the subjects then more closely approached and touched an actual snake. This can be considered the first and important empirical demonstration in the clinical context that *behavior* change can be obtained through human learning principles and language behavior therapy methods, by changing emotion. Early (1968) in social psychology, also employed PB's language conditioning methods to change positively the emotional response and thus approach behaviors, of students in a class, toward an isolate child.

The PB analysis added that changing the emotional value of words would also change their other two functions (reinforcing and directive). Let us take the case of a teenager who wants to quit school and get a job. A parent, counselor, or therapist, in describing in very positive words the advantages of educational achievements, and in negative words the disadvantages of lack of education, can change the emotional value of the teenager's considerations. And the change in emotional value of the alternative plans will change their directive (incentive) value. Hekmat (1974) showed that language conditioning that changes the emotional value of a word will also make that word into a reinforcing stimulus.

The important principle involved can be generalized to state that *what the individual will find reinforcing can be changed in verbal psychotherapy.* The PB analysis further indicated that various human problems involve changing the things that elicit an emotional response in the individual and hence are reinforcers and incentives for the individual. For example, because children elicit a positive sexual response in the pedophile, he approaches them and is reinforced by his contact with them. The problem can be reversed if children cease to elicit a sexual emotional response in the individual, as Raymond (1960) showed with a sexual fetish, using primary conditioning. PB development shows that emotional change can be effected through language interactions in psychotherapy, potentially in a more effective, broader, more profound manner than that which can be produced through primary conditioning.

Generally, people with problems of sex identity have sexual emotional responses to the wrong (culturally defined) sex objects. As another example, the person who has an anxiety disorder suffers, in part, because she has negative emotional responses to inappropriate types of stimuli. The depressed person is "depressed" because she lacks stimuli that elicit positive emotional responses and has too many stimuli that elicit negative emotional responses. The sociopath, on the other hand, has a problem in that her words and the words of others—words that would lead to not doing certain things—do not elicit the negative emotional responses they should. And there are many other clinical problems that involve deficit or inappropriate emotions. Such problems can be treated by changing emotional responses or by creating new ones. The most effective and general way of producing such changes can be through use of language.

Psychological behaviorism, moreover, because of its theories of language and emotion, can incorporate and interrelate other existing behavior therapy treatments into its explanatory framework. Systematic desensitization, for example, may be considered in these terms. Desensitization involves establishing a list of words that elicit negative emotional (phobic) images in the patient. The words are ordered and then used to evoke the images progressively, with weakly feared images coming first. The client must remain relaxed while experiencing the image. This relaxation experience amounts to extinction trials, in which the emotional response to the images is lessened by repeated presentation (evocation). "It is important to note that it is no different in operative principles to have a person relax when considering anxiety producing topics in systematic desensitization than it is to have the individual speak of anxiety producing topics in the 'non-threatening,' relaxed interaction of client-centered therapy—regardless of the differing theoretical frameworks" (Staats, 1972, p. 174). The same may be said of rational-emotive therapy. An objective is to change the individual's irrational emotional responses to stimuli, and this is done through language interactions with the therapist—following, it is suggested, the principles of language conditioning. The major point here, however, is that the ways the individual's general emotional responding can be changed in psychotherapy constitutes one of the central aspects of clinical treatment. We need to obtain a deep understanding of what is involved, and psychological behavior therapy (PBT) offers the principles and concepts by which to do so.

The same is true of the other language repertoires. Another example in the language behavior therapy analysis is that of the verbal-motor repertoire.

> . . . [V]erbal instructions can serve to produce new learning, new behavioral skills, in the individual. . . . There are types of psychotherapy that extensively employ verbal means to elicit instrumental responses in the individual (Ellis, 1967; Thorne, 1950) and assertive training includes this mechanism. (Staats, 1972, pp. 169–170)

This is true of social skills training, sex therapy, and the various areas of cognitive behavior therapy that involve verbal instructions. Words (in the verbal-motor repertoire) are used in a wide number of clinical treatments for the purpose of eliciting (directing) the patient's behavior.

One more example will be given here of a human learning principle involving language that is relevant for the consideration of psychotherapy. The principle is that the individual's own words will have the same effect on the individual's behavior as will the words of someone else. An early PB analysis of a violent episode in a schizophrenic involved his delusion—a complex of language responses—that mediated his overt behavior (Staats, 1963a, p. 387). The same behavioral mechanism is involved in activities described as problem solving, reasoning, planning, and intention (purpose), whether these are normal or abnormal. Such acts involve the problem (life) stimuli that elicit verbal-labeling responses in the individual. These verbal-labels themselves elicit verbal-association responses (that is, the individual's knowledge of the topic), and the verbal associations finally elicit the overt problem solving behaviors. (See Davis, 1973, pp. 55–56 for a summary of the PB theory of problem solving.)

It is relevant here to note that one of the prominent cognitive behavior therapy approaches is based on a similar analysis of problem solving. D'Zurilla and Goldfried (1971) take the position that clients—individuals with problems—have deficits in their problem-solving skills. Thus, a primary goal of therapy is to teach the patient those skills in a verbal psychotherapy type process. In the PB view when the individual inappropriately reasons, decides, problem-solves, plans, and so on, and displays inappropriate behavior as a consequence, this involves the individual's language-cognitive characteristics. Changing those language-cognitive repertoires ordinarily is most efficaciously accomplished in verbal interactions such as psychotherapy. More will be said of this in treating the personality level of study.

A very closely related "cognitive behavior therapy" approach is that of "coping skills techniques" and "stress-inoculation training" (see Meichenbaum, 1977). The conceptual foundation of the approach is that there are skills—repertoires—by which individuals may mitigate their anxiety, pain, or stress responses. The skills include calming self-talk (Meichenbaum, 1977), techniques of relaxation (Suinn & Richardson, 1971), use of positive imagery techniques (Turner & Clancy, 1988), distraction techniques (McCaul & Malott, 1984), and positive self-evaluation (Meichenbaum, 1977). These techniques actually involve the use of language interactions with which to train the client to language repertoires that elicit positive emotional responses or that get the individual to perform responses (like attentional responses) that lessen negative emotional responses.

Psychological behaviorism provided a basic behaviorism that justifies (and projects) such cognitive–behavioral methods. Many cognitive behaviorists, however, take their basic behaviorism from radical behaviorism and combine those principles with inconsistent cognitive concepts, thereby producing eclectic combinations. While these works are individually valuable, they break themselves away from a unified conception and instead produce multiple rivalrous therapies. Moreover, an eclectic theory of cognitive behaviorism is not generally heuristic. Psychological behaviorism, in contrast, provides a framework within which the various cognitive and cognitive behavioral methods can be understood and extended, within a consistent and heuristic behavioral set of principles.

Radical behaviorism did not produce a work considering verbal psychotherapy until many years later (see Hamilton, 1988). It is only at the present moment that some behavior analysts (Dougher, 1993; Dougher &

Hackbert, 1994; Hayes & Wilson, 1994; Kohlenberg & Tsai, 1994) are first beginning to adopt the interests, procedures, and phenomena of language behavior therapy and cognitive and cognitive–behavioral approaches. To do this they are creating an eclectic theory language that has a behavior analytic flavor, but is actually non-behavioral. The result is a convoluted methodology that criticizes concepts in cognitive approaches but develops the same kinds of concepts itself. For example, Dougher (1994) accepts (inconsistently) the use of desensitization, drugs, and instructions, as a means of treating a problem of anxiety, but he does not accept the concept of anxiety. He thus rejects use of the concept of reducing anxiety (as employed in Ellis' rational-emotive approach), introducing rather the concept that it is necessary "to depotentiate disruptive contingencies" (p. 249). Thus, a concept of anxiety, which can be given good behavioral definition, is rejected in favor of introducing a radical-behaviorism-sounding concept and principle that have no behavioral definition. Dougher (as is the case with other behavior analysts) is an outstanding behaviorist and needs a more advanced basic behaviorism and theory methodology with which to conduct his important work.

The general point is that important developments in clinical psychology should be unified with behaviorism. That requires use of a behaviorism that has the tools for the job.

Projections of the Human Learning/Cognitive Level

Psychological behaviorism's analyses, backed up by human learning study, indicate that behavior can be changed (1) directly in psychotherapy through the therapist's verbal instructions; (2) indirectly by changing the patient's emotional responding; and (3) indirectly by changing the individual's own "cognitions," that is, language repertoires. In the present view, traditional psychotherapy, radical behaviorism, cognitive, and cognitive–behavioral approaches lack concepts and principles by which to analyze what occurs in psychotherapy. That leaves psychotherapy as an art rather than a science.

It is time that the field systematically study psychotherapy, within a theory framework that has principles and concepts with which to do so, derived from the basic principles of conditioning. PB provides a theory framework for that purpose, as well as prototypical empirical developments. PB says that psychotherapy is a language process in which the interchange of words by the patient and the therapist results in changes to the patient. Various advantages will stem from knowing explicitly what goes on in psychotherapy, as well as the principles involved. By means of that knowledge it will be possible to train psychotherapists in a standard, effective manner, as a science rather than an art. The more analytic knowledge will also offer other advantages, such as providing a means of deciding for what patients psychotherapy is or is not relevant. For example, the PB conception indicates theoretically that psychotherapy is not appropriate for subjects who do not have the requisite BBRs. On a practical basis it has been found that psychotherapy does not work well for those diagnosed with such things as schizophrenia, mental retardation, or antisocial personality disorder. PB indicates why, namely, that such individuals lack the language-cognitive and emotional-motivational repertoires to engage in and/or profit from the language exchanges that occur in psychotherapy. *Such an analysis suggests, heuristically, that tests of the language and emotion repertoires could be used diagnostically, as a means of deciding who will and who will not profit from psychotherapy.*

The PB position is that verbal psychotherapy is the use of language with which to change the individual's BBRs, that is, her experiencing, learning, and behavior. Key to study of psychotherapy is the human learning/cognitive level that provides the principles of how language functions.

THE CHILD DEVELOPMENT LEVEL

It is important to recognize that the field of child behavior therapy and the field of developmental disabilities in behavior analysis have been based, in good part, on extending the basic level of study to analyses of children's behavior problems. With respect to simple behaviors—for example, excessive crying, lisping, temper tantrums, refusing to go to sleep at night, acting-out in class, and aggressive or destructive behavior—a simple analysis in behavioral terms is sufficient. PB began its work with children employing the basic principles of conditioning and, as was indicated in the earlier section, there are many important studies in the field of behavior therapy that have the same foundation. Methods of study and programs of training have been devised within this framework that are valuable to both practitioner and parent.

But many problems of child development involve complex repertoires, not just simple behaviors. Skinner (1957) made an important contribution in suggesting that certain types of verbal behavior are operants. Ferster (1961) elaborated that, to indicate that autistic children did not use tacts. These accounts, however, did not indicate the large repertoires and the complex processes of learning involved. Furthermore, an analysis of the learning conditions is necessary to serve as a basis for empirical (including applied) development. Especially, the account of how the learning can go awry provides an explanation of behavior disorders, as well as a basis for treatment. It is that explanation that can be used for prevention. PB dealt in depth with how the parent can teach the child new words by using reinforcement, and also with how the child learns the verbal-imitation repertoire, which is central in further word learning (Staats, 1963a). PB indicated how deficits and inappropriacies in learning can underlie the development of behavior disorders, including autism (Staats, 1963a) and, in 1958, PB work began using its token reinforcer system to work on language deficits in dyslexia. Several years later this framework was further advanced by Lovaas, Berberich, Perloff, and Schaeffer (1966) in a study involving training of verbal imitation to autistic children that established a tradition of research. Behavior therapy programs (see Schreibman, 1994) have been devised for training autistic children in the verbal-imitation responses and then have used these responses to further train the child to verbal-labeling responses. The work in this area is the most advanced in behavior therapy with respect to dealing with complex behavior problems in children.

But this work has been carried out in the radical behaviorism tradition and thus has not been concerned with general questions of child development, for example, questions of the need for, and the content of, the general study of child development through learning. It is also the case that the traditional field of child development is not behaviorally oriented and does not provide the necessary foundation for the study of child learning. There is thus not a well-developed behavioral field of child development for behavior therapy to draw upon. The practice of behavior therapy needs knowledge of the various BBRs the child must acquire, the conditions of learning that are involved, the cumulative-hierarchical learning processes, how those processes can go awry, the effects that this has upon the development of the child, how to detect when the process is going awry, how to prevent that, and how to treat the various anti-learning problems that have already occurred. In each case there are large areas of study to be established. This knowledge is needed by the practitioner for transmission to the parent.

The point is that a general field of study is needed, with respect to normal children, as well as in the treatment of children with problems. Moreover, the content of what is studied must be elaborated in various ways. For example, with respect to language, Skinner's theory of verbal behavior (1957) is lacking. That large repertoires are involved that are learned is not addressed. The PB theory of language, to illustrate, describes repertoires, including the verbal-motor, verbal-emotional, and verbal-image repertoires, that are not treated in radical behaviorism. These analyses provide a framework calling for systematic development in the programs dealing with autistic children. The verbal-motor repertoire, for example, is centrally important in the child's acquisition of the other repertoires. It should be taught first when the child has language deficits.

Moreover, other important concerns are being overlooked because of restriction to Skinner's theory. For example, as has been indicated, it is generally recognized that autistic children typically do not show normal affectional responses to parents. Without an understanding of emotional conditioning and how emotion directs behavior, the radical behaviorism approach to treating this problem was to reinforce the *motor behavior* of approaching an adult. The child was given electric shock until the child climbed into the trainer's arms (Lovaas, Schaeffer, & Simmons, 1965). But the *behavior* is not the crucial problem; the problem is that the child does not have a strong positive emotional response to the parent, as most children do. Shocking the child, moreover, will only worsen that problem. The child needs appropriate *positive classical conditioning* in order to love the parent. Treatment of autism needs to address the deficits in such children's emotional-motivational BBR, and that demands knowledge of what the normal child's emotional-motivational BBR consists of, the principles by which this BBR is learned, and the *conditions* under which the BBR is learned—including the parents' role in that learning. That is what is needed by parents who wish to prevent their children from having deficits in the emotional-motivational BBR. And that is what is needed by the professionals and parents who must work with the child to repair deficits in that BBR.

We cannot fulfill our objectives of treating children, or teaching parents how to do so, without general knowledge of child development and a theory of child development. Unlike the traditional position (see Eysenck, 1960a, p. 11; Lovaas, 1966, pp. 111–112), PBT calls for development of a level of study of normal and abnormal child development through learning. Is it the responsibility of the field of behavior therapy to establish that basic field? The answer is yes if behavior therapy cannot prevail upon the traditional field of child development to do so. This conception will be supported in further discussions.

THE SOCIAL INTERACTION LEVEL

In the multilevel framework of psychological behaviorism it is important to study the manner in which humans are stimuli for each other and respond to each other. Moreover, this level of study, and its concepts and principles of social interaction, should be an important foundation for psychological behavior therapy, as will be illustrated.

Therapy as a Social Interaction

Psychotherapy is a social interaction between two people. To Freud's credit, within his system he displayed interest in the relationship between client and therapist. The psychoanalytic concepts of transference and countertransference emerged from that interest. The concept of transference is that the patient's feelings, acquired with respect to some central figure—typically a parent or lover, with whom there has been emotional conflict—is transferred to the therapist. It is important to get the patient to understand her transference toward the therapist.

Radical behaviorism and behavior therapy (see Eysenck, 1952), in wholesale rejection of psychoanalysis, have neglected to analyze its parts, such as transference. PB's view is that it is necessary to evaluate the elements of knowledge individually, not to reject *en masse*. As I have indicated (Staats, 1975), the concept of transference reflects both productive and unproductive characteristics of psychoanalysis. While psychoanalysis contains many errors, it was productive to note the phenomena of transference—that the individual's past experience with people has general effects. The task, then, is to utilize the phenomena of transference within a better set of principles. In PB theory, as an example, the patient and therapist have emotional responses to each other, depending upon the nature of their emotional-motivational BBRs, and this influences their behavior to each other. Because of stimulus generalization, how we learn to respond to our mothers will be reflected in how we respond to other women, including therapists. A patient, for example, who has learned to complain about a variety of problems because the parent has reinforced this type of language behavior, will also complain to the therapist who has features that are like the parent. With respect to the sensory-motor BBR, a woman who has learned to be seductive to men who are in an authority role, will behave in that manner to a male therapist who fits that role. Emotionally, a man patient who has a positive emotional response to intelligent, strong women will have such a response to a female therapist with those qualities.

Behaviorizing such concepts in PB places the study of psychotherapy in a more elaborate theory language than that of psychoanalysis, a theory language that has been established on the basis of systematic, elaborate, and explicit empirical evidence, with various methods for research. And this behaviorizing has implications, centrally, that psychotherapy involves a social interaction. Behavior therapists should understand the nature of psychotherapy as a social interaction, and this calls for systematic attention by the field. Not all patients are equally helped by psychotherapy, and a question that arises concerns the variability that can occur as a function of social interaction variables. For example, unusually good results are being reported for EMDR (Eye Movement Desensitization and Reprocessing) in which eye-movements are employed (see Hekmat, Edelstein, & Cook, 1994; Lohr, Kleinknecht, Conley, Cerro, Schmitt, & Sonntag, 1992). The therapy procedure has the aura of medical science procedures, and many patients (and therapists) have a positive emotional response to (confidence in) such procedures. Any increase in the positive emotional response of the patient to the therapy or therapist will enhance the control of the procedural stimuli in the therapy. Such a patient will consequently show greater improvement than a patient with a neutral or negative emotional response. These expectations could easily be studied, and the findings could help explain the success of such therapy as EMDR, as well as individual differences in response to therapy in general.

That is but an example. Social interaction in psychotherapy should be generally studied. What kinds of therapists go best with what kinds of patients and what kinds of problems? When is it more advantageous to have a female therapist or male, an older person versus a younger person, and so on? What can the therapist do to maximize social interaction variables in treating patients? How do the patient's ways of responding to the therapy interaction indicate the nature of problems the patient has with social interactions generally? It can be expected that the knowledge that results from studying such questions will be helpful to the practicing psychotherapist. An approach to psychotherapy that sets itself in a science framework that includes the study of social interaction must be expected to have advantages over an approach that does not. PB suggests that behavior therapy be set in such a framework.

Family Psychological Behavior Therapy

Recently, Gross (1992) examined the field of family therapy, and considered it to be in a state of crisis because of its theoretical disarray. He states that "Family therapy lacks a unified theoretical base" (Gross, 1992, p. 42), pointing out that, "Although most family therapists base their work on systems theory . . . , this approach has many limitations when it is related to human behavior" (Gross. 1992, p. 42). It lacks a theory of abnormal behavior and its development within the family, as well as a theory of how the family interactions have influenced that development. And it lacks a theory within which to integrate research studies of families, theoretical concepts and principles from models of family functioning, and developmental models of the family. "[S]ystems theory does not possess integrative concepts" (Gross, 1992, p. 43). Gross suggests that behavioral family therapy is a confused mixture of systems theory and behavior theory (Fallon, 1988), and that cognitive–behavior family therapy (Ellis & Harper, 1975) is limited, concerned only with irrational beliefs. Theories in this field are said to be practical guidelines, not unified theories. His solution is to develop "an overview of paradigmatic family behavior therapy . . . , based on the principles of paradigmatic [psychological] behavior therapy (Staats, 1990)" (Gross, 1992, p. 39).

> [The] theoretical framework . . . attempts to relate personality functioning
> with social and abnormal behavior in families on the basis of language processes
> and principles. Whereas this approach gives attention to the involvement of

personality repertoires in family functioning, other family therapy approaches seem to neglect the influence of personality on social behavior. As social environments are regarded as possessing affective, reinforcing, and directive properties, they may contribute to the development and maintenance of abnormal behavior. Furthermore, such behavior may influence social environments. Thus, PFT [paradigmatic family therapy] examines the bi-directional influence of individuals and social systems on each other. PFT also incorporates a clinical framework that can be linked with various family therapy techniques. PFT aims to relate unified therapeutic procedures with a comprehensive theory of family problems. (Gross, 1992, p. 39)

In addition to his theoretical analysis, Gross outlines the PFT approach to family therapy to consist of six steps. The first step is introductory and involves getting acquainted with family members and establishing a beginning schematic of them. The next step involves identification of the problems that bring the family to therapy. It may be added that this is a central process, since the different family members will have different views. Having those expressed and reaching a consensual view, which can be an elaborate process, can then provide the basis for Gross's next phase, that of setting goals for the therapy. Considering the goals then leads to the further conduct of the therapy into the action phase. Fully conducted PFT would include a feedback (or follow-up) phase, including evaluation.

> PFT borrows from and attempts to relate to other therapeutic techniques. In addition, it provides techniques such as family awareness, whereby persons learn to be sensitive to the workings of the family. . . . Therapeutic change in family functioning would be indicated by the modification of specific behaviors as well as changes in the broader and more stable dimensions of family functioning.

> Finally, the aims of PFT are to decrease the number of negative behaviors in the family, and to replace those behaviors with positive ones. These positive behaviors, such as social skills, may help family members to solve their own problems in the future. Thus, interaction could facilitate problem solving rather than escalating conflict. (Gross, 1992, pp. 58–59)

The PB antecedents to the behavior modification interest in training parenting skills has already been described. That research tradition has elaborated (see Danforth, Barkeley, & Stokes, 1991) and should be integrated into Gross' paradigmatic family therapy.

Psychological Behavior Therapy and Community Psychology

The focus of individual psychotherapy is on the person. Although it may be recognized that individuals develop their problems in a social context, the treatment is directed toward changing the individual. Group therapy involves a group, but it attempts, nevertheless, to treat problems of the individuals in the group, so the focus is still on the individual's change. Family therapy may take into account the nature of the family and problems of the family, and the goals may be to ameliorate those problems. So this represents a further step that involves the family as a group. Community psychology goes further along that dimension to a concern with society along with the individual (group or family), in terms of original cause as well as in terms of treatment. "[Community psychology] throws off the constraints of the doctor–patient medical model—the idea that mental disorder is a private misery—and relates the trouble, and the cure, to the entire web of social and personal relationships in which the individual is caught" (Smith, 1968. p. 19). Community psychology shifts focus from changing the individual to consideration of individual's and group's problems within the social milieu, using social agencies by which to effect change.

Impetus for community psychology arose with the decision to return patients to their communities rather than hospitalizing them in large state institutions. That did not solve the problem, of course, and agencies such as half-way houses, community mental health centers, crisis intervention and suicide-prevention centers, and other public agencies were established to treat those with problems. One good outcome of the unsolved problem of treating those with severe behavior problems is a focus on prevention of problems of behavior. Giving children in disadvantaged homes compensatory training in preschool is an example. Another interest is in identifying problems for treatment at an early time.

It can be seen from these few words that there is great harmony of viewpoint here with PB, which focuses on the cumulative-hierarchical learning of the BBRs and thus on the environment. And PB focuses on the present life circumstances as the other determinant of behavior, including behavior problems of a social as well as individual kind. PB analysis indicates that a mental hospital represents a poor method of treatment. Individuals are psychotic because they have devastating deficits and inappropriateness in their BBRs. Placing such individuals together, where they represent the primary social environment for each other, is a poor idea, because patients lack the BBRs needed to provide the learning conditions for each other that would constitute therapy. Brief interactions with hospital staff cannot make up for that social deficit.

More centrally, many times the deficit and inappropriate conditions that produce behavior problems are actually societal in nature. For example, in our society there are thousands of children raised in deficient homes and deficient communities.

> [T]he language-intellectual training of disadvantaged adults has left them with gaping deficits that are then passed on to their children. For example, the disadvantaged parent's language is very poorly developed. It is ungrammati-

cal, ungainly, sparse, and minimally functional. . . . Individuals with such poorly developed language would have great difficulty with most academic learning. They would also be incapable, without some additional input, of training their children to better intellectual skills than they themselves have. (Staats, 1971a, p. 331)

This statement was part of a chapter outlining the "social implications of the [PB] learning conception" (Staats, 1971a). It states that children raised in American ghetto conditions cannot get the social environment they need at home, and they cannot get it from their peers, because most of the children have the same deficit and inappropriate environments. So they all have the same problems of BBRs and consequently cannot get what they need from being in a good school. But there is a vicious circle involved. Their schools are poorly supported and the student population is largely composed of children with the same deficits. So they are not good in terms of the academic atmosphere and standards.

What is involved is a perpetuating social problem, passed from one generation to another through learning, not through genes as the traditional "biological" orientation suggests (see Herrnstein & Muray, 1994). Until society makes the decision to intervene in that perpetuating cycle, the problem will continue to exist in every generation.

> The preceding would suggest that one way to break into this vicious cycle would be through training and support of the disadvantaged parent. . . . Rather than giving inadequate welfare payments, society [could] provide a suitable living to the parent who undertakes [i]nstruction in child-training principles and methods of the type described herein [as well as in] intellectual training of various sorts. (Staats, 1971a, p. 331)

This is the PB answer to the contemporary disillusionment with welfare. Cutting welfare and forced work will not solve the problem of the generational "inheritance" of learning deficits. Putting additional money into schools would not be sufficient, for school success depends on the entering child's BBRs. The *only* remedy will be the correction of the BBR deficits that parents pass on to their children. A successful program must involve educating the parents and providing supporting day-care for the children that will also provide needed training. This will take public funding, but it will be funding that has an end, and it will show savings in lessened expenditures for police forces, prisons, and other public agencies. Moreover, in the long term it will be economical. A large expenditure up front would cure the social problem. The funds that are currently spent just "maintain" the problem. Continued generation after generation, the problem will cost much more, and contribute to an ineffective, non-competitive society as well.

Psychological behaviorism recognizes that many human problems are "social problems," that is, they emerge from the problems of society and will only be dealt with by changing society. The problem may reside in the deficit and inappropriate environments extended to groups of children—such as minority groups, the poor, the ignorant—as well as children with parents with personal problems of various kinds. Sometimes the problem resides in S_2—as is the case when the individual is competent but cannot secure employment. Such conditions may yield criminality, for example, when crime provides the best opportunities or the only opportunities. Social problems may also be compounded. For example, poverty helps produce drug use, criminalization of drugs then creates an illicit market, a criminal class of suppliers and merchants, the strengthening of gun usage, and political corruption, all of which make the problem more difficult. As another example, when a religion prevents its officials from normal sexual expression those religious officials may be driven to seek expression with children that is a problem to society. There are many implications for community psychology and for the solution of social problems to be drawn from the PB conception of human behavior and from PBT.

One last point: Community psychology and PB coincide also with respect to prevention. The societal intervention proposed, with respect to the generational perpetuation of an underclass, constitutes an example of social prevention. PB's emphasis on learning ensures that prevention is a general aim, as will be further exemplified in the abnormal psychology level of study.

THE PERSONALITY LEVEL

There was a time when PB's work with complex functional human behavior was opposed by some radical behaviorists because most "operant research with humans . . . tended to involve only simple responses such as knob-pulling and button-pressing, and simple controlling stimuli" (Staats, Finley, Minke, & Wolf, 1964). But in behavior therapy now there is a growing use of various concepts introduced by PB—like deficit and inappropriate emotional, language-cognitive, and behavioral repertoires—in the analysis of behavior disorders (see, for example, Bellack & Mueser, 1994), even by those who are in the radical behaviorism tradition. There are programs to train social skills, assertiveness skills, problem solving, in addition to those that deal with simple behaviors. Earlier, when the experimental analysis of behavior methodology was the orthodoxy, first "functional analysis" had to be made acceptable, and then it too became an orthodoxy.

In the 1970s PB opened its call for the study of personality. "It is suggested . . . that a personality level is necessary in behavioral theory, . . . that the individual learns enduring personality repertoires that determine his general behavior, . . . and . . . that behavior therapy must begin to include analyses of personality repertoires and methods of changing such repertoires" (Staats, 1971a, p. 165). When the PB call was published in a behavior therapy journal, it met behavior analytic rejection (see Tryon, 1974). Even today, despite the fact that concepts equivalent to the BBRs are being employed in the field, there is still a strong radical behaviorism rejection, including the claim that PB's concept of personality, despite its behavioral definition, should be rejected because it is an intervening variable (see Plaud, 1995; Ulman, 1990).

That leaves the field of behavior therapy severely truncated. That is, cognitive theories and cognitive-behavioral theories of behavior therapy are widely used in the field, and they employ personality concepts. For example, Beck's (1967) theory is that depression comes from a "negative triad" of distortedly negative cognitions of the self, the world, and the future. These negative views are seen as the result of a memory problem that selectively exaggerates negative events and minimizes positive events, as well as attention selectivity that notes negative but not positive happenings. In addition, depressives are seen to engage in arbitrary inferences and selective abstractions and to overgeneralize and personalize their experience in ways that enhance the negative and decrease the positive. There is evidence that supports these cognitive personality characteristics (see DeMonbreun & Craighead, 1977; Heiby, 1981; Loeb, Beck, Diggory, & Tuthill, 1967; Wener & Rehm, 1975). The therapy follows its conception. "Cognitive therapy is an integrated set of cognitive and behavioral interventions designed to identify, evaluate, and change erroneously negative beliefs and modify maladjustive information processing styles" (Hollon & Carter, 1994, p. 92). The therapy uses techniques such as self-monitoring of behavior and mood which establishes a correlation between immediate situations and emotional response. The self-monitoring also provides information by which to plan a program to get the individual to be more active in conducting life affairs and channel the individual into more positive circumstances. Another step involves "identifying beliefs related to negative affects and behavioral passivity" (Hollon & Carter, 1994, p. 95). The next step involves evaluating the accuracy of the client's beliefs. Clients are trained to consider what the evidence is for the belief, whether there is an alternative explanation for the event, and what the real implications are if the initial belief is true. "General beliefs, referred to as underlying assumptions, typically constitute basic world views that are rarely recognized [before treatment] as idiosyncratic" (Hollon & Carter, 1994, p. 97).

There are several points to be made in this context. The first is that these treatment procedures are harmonious with the language behavior therapy that PB proposed in the early 1970s (Staats, 1972). The reason is that the theory involved, although it is generally considered to be "cognitive" in nature, is coincident with and could be behaviorized by translation to PB concepts and principles. (I recall a letter from Beck following my 1972 publication that recognized such common interests.) Very early PB analyses conceptualized in behavioral terms how language-cognitive distortions could lead to emotional and behavior problems. "[It] is important that the child acquire a veridical language system . . . the individual's solution of his social-personal problems will depend upon his language system (Staats, 1963a, p. 387). One example of an individual's "distorted beliefs" and how they can cause abnormal emotional experiences and behaviors involved a description of a paranoid episode. A learning analysis was made of how the individual learned inappropriate verbal-labeling and verbal-association repertoires that led to abnormal behavior. "[M]any cases of psychopathology involve idiosyncratic language which mediates inappropriate behavior" (Staats, 1968a, p. 189).

> Moreover, the emotional quality of the words in one's self-concept is very important. One's "happiness" with himself (the extent to which he receives positive emotional experience) will in part depend upon this aspect of the self-concept. . . . It is thus crucial that the individual's labeling and reasoning sequences are veridical. . . . The importance of the individual's language repertoire in his thinking, reasoning, planning, and decision making, and hence in his actions, cannot be overemphasized. . . . [T]hese language repertoires have been learned . . . and can be changed . . . in therapy. (Staats, 1972, pp. 180–183)

But why is it important to behaviorize cognitive and cognitive–behavioral theories of therapy? The reason can be seen with Beck's theory. As valuable as the therapy is, and hence the conception associated with it, it is not a scientifically constructed theory. Although using the term *information processing*, for example, the theory is not connected in any meaningful way to information processing theory, as in generating experiments. The same is true of other "cognitive" terms such as beliefs, worldview, and selective memory. The fact is that cognitive theories in behavior therapy are constructed solely on the basis of their clinical observations and work. The theories are only couched in the general language of cognitive psychology.

The present position is that the cognitive and cognitive–behavioral theories should be put into the PBT framework, their concepts and principles translated in a systematic theoretical endeavor. Doing so would provide a common language that would unify the various theories, and there are many. Doing so would also bring the knowledge of the various levels of study of PB into supportive connection with those theories. And doing so would have heuristic scientific products. As exemplified in the human learning level discussions, PB's analysis of the language-cognitive repertoires provides concepts and principles for analyzing what happens in verbal psychotherapy, including the cognitive and cognitive–behavioral therapies.

Normal Personality Study in Understanding the Abnormal

Behavior therapy (like abnormal psychology), because of its clinical locus, focuses its interest on clinical problems, not on the study of normal behavior and personality (BBRs). The PB position is that this constitutes a problem for any clinically based approach. That weakness underlay the criticism of psychoanalysis—that it was based on a biased sample of neurotic women in Vienna. Restriction to the study of clinical problems, regardless of the approach and subject sample, results in incompleteness. Let me elaborate. When we see a behavior and consider it abnormal, we can do so only because we have been exposed to what is normal. That is really what underlies the recognition that what is defined as "abnormal" is relative to culture, class, time period, and so on. It is knowledge of normal behavior that tells us what is abnormal.

This position has important implications for behavior therapy. It says that we cannot expect our knowledge of human behavior to be clinically driven, for that restricts us to only part of the domain of study. Let me give an example. In traditional psychology there has been study of dyslexia for years. Dyslexic children, for example, are given psychological tests—like tests of perception and reading level—to establish what their characteristics are. The idea is that the disorder is caused by some aberrant biological-mental characteristics of the child. These various studies, however, are conducted without knowledge of what a normal reading repertoire is, how it is acquired, what it enables the individual to do, what the child has to have before training in the reading repertoire can be successfully conducted, and how and in what ways the *process* of learning to read can go awry. How can the disorder be understood, a therapy be devised, and prevention be planned, in the face of that ignorance? Attempting to study dyslexia without knowing these things is like sailing without a compass.

A theory of dyslexia must be set in a general theory of language and reading. And the same applies to behavior therapy theories. Clinical theories, such as those of Beck and Ellis, valuable as they are in specific areas of treatment, do not indicate what personality is or analyze their personality (cognitive) concepts into more basic principles and place them into a larger theory framework. Thus, the theories cannot indicate well the genesis of the behavior disorders with which they deal. Moreover, the lack of theory development has other outcomes. For example, what are the relationships of the behavior disorders dealt with in the different theories? What are the relationships among (1) the depressed person whose ruminations about what has happened accentuate the negative and minimize the positive; (2) the person who "employs a defense mechanism" in order to minimize negative statements from others and oneself and thereby prevents herself from dealing with her problems; (3) the paranoid schizophrenic with delusions of grandeur; (4) the manic person who makes plans in which every possibility comes out unrealistically well; (5) the obsessive person whose worries about upcoming events elicit anxiety; and (6) the sociopath who swears she will never do again that which she has already done various times and will do again at the first opportunity? What is similar about such cases? And what is different? Are they to be explained in the same set of principles and concepts and causal conditions? Can they be treated with the same therapy? Or do the differences involved demand different types of therapy and different types of theories?

If there are similarities and differences in the characteristics of the disorders involved they can only be seen through underlying, more basic, principles and concepts. PB can analyze the several disorders using the same concepts and principles. Such an analysis can indicate what is alike about the cases and what is different. And that analysis will serve various purposes. For one thing it will dispel the need for constructing a different conception and therapy for every different type of problem behavior. At present the field of behavior therapy is broken up by different theories, whose difference lies mainly in the fact that the theories were worked out in the context of different problems. There are behavior therapy theories of the anxiety disorders that are different from each other and different from the behavior therapy theories of depression, schizophrenia, and the personality disorders. The anxiety disorders and depression are considered within the same theory framework in PB and the similarities and differences involved can be seen. The PB analyses of these disorders also reveal that such clients have functional language-cognitive BBRs (although they have inappropriate aspects of those BBRs). In some of the above-mentioned disorders, because of the presence of functional language repertoires, forms of language (cognitive) psychotherapy can be employed. In other cases the deficits and inappropriateness in this repertoire negate the use of a language (cognitive) form of therapy. The point is that it is the theory of normal language-cognitive BBRs (among other things) that provides the basic foundation for understanding the different disorders, the relationships of the disorders, and the types of treatment that are appropriate for the different disorders.

The behavior therapies and theories of Beck, and Ellis, and Barlow, and Bellack, and Lovaas, as examples, are not general theories, and they are not placed in a general theory. Thus they apply conceptually and in practice only to specific problems. To illustrate, what does Beck's cognitive therapy have to say about the developmental disorders? How can it be used to treat developmental reading disorder, autism, conduct disorder, and such? What does such a cognitive theory have to say about early intervention and the prevention of such disorders, even the disorder on which the theory focuses? On the other hand, what do Lovaas' work with autistic children, classroom-management techniques, and behavioral toilet training methods have to do with the cognitive therapies that treat anxiety disorders and depression? Because the theories are not part of a general theory, they may even be grouped into antagonistic positions, which detracts from the power of the field.

What these examples tell us is that the field of behavior therapy—with its many interests, techniques, assessment instruments, therapies, and theories of behavior problems and behavior disorders—needs an overarching theory that includes the study of normal personality and a theory of normal personality. When a behavior therapy theory addresses only a narrow band of problems or disorders, this informs us that the behavior therapy and its theory are not general. Rather than incorporating other behavior therapies and theories, this behavior therapy is destined to be incorporated into a more comprehensive theory framework.

The relationship of clinical theory to basic principles is or has become tenuous in various cognitive and cognitive–behavioral therapies. Let me suggest that this is a real, rather than purely esthetic, loss. To illustrate, cognitive therapy is based on language, between therapist and client. For that reason alone it is important to have a basic theory of language that instructs the therapy in the types of things that can be accomplished through language. As another example, if cognitive therapy has a goal of changing the client's personality characteristics, then it is important to have a theory (of personality) that systematizes what is involved. Moreover, if the cognitive therapy wants to change the client in the belief that those changes will change the client's behavior in the life situation, then the theory employed must indicate how the individual's personality characteristics that are changed in the therapy affect other aspects of the individual's behavior. Only with such specifications in theory is there a framework for generating the various types of research that are needed in a scientific approach, as well as for making clinical progress.

The Theory of Personality Is a Basis for Treatment

Traditional therapies describe personality concepts, and problems of personality, as a foundation for treatment goals. Psychoanalytic theory, with a specific personality theory, had specific goals. Client-centered therapy did not accept the psychoanalytic theory of personality, thus it did not accept the goals or methods of psychoanalytic theory. With really a very simple and general theory of personality, client-centered therapy projected a more simple and vague goal, that of self-actualization, and a therapy with correspondingly simple features.

The theory is central in the therapist's understanding of the patient, the patient's problems, the resources the patient has, the environmental conditions acting on the patient, as well as the measures that can be employed to help the patient. A therapist who considers homosexuality as the expression of a genetic condition will approach a patient presenting homosexuality as a problem in a different manner than will a therapist who considers homosexuality to represent a problem of working through the oedipal conflict, than will a therapist who considers that some undefined "learning history" may have played a role, than will a therapist who considers homosexuality to be the result of specified learning with respect to the BBRs, especially the sexual aspects of the emotional-motivational BBR, or to a therapist who has no conception of causation of the "problem." One may agree with what client-centered therapy does in practice—if one's theory of personality is poor, it is better not to attempt to change personality. Error in theory is likely to lead to error in treatment. But, recognizing this, it is straightforward to realize that the richer and the more accurate the theory of personality on which the psychotherapy is based, the more valuable it is as a tool for the clinician.

The PB elaboration of the BBRs, in a way that establishes a systematic theory of personality, provides avenues toward deeper and more general understanding of the nature of the enterprise. That is why behavior therapy needs basic fields that systematically specify the various BBRs of which personality is composed. This must include accounts of how those BBRs are learned and, as a consequence, of how those BBRs can be created and changed through learning. Those accounts will then serve as the basis for constructing programs of therapy by which to treat clinical problems that spring from deficits and inappropriateness in the BBRs.

Let me take intelligence as an example. Cognitive behavior therapy and behavior analytic clinical approaches do not actively research intelligence, study what it is, how it is learned, how it functions, and how it can be changed through a training program. There are no behavior or cognitive–behavior treatments for the lack of intelligence. Yet behavior therapists and behavior analysts confront problems involving deficient intelligence. As has been indicated, PB has studied repertoires that compose intelligence, as well as how they are learned and how they function. Experimental-longitudinal research with young children demonstrates the manner in which children can be trained in such language-cognition-intelligence BBRs. Mental retardation has been analyzed in terms of deficits in these BBRs, and autism as well. Lovaas (1977) and others have also showed that autistic children can learn some of these repertoires. Staats and Burns (1981) have shown explicitly that intelligence can be changed through training in language-cognitive basic behavioral repertoires. These various works constitute ample support for the PB position that intelligence problems can be treated in behavior therapy. With the necessary development of research, to expand the knowledge base—and this means extensive development—behavior therapy could offer general treatment for developmental "cognitive" disorders, including mental retardation.

There are treatments in behavior therapy of social skills, assertive skills, and such. These involve complex repertoires. To know what they consist of is essential in establishing treatment programs. Would it not make sense to study how social and assertive skills relate to extroversion, and how lack of such skills relates to introversion? In this manner behavior therapy could utilize the knowledge of introversion–extroversion that has been developed in the field of personality measurement. Would it not make sense to analyze the repertoires that are involved in each case? Would it not make sense to study how those repertoires are learned and how problems in those repertoires can be prevented, in the early training of desirable features? The general point is that the PB personality theory provides a framework for generally considering all of the "traits" of human behavior that are considered desirable and undesirable in our society, adjustive and maladjustive (and that, in the problematic state, are presented to the clinician). Such a personality theory, as it is elaborated, can be expected to serve as a foundation for an advancing behavior therapy that is capable not only of dealing with specific behavior problems, but also with the various personality traits, and problems of those traits, not only after problems have developed, but also in providing prevention possibilities. When a clinical problem arises that involves a particular personality trait, development of the PB type of theory can be expected to provide the clinician with understanding of the composition of the personality trait, how it is learned, and how the trait can be changed.

The major point here is that the field of behavior therapy cannot limit itself to clinical study and clinical interests. There is a basic psychological science—including the study of personality—that must underlie behavior therapy. That connection to a basic science must be systematically created. It does not now exist. The field of behavior therapy today is represented by the Association for the Advancement of Behavior Therapy, which is largely limited to clinical level study. The Association for Behavior Analysis (ABA), which includes interests in the basic level of study, is currently restricted in practice to Skinner's radical behaviorism and, as such, does not include the various levels of study relevant to behavior therapy, including that of personality. Behavioral psychology has not been put together—organizationally or conceptually—in the manner necessary to systematically face its purview, and the lack of an area for the study of personality is one of the most important weaknesses.

THE ABNORMAL PSYCHOLOGY LEVEL

Abnormal psychology taxonomic systems provide valuable information for clinicians. For example, clinicians can find the various behaviors of a patient represented as a particular disorder, yielding the basis for diagnosis. In such a case there may be corresponding suggestions concerning the etiology of the disorder and recommendations for general methods of treatment. The abnormal psychology is also useful in training a student to be a clinical psychologist or psychiatrist. Someone with no experience in abnormal behavior can learn a good deal from traditional taxonomic works that describe types of abnormal behavior, as well as suggestions concerning causes and treatments.

To the extent that an abnormal psychology provides a basis for diagnosis, it also provides a basis for the construction of tests to aid in this task. And the abnormal psychology also provides the foundation for research. Geneticists, physiologists, biochemists, pharmacologists, and anatomists, as well as psychologists, can look for differences between normal individuals and patients in a particular behavior disorder classification. The particular abnormal psychology serves as the basis for education, theory construction, treatment, and research.

The Behavioral Abnormal Psychologies

Prior to the original PB abnormal psychology (Staats, 1963a, chap. 11) there were no systematic behavioral taxonomies. Radical behaviorism, consistent with its restriction to its own experimental analysis of behavior methodology, had no means of using the knowledge of abnormal psychology. Neither did social learning theory (see Bandura & Walters, 1959; 1963); and when such an abnormal psychology was presented (see Bandura, 1968) it was an adaptation of the 1963 PB conception. That PB behavioral taxonomy of the behavior disorders unified observations of traditional abnormal psychology along with its behavioral analysis, to introduce new categories, concepts, and principles. This was a general conception and it suggested that the various behavior disorders could be so treated.

Following the PB work (plus the various behavior therapy studies that had accumulated in the interim) Ullmann and Krasner (1968) published a book that attempted to deal with abnormal behavior within the framework of radical behaviorism. Although the book had valuable parts, linking the work with radical behaviorism was a step backward, subtracting concepts and principles. Limited by the principles used, only traditional descriptions of the behavior disorders were presented along with the behavior modification studies with patients with those disorders. Little analysis was made of what the disorders consisted of behaviorally, or what caused them. The combination of traditional psychopathology classification with radical behaviorism work was eclectic, not unified.

The PB framework theory of abnormal psychology (Staats, 1963a, chap. 11; 1975, chap. 8), however, with its exposition of the three basic behavioral repertoires, provided new ways for analyzing the behavior disorders that are harmonious with contemporary developments. Street and Barlow (1994), as an example, consider emotion in their behavioral treatment of the anxiety disorders. Bellack and Mueser (1994) consider schizophrenia to involve deficits and inappropriacies in thought processes, affect, and behavior as did the PB analysis. There are behavioral conceptualizations of depression (Ferster, 1973; Lewinsohn, 1985; Rehm, 1977) and conduct disorder (Kazdin, 1994) as well as behavioral accounts of other areas (see DuPaul, Guevremont, & Barkely, 1994; Hollon & Carter, 1994; Kazdin, 1994; LoPiccolo, 1994; Schreibman, 1994; Whitman, 1994). These theories, for the most part, are placed within the radical behaviorism framework, but concepts and principles are employed that are like those in PB. Let me also suggest that, valuable as these theories are, in retaining characteristics of radical behaviorism, they are incomplete in stipulating what the disorder is and, especially, how it comes about, and how it has its effects. Using radical behaviorism as a basic framework does not provide an interest in how complex human behavior is learned. Part of the incompleteness, however, is a result of taking a therapy viewpoint rather than the more basic abnormal psychology interest.

Finally, there is a tendency to focus on parts of disorders and to be little concerned with establishing large-scale unified theory (see Heiby, 1987). For example, Rehm's (1977) theory of depression concerns the individual's lack of self-reinforcement. Ferster's (1973) theory treats the loss of reinforcement, ratio strain, and punishment of nondepressed behavior. Seligman (1975) considers the independence of response and reinforcement in producing depression. Lewinsohn (1974) concludes that loss of reinforcement, the reinforcement of depressed behavior, and poor social skills to be causes. Beck (1967) considers cognitive dysfunctions to be the cause. The point is that these theories, each dealing with its part, arise and continue to exist in isolation from one another—because they lack a framework that calls for unified theory construction. Thus, none looks at the large picture—such as how behavior therapy (and their particular theory) should relate to the field of abnormal psychology—or lays out a program for constructing or using an abnormal psychology. Rather, the behavior disorders are dealt with separately and partially, without setting forth the general nature of the endeavor.

Lacking a behavioral abnormal psychology, behavior therapists/analysts, without realizing it, accept traditional psychology positions. For example, the treatment of mental retardation in behavior therapy relies on behavioral methods, but the disorder is conceived of in the same vague biological terms as in traditional abnormal psychology (see Whitman, 1994). The same is true with respect to autism (see Lovaas, 1966, 1977). Again, this amounts to eclectic inconsistency and constitutes weak theory.

PBT and the Abnormal Psychology Level of Study in Behavior Therapy

Abnormal psychology has been discredited for many behaviorists because its diagnostic categories imply mental-biological causation. Moreover, traditional diagnosis does not itself yield knowledge concerning treatment. Traditional abnormal psychology, strangely, is rejected as an endeavor, but is also used at the same time. In contrast, the PBT position is that abnormal psychology's behavioral descriptions are valuable, basic to the field of behavior therapy. What is needed is a behavioral abnormal psychology, where the behavior disorder categories are given a psychological-behavioral analysis. Such an abnormal psychology can provide the foundation for behavior therapy research, assessment, and treatment developments. This can only be exemplified here.

Let us take the PB abnormal psychology of autism that was summarized in the preceding chapter. Because the approach emphasizes the breakdown in the autistic child's learning of the BBRs, it provides an emphasis on prevention that is lacking in approaches that look to radical behaviorism for the basic conception. The PB theory of autism says that behavior therapy needs to develop measures by which autistic children can be discovered early. When a child is brought in and receives a diagnosis of autism that means that the problem has existed too long, long enough for serious deficits in BBR development to have occurred, and long enough for seriously inappropriate BBRs to have been learned, especially the anti-learning BBR. Many parents of children who are diagnosed as autistic seek help without being able to get advice on how to deal with their child. PB says that autism does not spring out full-blown; it has a history of some years. Professionals have lacked abnormal psychology/psychological assessment tools by which to pick up the problem before it has become full-blown. And they have not had the knowledge by which to educate the parents to improve the incipient autistic child's learning. *Prevention requires a full theory of autism.*

The PB abnormal psychology of autism thus calls for extensive developments. For example, in terms of assessment, PB calls for new procedures that involve observing the parent–child interaction as a means of seeing how the training environment is deficit and inappropriate. That is necessary as the basis for planning a program to train the parent to rectify those conditions and turn the training environment in a positive direction. Such directives for the development of assessment and behavior therapy—which are meant to apply to all disorders—do not emerge from traditional conceptions, which infer biological causation; or from an eclectic behavior therapy; or from radical behaviorism, which is unconcerned with etiology and focuses on treating the "behavior problem" after it has surfaced.

To provide an additional illustration, let us take the PB theory of depression, for it also has various implications. As an example, in the theory it is said that a narrowly developed emotional-motivational system can make the individual vulnerable to depression, because when an environmental loss (or trauma) occurs there are few positive emotional stimuli to act in counterbalance. For one thing, behavior therapy needs to research this analysis. To illustrate, there are various tests that measure the emotional-motivational BBR (like interest inventories) that could be used to measure differences between depression-vulnerable people and normals. Those with a narrow range of interests should be more vulnerable to depression. If it is the case that narrow interests are a risk factor, then abnormal psychology will call for the study of how interests are learned, how they can be measured with respect to depression vulnerability, and how they can be modified. More generally, the PB theory of depression states that the disorder involves various sites of causation, including the formation and compounding of the negative emotional state. For behavior therapy that means that each of these sites must be studied in order to provide the basis for assessment and treatment procedures.

The construction of a psychological-behavioral abnormal psychology should become one of the subfields of behavior therapy. This psychology must analyze behavior disorders in terms of the BBRs involved, the original learning of the BBRs, the effects of the BBRs on behavior, and the effects of the behavior on the social environment and, hence, back on the individual. This psychology must also analyze the effects of the current situation on behavior. In addition, the field must link its special concerns—the diagnosis (assessment) of behavior problems and the treatment of those behavior problems—with the general knowledge of behavior problems that is the purview of abnormal psychology. That means establishing instruments to aid in diagnosis (measuring the BBRs and the current life situation, and such) of specific behavior disorders. And that means establishing the treatment methods that are most effective with those behavior disorders.

The PB position is that an abnormal psychology that analyzes what the disorders are in behavioral (BBR) terms, that specifies how they are learned, and how they work their effects on behavior, in conjunction with the present environment, is a central part of the psychological-behavioral clinician's knowledge. With such a theory, diagnosis becomes that of indicating the deficits and inappropriateness of the BBRs and deficit and inappropriate current life conditions. And this analysis then generally provides the basis for developing lines of treatment and research—that is, that deal with changes in the BBRs and in the current life environment. The more detailed and comprehensive the abnormal psychology the better tool it provides the clinician.

The PB abnormal psychology in its prototypical form is intended to serve as a foundation for the psychological behavior therapy clinician or researcher. With its multilevel theory development it provides concepts and principles for communication across the various behavior disorders. Analyses of the disorders in terms of PB concepts and principles provide understanding of the disorders. When a diagnosis is made in terms of the PB abnormal psychology, the diagnosis will suggest or specify the etiology and treatment of the disorder, in a way that is absent in traditional abnormal psychology. That is, the description of the disorder will indicate the deficits and inappropriacies involved, how they were learned, and how they can be changed. PBT is still prototypical in this area, a framework, indicating an important direction of needed development of behavior therapy.

THE PSYCHOLOGICAL MEASUREMENT LEVEL

The field of behavioral assessment has made important advances and produced a number of valuable instruments. But, as has been indicated, the field of behavioral assessment has remained at odds with the field of psychological measurement. That alienation springs from the recognition in behaviorism, that while tests categorize people—as retarded, paranoid, and so on—they supply little knowledge by which to conduct treatment (see Spence, 1944; Staats, 1963a). For example, the child who does poorly on an IQ test is categorized as a mental retardate. The adult who scores highly on the PA scale of the MMPI is categorized as paranoid. But such tests do not indicate what is measured, what the causes are, or what specifically must be done to rectify the problem involved.

At present, behavior therapists, because of adoption of radical behaviorism as a basic theory, use psychological tests, but eclectically (see Craighead, Craighead, Kazdin, & Mahoney, 1994), and in the same manner as do traditional clinicians, that is, without deriving treatment specifications or deepening their understanding. For example, it is the total score of the intelligence test that is used by the behavior therapist, and in the traditional way, as in deciding whether or not a child is mentally retarded and should be placed in a special education class. The test is not used as a basis for behavioral treatment of the retardation and tells nothing about the specific deficits of the child.

The reason that traditional tests do not have treatment directives is because they do not analyze in behavioral terms the traits they are supposed to measure—such as paranoia, intelligence, introversion, dependent personality, sociopathy. The tests do not indicate specifically what the causes are of such traits, biological or learning. And the tests do not indicate how the traits function to determine the individual's problem behavior. How is it that the "paranoid trait" makes the person have life problems?

Nevertheless, it is not the PB position that psychological tests should be rejected because they do not provide these types of information. For they do provide important information. What is needed in behavior therapy is an addition to the knowledge already provided by tests, to supply what is needed by the clinician. That can be done via the PB type of analysis of psychological tests. For example, for clinical practice intelligence tests should be behaviorized—that is, the behavioral constituents of the intelligence test should be specified. PB says that using only total scores—for example, total scores on an intelligence test or on the MMPI—is very limited. The total IQ score can tell one only grossly that the child has intellectual problems that will interfere with school learning. But such use of the intelligence test overlooks the most important information contained in the test. *PBT says that it is the items on the test that contain the specific information regarding the child, indicating what aspects of the child's BBRs are deficit.* What needs to be considered are the *items* that measure the child's verbal-motor repertoire, the child's verbal-labeling repertoire, the child's number repertoire, writing, copying, and related skills, and so on. The same is true for all the tests that are used clinically.

Behaviorizing a test is not done by word magic, of course. It is only possible to analyze the items on an intelligence test in terms of the basic language repertoires because those BBRs have been specified in theory and research. Behaviorizing a test demands that type of analysis, based upon that type of basic knowledge. When that analysis has been done for all of the items on intelligence tests, then it will be possible for the behavioral clinician not only to look at the total score of the intelligence test, but also at the individual items. Each item, having been analyzed to indicate the repertoire(s) it measures, will contribute knowledge of the nature of the child's BBRs. Since there is overlap in the BBRs that items measure there could be grouping of items to yield subscores. That will tell the clinician the child's strengths as well as the repertoires that are deficit. When all such items have been behaviorized it will be possible to construct summary measures of the strengths and deficits in the various BBRs involved. This is a call for a large new research area, as has been indicated.

The same thing is true with respect to treatment. The intelligence test—even after it is behaviorized—will provide no information with respect to a treatment program for the child, unless research has been done to establish how to treat deficits in the various BBRs. That is, knowing that the child has a deficit verbal-labeling repertoire will be no help in treatment, unless one also knows how to train a child to remediate that deficit. Staats and Burns (1981) showed that training in learning to say the names of letters, and to copy them, provided the child with repertoires that enabled the child to do well on the Geometrics Design part of the WPPSI (Wechsler, 1967). That research provides knowledge by which to rectify the deficits of children who do poorly on the Geometrics Design test. This same study showed how to remediate children who have deficits in the number concept and arithmetic skill area. And the study showed that children's conceptual ability could be improved by verbal-labeling training. That type of research, extended to the various items on intelligence tests, would provide methods by which the behavior therapist could treat intellectual deficits that occur in mental retardation and childhood autism.

Psychological behavior therapy actually establishes a framework that calls for developing a great research field, that involved in behaviorizing the field of psychological testing, and in establishing the methods for clinically treating the deficits and inappropriateness in the BBRs that are established by tests. Because of their construction, psychological tests contain basic elements of knowledge concerning the repertoires that compose the traits they measure. That knowledge, however, is inchoate, shapeless, and unmeaningful. That knowledge needs to be elaborated by the types of analysis and research that PBT describes. When this type of work has been done the clinician will have very powerful knowledge. This is what the PB framework calls for.

But PB Psychometrics Is Not Presently Available!

This discussion proposes the development of a large field of study to give psychological tests new powers. But what is the behavior therapist to do today? How can PB be a help? Let me answer this by saying, first, that PB's conception already provides a useful framework for considering problems of human behavior. That framework is rich in basic principles and in exemplar analyses. That framework indicates how to analyze human behavior and problems of behavior. And that framework generally exemplifies how items on tests can be analyzed.

This framework is there now for the clinician herself to employ to construct an analysis of the tests that she uses. Most clinicians employ a group of tests, not all of the hundreds of tests that are available. It is typical for the clinician to gain a great deal of experience with those tests regularly used. This means the clinician has the opportunity to relate the test scores to the characteristics of the people involved. The behavior therapist, however, in doing so, usually uses an informal mixture of traditional and behavioral concepts and principles.

It is suggested, rather, that the systematically constructed PB framework be used in working with traditional psychological tests. The behavior therapist needs to study the items of the tests that she uses repeatedly and make a PB behavioral analysis of those items. The therapist can then employ the range of behavior therapy procedures available for treating the deficits and inappropriacies in the BBRs as indicated in each specific case. And the behavior therapist can be concerned with validating the effects of that treatment on the patient's performance. Until PB analyses of the items of psychological tests have been done more widely—which will require many studies—the individual behavior therapist must make her own analyses of the tests that are employed.

THE NATURE OF THE MULTILEVEL PSYCHOLOGICAL BEHAVIOR THERAPY APPROACH

PB Provides a Conception for Behavior Therapists

The substance and methodology of PBT give it general characteristics that are important to consider. All therapists, including behavior therapists, need an overarching theory that provides them with a conception of human behavior. They use their conceptions in analyzing different clinical problems. Behavior therapists—clinicians as well as researchers—also need a theory that allows them to understand in a unified way the relevant research in their own and other fields of psychology. And behavior therapists need a heuristic theory that provides new directions for treatment, assessment, and research activities. It will be suggested that the PB theory that has been advanced here is such a conception for behavior therapists, and for the field of behavior therapy. With this theory the various aspects of behavior, cognitive, and cognitive–behavioral therapy—as well as elements of traditional psychotherapy—can be behaviorized into a consistent, specific, systematic theory with range and depth. PB should be compared with the other conceptions in behavior therapy in this respect. In this as in other respects, PB is a framework theory that calls for development.

PBT's Multilevel Approach and the PB Model of Human Behavior

There are types of problems in behavior therapy that are ideally suited for the straightforward application of basic principles of conditioning. As examples, take the child with otherwise normal behavior who lisps, has temper tantrums, or is not toilet-trained. The use of established training procedures are sufficient. But there are other problems of human behavior that involve complex learning causes that have resulted in complex deficits and inappropriacies in the BBRs that produce social problems that in turn effect additional negative learning. Such complex problems require an analysis including concepts and principles from the human learning, child development, social interaction, personality, psychological, and abnormal behavior levels of study. Simply knowing the principles of reinforcement and classical conditioning, behavior therapy/analysis studies, and traditional clinical knowledge, in an eclectic cognitive–behavioral mix, is not sufficient for the analysis of complex problems of human behavior.

Let us take a case that has been mentioned already, of a four-year-old child with no language and consequently no social behaviors, as well as uncontrolled behaviors of various kinds such as acting bizarrely to attract attention, to break-up boring situations, to get what is wanted, and to avoid learning situations. He also had toilet accidents, resisted going to bed, and was generally uncontrollable. Psychiatric opinions had labeled the child as emotionally disturbed and autistic. All of the levels up to and including the verbal psychotherapy of the PBT level were employed in analyzing and treating this case. The mother was interviewed and her child-rearing practices observed. The child was observed in a preschool setting to which the child was admitted. The child exhibited glaring language-cognitive deficits on an intelligence test. The PBT treatment focused on the deficits in the basic behavioral repertoires rather than the inappropriate repertoires. The latter were considered to emerge essentially because of the deficits in the former. The analysis indicated the child's problems would be largely solved by learning normal BBRs that would replace the inappropriate BBRs. The child was thus given training in the language repertoires, especially the verbal-motor repertoire and the verbal-labeling repertoire. This training used the token-reinforcer system for working with young children and the training procedures worked out at the child development level of study. The mother (who was laconic and provided little informal training in language) was instructed in how to provide that training. And the mother was trained on how to interact with the child benignly in effecting toilet training, going to bed at night, not reinforcing crazy behavior, and such. How to improve the mother–father relationship with respect to training the child was also treated. Very important was the parent's conception concerning the child's problem—which was that the child was crazy and essentially not subject to learning.

The outcomes were closely related to the treatment which lasted seven months. As the child acquired the language-cognitive BBRs the child's behaviors improved as did the child's interaction with other children. For example, the child was able to establish a relationship with a playmate at home on the basis of his newly acquired ability to interact verbally. The changed training environment at school and at home contributed to the repair of the child's language deficits and to correcting the negative emotional response to learning situations. That is, progress occurred in replacing the child's anti-learning BBR with normal BBRs. The parents' conception of the child was changed through verbal psychotherapy and through observing that the child could learn and was controllable. The point is that this case demanded the knowledge of the various levels of study of PB. Simple training in behavior analytic principles or in behavior therapy works would not have sufficed in analyzing and treating the child's problems, the parents' problems, or in using verbal psychotherapy type methods for changing the latter.

Leduc (1988), who leads the development of PB in the French-speaking community, has advanced PBT methods in treating a case of a six-year-old feral ("wild") child who had been raised in extremely deprived circumstances (by an alcoholic, mentally retarded prostitute). Her language-cognitive BBR was that of a child of 18 months, consisting only of single words, with response only to a few commands. Her Wechsler Intelligence Scale for Children (WISC-R) IQ was 54. Confined to a box for long periods, her sensory-motor BBR was deficit, and she had inappropriate repertoires such as temper tantrums and tearing her hair out. She also displayed autistic behaviors, narrow interests and fixations, such as playing with water from a spigot for long periods. The child was removed to a day-care center, with mostly autistic children, in a psychiatric hospital.

Leduc employed the human learning, child development, personality, psychological measurement, and abnormal psychology levels of PB to analyze this case. The focus of the therapy was to repair the language-cognitive BBRs of the child using the methods of PBT based on its experimental-longitudinal research. She received language training and concept training, and training in reading and number skills. Thought to be incapable of learning by the staff of the institution, the following corroborates Leduc's analysis that placed the problem in the child's original deficit learning environment.

> Dominique is now very close to her chronological age in the areas of language and concepts. In reading she is about to complete second grade; she decodes and has a good understanding of what she reads. Her number abilities are those of a child at the beginning of the second grade. She is beginning to write in cursive writing. (Leduc, 1988, p. 12)

The examples have involved children. But the points hold also for adult cases. The behavior therapist of the new generation needs to know the human learning, child development, social interaction, personality, psychological measurement, and abnormal behavior levels of study. The concepts and principles provided at these levels are necessary for analyzing problems and devising treatments, as well as for projecting research.

Various additional issues have arisen in the context of clinical treatment, either in traditional or behavioral frameworks, or sometimes in disagreements between the two. Some of these can be employed in characterizing PBT.

Directive or Non-Directive

At one time Rogerian therapy was called "non-directive," to distinguish it from therapies in which the therapist was in the role of an expert delivering prescriptions to someone less expert. The idea was that only the client could exhibit and know her own true nature, given an accepting environment—which was the therapist's responsibility to provide. Any direction from the therapist would reflect *her* nature, not the client's.

In the PB view this dichotomy touches on a relevant characteristic. To begin, our early applications of conditioning principles constituted a model. The model was that of the animal laboratory, which involves manipulating environmental events that produce effects on the animal's behavior. This model, when employed to envision clinical treatment, suggests manipulation of environmental variables in order to change behaviors according to the behavior therapist's plan. The term *behavior modification* captures this quality. It was that implication that engendered opposition to the term.

Does the use of conditioning methods "de-humanize" clients, and should such therapy thus be rejected? Not in PBT's multilevel approach. There are cases when the problem calls for introducing environmental manipulations that will change the client's behavior. This involves treating the client as though the individual is not capable of being dealt with on a higher level. But that indeed is true in some cases. It is not possible to deal with a two year old, who has learned some undesirable behaviors—such as temper tantrums, or making a fuss at bedtime—by verbally asking for a change in behavior, or by reasoning with the child. The child's language repertoires, by which to affect the child's behavior through language, have not yet been learned. Language deficits in schizophrenia and sociopathy may also make treatment through language interactions unfeasible. In such cases environmental manipulation may be necessary.

On the other hand, let us take the case of the highly educated, successful, articulate and normal individual who has achieved a rich life but who still has unhappy feelings about her relationships with her siblings and mother and father and the family interactions. Having an opportunity to spend time describing family events and personal reactions, in an accepting, warm, unrestrictive therapy relationship may indeed result in changes in the client's conception regarding the family and herself, changes in emotional responses and happiness (emotional state), as well as changes in the client's behavior, and changes in the family members' response to her. This can occur with no planned direction by the therapist as in non-directive therapy. The changes will occur according to specifiable behavior principles, although they may not be intentionally manipulated.

The multilevel approach of PBT recognizes that there are various kinds of human problems, with people who have various personality characteristics, people who are established in various types of environments. Those various problems call for various kinds of treatments, involving various combinations of the levels of knowledge involved in the approach. Thus, treatment can vary from directive to nondirective, within the consistent set of principles.

The trick, of course, is to understand the nature of those treatments in basic terms, so they can be developed scientifically, as well as by clinical artistry. The point is that PB, because of its multiple levels, offers principles and concepts by which to understand and develop various types of therapies, without the mutual exclusiveness that results without a unifying theory.

Treating Symptoms or Causes

In the preceding chapter the principle of compounding was introduced, which is that the individual's personality repertoires and life conditions (such as loss of employment) may result in an emotional state and consequent behaviors that exaggerate what would be a reasonable emotional response. As was indicated, once the exaggerated negative emotional state is reduced, a swing back to a normal response to life conditions can commence. When the dysphoria is reduced, then the individual does not say such negative things, the individual's incapacities are then reduced, the individual is not responded to so negatively, the dysphoria is thus further reduced, and so on. That process that begins undoing the exaggeration can be the action of a drug that reduces the dysphoria the depressed person experienced from the environmental (job) loss.

Remember, however, central in the depression are the individual's BBRs, including the negative verbal labeling, the lack of assertiveness, and the poor job-seeking skills. The drug will not affect the individual's BBRs. In that sense the drug treatment is symptomatic. For the individual is still vulnerable to exaggerated response to negative environmental occurrences. If during the drug treatment the patient has made no BBR changes, and the environmental problem still exists when the drug is withdrawn, the patient will experience the negative emotional state again and the resulting compounding.

Let us say, however, that the drug treatment has been combined with other treatment. Let us say the client has been given psychotherapy that changes the individual's negative verbal-labeling repertoire and such. Also, without the crippling dysphoria, she has received job counseling and has been guided to look for work, make plans, reconstruct goals, and to learn she has abilities to do so. Let us say that these things, in addition to the drugs, have improved what she says about herself, hence reducing the dysphoria on a more lasting basis. With such changes she may be able to withstand withdrawal of the drug. For to successfully treat a person's vulnerability to depression it is necessary to change the BBRs that lead to exaggeration of the negative emotional state in response to life's buffets, failures, and demands. The implications of the PB theory are clear, that is, that drug treatment should be coordinated with psychological-behavioral treatment. Treatment may also demand dealing with the environment to make it less negative, when this is pertinent and possible.

The view that "Cures are achieved by treating the symptom itself. . . . Symptomatic treatment leads to permanent recovery" (Eysenck & Rachman, 1965) has set up an opposition to traditional therapy. The PBT position is that the behavior itself in some cases is the problem. But in other cases the proximal cause of the behavior problem may reside in the individual's personality repertoires or the social environment or, less proximally, in the client's past. Manipulation of conditions that change the behavior without changing the causative conditions can be symptomatic and not effective. The "school phobic" child who goes to school because of a contingency contract that yields reinforcement will not be "cured" if the real problem consists of deficit language-cognitive BBRs that prevent her from doing well in school, or of sensory-motor deficits that make her the butt of teasing in gym class, or of a gang of schoolmates who menace and mistreat her. Behavioral treatment that does not make an analysis of the various causes of the problem behavior may indeed be symptomatic.

Ahistorical or Historical

As already indicated, Eysenck (1960a) criticized psychoanalysis in part because it was historical. In the present view that was "throwing out the baby with the bath water." That psychoanalysis attempted to consider child development was a strong plus; the problem was it dealt with historical events poorly. Radical behaviorists have also expressed lack of concern with the origins of behavior problems (Lovaas, 1966). PBT considers important the conditions of the client's original learning of the BBRs. Knowing about past conditions may be essential in understanding the behavior problems of the individual and treatment may involve "repairing" the effects of the past learning in the psychotherapeutic exchange.

Let me extend the principle with respect to child and family behavior therapy. It is a mistake to deal only specifically with a child's reporting problem, as something to be taken care of by application of a behavior principle. A child's problem is always a problem of learning (even when the limitation is biological). If the child has an inappropriate behavior it can only be because training conditions of the social environment have included inappropriate elements. If the child (without biological limitations) has a deficit in behavior it is because the social environment has not arranged training circumstances to produce development of that behavior. Moreover, a training environment that has been awry in one way is more likely to be awry in others.

The behavior therapist needs knowledge concerning the learning of the BBRs generally, to be able to specifically and generally analyze actual and potential problems of training. The therapist who knows about the child's development through learning and how the parent can promote it may have very valuable preventive-treatment services to offer. The behavior therapist should have as full understanding as can be gained of how behavior problems develop in order to consider the individual's general, as well as specific problems. Such knowledge would, for example, enable behavior therapists to identify potential cases of autism. Behavior therapy must develop its interest in analyzing child learning.

Multimodal or Single Technique Therapies

A strict radical behaviorism approach to therapy rests upon the principles of reinforcement and techniques of application—such as contingency contracting, token reinforcement (token economy)—that have come to be accepted. Such an approach does not use systematic desensitization, rational-emotive, cognitive–behavioral therapies, or any verbal psychotherapy. In practice, however, most behavior therapists, even those who are behavior analysts, combine techniques in an eclectic way.

The PBT levels of study, in contrast, provide the basis for a multimodal approach that is "principled" rather than eclectic. Thus, PBT provides the conceptual basis for combining conditioning procedures with psychotherapy, depending upon the demands of the case. PBT, because of the breadth and depth of its underlying theory, is intended to serve as the framework for dealing with all types of human problems—including existential problems as well as those in abnormal psychology taxonomies. Sometimes the problems are limited and apparent, such as a child without toilet skills. Sometimes the problems are complex, such as a general dissatisfaction with one's life. It may be that the nature of the problem is only revealed after engaging in therapy sessions. The therapist may first have to establish what the problems are in the client's BBRs through interviews and through using assessment and psychological test instruments, not through the client's version of the presenting problem. The nature of the current environment may be involved in the problem, perhaps in complex personal relationships—that may have to be uncovered. Treating the problem may involve changing the individual's BBRs, or changing elements in the current environment. This may involve work only with the client. But it may involve work with couples, with families, with social agencies, or call for social change.

Are the constituents of a radical behaviorism approach too restrictive? What about the new interest in "functional analytic psychotherapy" (Dougher & Hackbert, 1994; Kohlenberg & Tsai, 1994)? Well, for one thing, this interest in psychotherapy is arising with a more than 20-year lag and does not originate from radical behaviorism. Moreover, the methods that Dougher and Hackbert employ, for example, are no different than those used in Rogerian psychotherapy, or Ellis's rational-emotive therapy, or PBT's language behavior therapy, when the principles involved are analyzed. They are verbal psychotherapy methods which, in each case, include decreasing the client's negative emotional state. Rogerian therapy decreases negative emotionality by the extinction that occurs through warm acceptance and the resulting catharsis; Ellis by discussions indicating to the client that the negative emotional state is irrational and by pointing out a more positive way of thinking; PBT by changing language patterns in order to elicit more positive emotions; and Dougher and Hackbert do the same by telling the client not to worry about having the negative emotional state because the state is natural and expected. All of them get the client to speak (think) more positively about her state of affairs. But only PBT analyzes what is done in terms of more basic principles. The manner in which "functional analytic therapy" (see Dougher, 1994) rejects other psychotherapies is inconsistent, since it is not itself derived from radical behaviorism knowledge and is no better founded than the clinical psychotherapies.

Psychological behaviorism therapy states that the various psychotherapies require analysis in terms of more basic principles and concepts and that PB provides the conceptual foundation for that purpose. When this is done—as Gross (1992) showed with family therapy—the reasons for the efficacy of the therapies will be understood and further development projected.

> If client-centered therapy could be founded upon a set of empirically derived, cause and effect principles, and methods of research introduced on this basis, it might be possible to develop the method to have the scientific advantages of behavior therapy. This is but an example, to open up the possibilities for investigation and to break down the boundaries of dogmatic separation. (Staats, 1972, p. 174)

There are great advances to such unification. It is time that our field begins to realize such advantages.

Separatistic or Unificationistic

In the above statement we can also see an early call for unification in the field of psychotherapy within behavior therapy, which PB elaborated in the context of recognizing that there are several hundred different psychotherapies, each a separate theory and method. "They don't listen to anybody else; t]hey don't read anybody else's literature[; i]t's quite an odd mishmash of things" (Marshall, 1980, pp. 506–507). This is a very ineffective way to run a scientifically based profession, actually like the state of the natural sciences some 500 years ago. Radical behaviorism has been no help in this problem, for radical behaviorism carries a deep characteristic of separatism and disunification (see Skinner, 1988) which appears in its applications. As an example, when Dougher (1994; Dougher & Hackbert, 1994) proposes a radical-behavioral therapy he does so by rejecting the rational-emotive approach. This is done as a matter of course, even though the two psychotherapies are really very much alike, and rational-emotive therapy preceded radical-behavioral psychotherapy and must, along with other therapies, have been functional in the development of the latter.

Psychological behaviorism, in contrast, asks how there could be several hundred psychotherapies without a great deal of overlap. If that commonality exists then our field is much less useful to the student, researcher, theorist, and applied worker (clinician) when that commonality is hidden in several hundred different theory languages. One line of advancement of behavior therapy that must receive attention is that of developing or using an overarching theory that selects the valuable parts of the various therapies and puts them into a common set of principles and concepts. It is suggested that, to serve such a unifying function, the overarching theory must have a rich set of principles and concepts. The set of conditioning principles offered by radical behaviorism is not rich enough. One of the features of the multilevel theory structure of PB is that by development of the basic conditioning principles over the several levels of study, the fund of principles and concepts is greatly elaborated, made richer and more general. With each behaviorizing analysis, of theoretical elements, phenomena, methods, therapies, psychological tests, and such, the theory grows more rich and more heuristic as a consequence. PB has been employed to analyze the elements of various therapies in showing that it can serve as an overarching theory with which to unify the different therapies. It is suggested that PBT theory be systematically used to analyze the various therapies and abstract their common concepts and principles in the process of incorporating their elements into a unified framework. Done systematically, this would add to a psychological behavior therapy intended to be broad, deep, and heuristic. Such work would advance enormously the value and status of behavior therapy and psychology.

The Behavior Therapy Relationship to Basic Study and to General Psychology

A perennial complaint in behavior therapy is the separation between basic study and clinical practice. That complaint arises because even the behaviorally oriented behavior therapies do not have a basic theory that connects them to basic study. For example, those interested in treating patient's worldviews, irrational beliefs, excessive memory of negative events, and many other clinical problems, using radical-behavioral psychotherapy, find no suitable principles or analyses in Skinner's behaviorism. Behavior therapy needs connection to more basic fields—such as human learning, child development, social psychology, personality, personality measurement, and abnormal psychology—that radical behaviorism does not provide. The basic theory for the field cannot be narrow.

A theory such as PB, with its multilevels, provides a means by which to connect to and use those more basic fields. When such a behavior therapy theory is employed there is no need for a basic-applied separation. At present the approaches in behavior therapy are not providing the needed bridges, even among the different approaches on its own level. Rather, cognitive and cognitive–behavioral approaches are generally placed in opposition to behaviorism (see Meichenbaum, 1977, pp. 143–144), meaning Skinner's radical behaviorism. That opposition is unnecessary, if psychological behaviorism is considered.

Psychological behaviorism says that cognitive, cognitive–behavioral, and radical behavioral approaches do not include in their purviews the bridging developments for developing behavior therapy. And they include materials that are obstacles. As examples of the latter in radical behaviorism, the superfluously detailed study of reinforcement schedules, the approaches called contextualism, emergent behaviorism, and interbehaviorism, the over-specialized and underanalyzed studies of stimulus equivalence, the limited and non-empirical study of rule-governed behavior, and the excessively convoluted theory of establishing operations have not produced new developments that are important to behavior therapy—although this is claimed (Dougher & Hackbert, 1994; Hayes & Wilson, 1994). Similarly, much of the theory of cognitive behaviorism—treatments of the philosophies of hermeneutics, and constructivism and allusions to information processing, connectionism, and attribution theory—are cited as though they are basic to behavior therapy (see Craighead, Craighead, Kazdin, & Mahoney, 1994), but they have never been used, or projected for use, in the research or practice of behavior therapy. These are all currently popular topics, so there is a press to include them, but there is no justification on the basis of past or present utility.

Psychological behaviorism suggests, on the other hand, that there are materials not currently being studied in behavior therapy that really are integral to the advancement of the field. These materials are present in each of the levels of study that has been dealt with. For example, the principles by which classical conditioning is related to operant conditioning are essential to understanding how emotion affects behavior. This needs systematic research which would provide an essential basic-applied connection underlying the various behavior therapy procedures that change behavior via changing emotions. Such study provides basic understanding of why emotion is of concern when we are interested in problem behaviors. There cannot be a basic-applied connection unless basic study is relevant. Also the human learning level of study has not been organized as a systematic field, and hardly considers the needed topics. The principles of social interaction are not systematically dealt with, which means they are not available for dealing with topics involving family behavior therapy and for introducing a "behavioral community psychology." Behavior therapy makes little connection to the field of child development, despite the centrality of this subject matter. The deficit that is caused from lack of a working connection to the fields of personality and personality measurement is catastrophic. And behavior therapy has not had a bridge by which to elaborate a heuristic, bi-directional connection to the field of abnormal psychology. Behavior therapy needs an overarching theory that provides a basis for these bridges to the basic levels of study important to behavior therapy.

The Methodology of Concept Definition

Skinner's (1948, 1950, 1969) behaviorism has been advanced as though its methodology is consistent (see also Sidman, 1960), with its terms operationally defined by experimental analysis of behavior procedures. The fact is that this methodology is consistent only as long as experimental-analysis-of-behavior phenomena are treated. When human behavior is dealt with (see Skinner, 1953, 1957) terms are introduced that do not follow that methodology. Take the concept of *private events* (Skinner, 1953). There are no behavioral operations that define that term. That enables behavior analysts (see Dougher, 1994; Dougher & Hackbert, 1994; Hayes & Wilson, 1994) to use the term private events to "explain" anything, in a manner that is not different than the mentalisms of traditional psychology. Dougher (1994) uses the concept as a means of criticizing the term anxiety as used in Ellis' cognitive–behavior therapy (see Robb, 1994). Strange as it seems, the field of radical behaviorism contains many terms that are not behaviorally justified. When Skinner used poorly defined terms he established a model for others to follow. Terms like *augmenting, establishing operation, shaping, rule-governed behavior, rules,* and *conditioning history* are used in a variety of ways without specific definition. The following is a good example of the type of faulty theory construction that occurs in behavior analysis. Dougher (1994) has criticized behavior therapy for using a concept of anxiety, along with the idea that reducing anxiety can provide treatment of behavior problems. His behavior analytic position is that anxiety does not determine behavior, environmental contingencies determine behavior. So, in treating a case of public speaking phobia, instead of the concept of reducing anxiety he would substitute the concepts of "disruptive contingencies" as the cause and "depotentiating the disruptive contingencies" as the treatment.

> One could, as well, depotentiate the disruptive contingencies in a variety of ways, rehearsing the paper while anxious, telling oneself repeatedly that it is not critical that one gives a good paper, . . . taking a Valium, engaging in relaxation training, etc." (Dougher, 1994, p. 249)

But by what means does Dougher convert rehearsing a paper, taking a Valium, and so on, into the environmental events that gave rise to the problem? There is no relationship between such events and the environmental events about which Dougher speculated. What rehearsal and Valium do change is the anxiety (emotional) response of the individual to public speaking (actual or projected). Because radical behaviorism lacks a concept of emotion as a causal process, Dougher invents "causal" terms with a radical behaviorism flavor. Just like Skinner's term *private events,* however, Dougher provides no empirical definition of his principle of *depotentiating contingencies.* The term is as vague and circular as any mentalistic term can be, lacking even the specification of an intervening variable.

The field of behavior analysis has taken Skinner's position, and what others have thought Skinner's position to be, as the authority with respect to theory. That position has detracted from the otherwise valuable works of important radical behaviorists such as Dougher. For Skinner did not have a good grasp of what theory is or what psychology needs as theory. There has thus been no systematic program in radical behaviorism for establishing theory in behavior therapy/analysis. PBT takes the position that empirical concepts and principles at each of the levels of study—as well as the animal level—must be introduced with the same empirical methodology. PB does not employ the intervening variable methodology (Plaud, 1995). In Hull (1943) and Spence (1944) the intervening variable *learning* was defined by conditioning variables on the antecedent side and response variables on the consequent side. Learning itself was nothing, just a term labeling the relationship between antecedents and consequents. However, PB's concepts are not like that. For example, the concept of the emotional response refers to a real event. The same is true of the BBR. This term stands for actual repertoires of learned behaviors that must be isolated and studied (defined) empirically. Centrally, however, we should understand that empirical definition is only *one* of the important parts of psychological theory construction concerns.

Framework Theory

A textbook or review chapter or article presents a summary description. The framework theory is also less than complete and, in that sense, can be considered a summary presentation. But these types of work are not to be confused. The review groups materials for didactic presentation. It contains minimal theoretical formulation. In contrast, the framework theory is incomplete because it is developed in detail only at selected places, having beginning developments at other places, and empty places in still others. But framework theory is real theory; it has the heuristic value of theory where it is developed in detail. It also has heuristic value where it has only begun development. And it has heuristic value in the empty places for the researcher who can extrapolate the theory's principles and concepts to new areas.

For example, PB's detailed analysis of language and its learning and function has been presented as a theory of what takes place in psychotherapy. That could provide a framework for a program of research on psychotherapy, such as in studying the various ways the individual can be changed through means of language for therapeutic purposes. As an example of an area that has a beginning analysis, let us take the development of the emotional-motivational repertoire in childhood. It has been suggested that behavior disorders, such as childhood autism, involve deficits and inappropriateness in learning the emotional-motivational BBR. That may be considered a beginning theory development that calls for systematic extension and research. Even more generally, the framework asks how the child learns interests—to playing with others, to appropriate sex identity and preference stimuli, to proper foods, to reading, to athletics, to helping others, to achieving, to others' opinions, and so on. These things are all important for the child's development and for continuing adjustment through adolescence into adulthood. This central area has virtually no development in psychological study. The framework theory provides a starting point.

There are other places in the framework theory that have little or no beginning analysis, perhaps no indication that there is a complete absence of development—where the theory could be employed. For example, no systematic theory has been constructed to unify the many concepts, principles, and procedures of treatment employed in the field of clinical psychology. There has been no theoretical structure by which to do this. But such a work would be enormously valuable for the student, the practicing professional, and the researcher. PBT, because of its comprehensive structure, could be used as the framework within which to carry out such a large work. But that PBT work has not been done. The PBT framework has various other empty places that constitute a call for development. Important aspects of PBT are its framework theory, character, the heuristic value of this type of theory, and the fact that works elaborated within the framework will be part of a unified structure.

THE BIOLOGICAL LEVEL: DRUGS AND PBT

Psychological behavior therapy can only be exemplified, and that includes each topic treated, including this section's concern with the use of drugs in clinical treatment. Drug treatment of problems of behavior is traditionally linked to biological explanations of human behavior. Let me use depression as the first example. The fact that drugs can be employed to treat depression suggests to some that depression arises because of some biological condition that the drug remedies. But in the PB view that is a gratuitous interpretation. The drug's success may result from a quite different type of causation, as has been indicated in describing the example of symptomatic treatment. Success of a drug in relieving depression may have nothing to do with treating some biological problem or deficit in the individual. In the PB view, also, the drug does not have its effect by changing the BBRs (the individual's personality), the environment, or the individual's past learning history. The drug has its effect by lessening the individual's negative emotional state, the dysphoria, and negative emotional responding. And that change, in turn, affects the individual's behavior. Moreover, that change, in turn, affects the individual's life situation, which acts back upon the individual (affecting her emotional state, her BBRs, and behavior, in a continuing interaction).

In the PB view it is incorrect to conclude that the positive effects of a drug prove that there was something wrong with the individual biologically to begin with, that some defect in brain anatomy or function caused the person to be depressed. To exemplify the PB position, it is quite evident that alcohol can make a person "happier," but that does not mean that the person had a biological defect to begin with that was making them unhappy. The person could be normally happy, with no hint of biological defect, before consuming the alcohol. Alcohol can simply give a high, as can other psychoactive drugs. The same logic applies to those with anxiety disorders. Successful treatment with drugs is not proof of prior biological problems. The ordinary way that behaviors (including emotions) are elicited is by a certain type of environmental input. It is possible, however, to get a behavioral output by directly affecting the brain in some way—electrically, chemically, by injury, and by drugs.

The use of drugs should be studied within the framework of how they affect the organism at the several sites in the PB theory, that is, O_1, O_2, and O_3, shown in the figures of the preceding chapter. Drugs can have their effects by changing how the individual learns BBRs, by changing the general operation of BBRs themselves, by changing how the individual perceives and responds to the environment, and by changing the individual's emotional state. Each will affect behavior. Effective drug action, in the PB view, ordinarily takes place through these behavioral mechanisms, not by curing biological problems.

The drug effect is not analogous to replacing or repairing a part in an automobile engine, such that the change produces a well-functioning mechanism from one that has been malfunctioning. Complex human behavior is the result of complex environmental experience in the complex interactive way that has been depicted. It is important that this conception be understood, for the biological-defect-and-cure conception cuts out the learning-behavioral conception that is the real cause of individual differences in human behavior and in problems of human behavior. PBT calls for a program of research to study the various ways that drugs have their behavioral effects through their actions at the various sites of causation that have been described.

The PBT position, thus, is that the biological level of study must also be added to the various levels that behavior therapy needs to address. Doing so provides a basis for projecting new directions of research on the clinical effects of drugs in treating behavior disorders. The types of biological study that are needed are not being produced in the traditional framework. As in the other cases, behavior therapists also need to understand how the biological level can be linked with the other levels of study in a principled, noneclectic manner. If drug prescription privileges come to be added to clinical psychology training, it will be even more crucial that behavior therapy have such a theory foundation.

THE NATURE OF BEHAVIOR THERAPY/ANALYSIS AND ITS POTENTIAL FOR DEVELOPMENT

The field of behavior therapy/analysis today has great power. That power derives from having arisen within the behaviorism tradition. For that tradition has as its purview central principles for explaining human behavior, the principles of learning/behavior, and a scientific (behavioral) research methodology. Any field that adopts that tradition will have power in the study of human behavior. Thus, behavior therapists/analysts have employed the principles and methodology in dealing with a wide array of human problems, constructing treatment procedures and measuring technologies as well as empirical means for assessing results. The products of those applications can be seen in the textbooks on the field (see Craighead, Craighead, Kazdin, & Mahoney, 1994), as well as in the impact that behavior therapy has had on the fields of clinical psychology and abnormal psychology.

But behavior therapy/analysis has employed the second-generation radical behaviorism for its basic principles and its methodological philosophy. Cognitive social learning eclectically adds to those constituents modeling (incorrectly considered as a basic principle), plus appended parts of other behaviorisms (including PB), as well as commonsense cognitive concepts. Neither of these framework theories is adequate for the task of guiding the development of the field. The result is an aimlessness that is clear to see (Staats, 1995b), and a grasping at what is popular in psychology, whether or not it pertains to behavior therapy. Thus, a recent textbook in the field (Craighead et al., 1994) presents such topics as information processing, hermeneutics, connectionism, social constructionism, and other cognitive topics, as though they are basic foundations—when these aspects of psychology played no role in the behavior therapy's development, and do not do so today.

Behavior therapy/analysis needs an overarching framework theory that makes the learning/behavior principles central, but that also provides additional principles and methods by which to establish linkages with the fields of psychology. No approach to clinical psychology—not psychoanalysis, Rogerian therapy, rational-emotive therapy, etc.—has established such linkages. Each, thus, can only serve limited functions, and must remain isolated and not fully general, even within its own sphere of interest. The same fate is in store for the field of behavior therapy that concentrates its development in only the clinical level of study, using the second-generation behaviorisms (and cognitive behaviorisms) that have been employed. That constitutes a limited scope of development, because it is based on a limited use of the potential of the area of science that addresses the principles of learning/behavior.

Behavior therapy/analysis needs for its development a multilevel theory that is behavioral in principle and method, and *maintains* its responsibility for the study of the principles of learning/behavior. But that theory must also connect in a close theoretical and heuristic development with the various fields of psychology. Behavior therapy needs knowledge developed in basic animal learning/behavior study, human learning/cognitive study, child development study, social psychology study, personality study, personality measurement study, and abnormal psychology study. Behavior therapy also needs to provide input into those fields so that they in turn study matters important to behavior therapy and to an understanding of complex human behavior generally. Behavior therapy/analysis will only achieve such developments if it adopts a theory framework that provides the necessary avenues for that development. Unified with an overarching, multilevel, framework theory such as PB, behavior therapy/analysis could not only connect to psychology's fields, and become more closely woven into psychology, but also serve as the vanguard in leading psychology in the manner promised by the original behaviorism revolution.

CHAPTER 9

A New Type of Theory: Formally and Heuristically

There are different methods of constructing theories—some of which have been considered generally in science. Theories differ, for example, in their formal features stemming from their construction.

FORMAL FEATURES OF PB

Logical Characteristics

Logical positivism's emphasis on axiomatization/mathematization of theory in the PB view established a standard of scientific theory for psychology that was misleading. Axiomatization/mathematization is valuable in certain special circumstances, for example, when the phenomena studied lend themselves to depiction in the precise language of formal logic and mathematics. However, for the modern disunified science of psychology—with its morass of theories, methods, and findings—the primary task of a unified theory is weaving together a consistent, principled theory that is logical and heuristic even though it is much more complex than can be represented in formal logic and mathematics.

PB is not axiomatized, but it follows throughout a logical, closely reasoned construction. It is possible to trace the statements at the advanced levels of the theory back to the basic principles in a clear manner. Several requirements are involved in constructing such a theory.

Explicitness and Analysis

One way that psychology theories differ is in the explicitness of their statement. Some make specific and explicit analyses, indicating clearly what the phenomena are, the causal conditions, as well as the principles that relate the two. When theories have this characteristic of explicitness we know what the theory states. We can make predictions from the theory, derive expectations, and change the phenomena by manipulating the causal conditions.

We can see the differences among theories in this respect. Typically, for example, theories that have been derived from naturalistic study will not explicitly stipulate the behaviors involved or the causes of the behavior. With complex occurrences the various events will not be analyzed and separated. Rather, vague concepts will be employed that refer to combinations of events that are not well identified. For example, Gregory (1992, pp. 157–158) lists more than 20 different definitions of intelligence. Traditional psychological theories are not the only ones that are not explicit. Bandura (1977b) uses the concept of modeling in such a variety of ways—not only for imitation, but also communication, verbal instruction, meeting standards, and reading—that modeling is a catchall category. Rather, each different phenomenon requires distinguishing its concepts and principles. Today in the field of behavior analysis there is disagreement on the definition of rule-governed behavior because it is a vaguely stated concept (see Burns & Staats, 1992). Piaget, as another example, uses analogy as though it is explanation in his theory construction (see Staats, 1975, pp. 567–570), in his concept of *assimilation*, in place of clearly specified basic principles of learning.

PB does not accept such methodologies. Instead it demands specific analysis and explicit concepts. As one example, the PB concept of intelligence is derived from the study of specific repertoires, how they are learned, and how they affect the later experience, learning, and behavior of the individual. The PB theory requires explicit concepts to stand for explicit events. Thus, in personality the concept of the BBR is different than the traditional concepts of the trait, the ego (id and superego), the self, the self-concept, self-efficacy, personal construct, need, personality type, cognitive style, schema, and so on. It is also different than concepts such as private events, learning history, shaping, augmenting, depotentiating disruptive contingencies, and modeling. Each of these ostensibly behavioral terms is a catchall term lacking explicitness and specification. Theory that is based on vague, unspecified terms can only vaguely address problems to serve theoretical, methodological, or empirical functions.

Intervening Variable and Internal Processes as Causal Agents

Modern radical behaviorism, following Skinner's original position (see Hayes & Brownstein, 1986) is that the task is to study how the environment directly determines behavior. Concepts of internal behavioral events are conjectured but are not treated systematically. The position is that emotions as well as thoughts (cognitions) can be considered as behavioral in nature, but not as causes of behavior. This position is considered to be in opposition to "mechanistic" views (Hayes, 1995; Hayes & Brownstein, 1986) and to the use of intervening variables (see Plaud, 1995; Ulman, 1990). Within this position traditional concepts such as personality, intelligence, emotion, mediating responses, attitudes, and many more are rejected as being intervening variables. PB is considered mechanistic because it analyzes into specific stimuli and responses more complex behavioral events. No distinction is made between the concept of intelligence in traditional psychology and the concept of intelligence that is analyzed into its behavioral components in PB. All non-indigenous concepts that refer to personal causation of behavior are rejected (see Dougher, 1994; Hayes & Brownstein, 1986). This position actually involves methodological confusion and inconsistency in theory construction. For example, Hayes criticizes the use of analyses that involve one of the individual's behaviors being the cause of another. But then he makes analyses that involve just such uses (Hayes, Zettle, & Rosenfarb, 1989), for example, when suggesting that private events explain how the individual behaves. That is, Hayes' concept of private events is apparently "kosher" because it is indigenous to radical behaviorism and is vague and unsystematic. Thus, what is involved is that it is acceptable to infer internal causal events when the concept is vaguely suggestive of some behavioral process, but not when the behavioral process is systematically defined in an explicit manner.

PB takes the position that there are internal behavioral events that have stimulus properties and thus can help determine the individual's behavior. PB considers this circumstance to represent a special problem for psychology, that is, that very generally events important in immediately determining human behavior lie within the individual, out of sight. The trick is to study those events as systematically as possible, not to refuse to consider those events or to do so only vaguely. It is systematic development that enables the internal event to be considered as a determinant of behavior. It is that development that provides a basis for doing something about such internal events in a way that has useful scientific outcomes. Without systematic development a concept such as the private event is not a useful "cause" in a behavior analysis. It is a concept that can be used to suggest that some question has been answered without actually doing so.

When personality is considered an intervening variable, as it is in cognitive social learning theory (Bandura, 1978; Rotter, 1954), what personality *is* is not specified. The concept of the BBR, however, is not an intervening variable. PB makes, and calls for, empirical definition of the contents of the BBRs, how the contents are learned, and how they have their effects on behavior. It is because PB provides such analytic definition that its concepts of personality, such as intelligence and the emotional-motivational repertoire, are not intervening variables. They are concepts that specify causes (the environment), the personality events, and the behaviors that are affected. Many of the BBRs involved in personality have not been identified yet. The theory thus calls for much additional theory, method, and empirical development. But the task is generally that of identifying actual repertoires, not inferred processes out of reach of observational specification.

Vagueness and the Radical Behaviorism Rejection of S-R Analysis

Part of radical behaviorism's opposition to analysis of complex behaviors into more elementary stimulus-response (S-R) constellations is relevant here. This position derives from the fact that in the second generation of behaviorism it was Hull (1930) who was interested in S-R analysis and Skinner was not. That difference was elevated into an orthodoxy in radical behaviorism. But that position today prevents radical behaviorists from being analytic in facing the task of studying complex behaviors and repertoires.

In the PB view this handicaps radical behaviorism, condemning both animal and human behavior theory to vagueness and lack of analysis. We can see this in the radical behaviorism concept that reading can be explained as texting, that is, as verbal responses under the control of written verbal stimuli. That simplistic, unanalytical conception can be contrasted with the PB theory of reading as a set of different types of repertoires that are considered in detail. In general, PB presents a clear and contrasting approach, that human behavior is not understood until it has been analyzed into the behavioral events of which it is composed, which are stimulus and response events. The better the analysis in this respect the better the understanding.

There are various additional formal characteristics of PB that should be compared to those of other approaches. The above have been described because they bear on points of issue that are the basis for contemporary separations among radical behaviorism, psychological behaviorism, and cognitive behaviorism.

HEURISTIC FEATURES

Although there have been various grand theories in psychology—the period preceding the 1960s was considered the "Age of Theory" (Koch, 1981) because the second-generation behaviorisms aimed to be such theories. As has been indicated, however, those theories did not address the various fields of psychology. PB, in contrast, has been constructed to serve as a real, heuristic theory, not just in one of its levels of study, but in each of them.

It is not easy to indicate through examples, but the PB program includes over forty years of using PB concepts and principles in analyzing each behavioral event the author encountered. That included the events encountered in personal (and professional) experience as well as second-hand experience as in reading research articles and news and magazine accounts. That reading cut across the various fields of psychology and the social sciences. Each of the analyses made in that manner became part of the developing overarching framework theory. The importance of that activity should be stressed. Theories based only on laboratory study, on what has been learned from dealing with some research area, and the special research derived from the theory, have a less rich foundation. Usually such theories do not address life behaviors. The more a theory is used in a broad-spectrum analysis of behavior, and extended and elaborated in this use, the more broadly and deeply the theory can be developed. This is a part of theory construction in psychology that is not systematically considered. It is also of interest to note that the more, and the more widely, the user of the theory makes analyses with the theory, the better she or he becomes in its use. My experience of these various types has been that there is no type of human behavior that cannot be analyzed within the PB theory, and in a manner that improves upon an analysis that has been made with another theory that is limited to study in a specialized area.

Some of PB's implications for development will be described. I have said that PB is composed of three types of theory, the individual specialized theories, the level theories, and the overarching theory. A word will be said of each of these.

The Three Types of Theory

The Overarching Theory

The overarching theory is heuristic in setting general directions of development. In this sense it functions systematically but broadly, for the scientist, clinician, or lay person. With respect to the psychological scientist, for example, the overarching theory is heuristic in terms of indicating the relationships of the fields and thus where to look in each field for the explanation of its phenomena. It is heuristic also as a guide for definition of the fields. Let us take social psychology as an example. One position is taken by Worchel, Cooper, and Goethals (1988), who define social psychology to concern general laws of social behavior. "[P]ersonality differences are not what concern the social psychologist; he or she is interested in determining the way in which *most* people interact" (Worchel, Cooper, & Goethals, 1988, p. 7). However, the field of social psychology is where much of the research and theory in personality takes place. The question that should be posed is how does the study of general principles of social interaction relate to the study of personality (individual differences in behavior)? As has been indicated already, the overarching PB theory provides a framework for personologists, social psychologists, and psychometricians to consider their levels of phenomena within the same framework of principles. This unification calls for studies showing how social interaction principles and personality principles are interrelated in determining behavior. Because social-personality phenomena generally are not analyzed in terms of more basic principles they are not integrated, but are considered different in principle (e.g., Tait, in press). For example, cultural determination of human behavior is frequently considered differently than personality determination—when in PB they are considered in the same learning terms in a manner that has heuristic implications.

The overarching theory also must be progressively developed to indicate those elements in the various fields that are to be considered. In addition, the overarching PB theory indicates (progressively) the range of problem areas to be studied in the science and provides principles, concepts, and methods by which to analyze and relate major phenomena studied in the various fields. When this vision is narrow, the work conducted within the overarching theory has that characteristic. The difference in the purview of radical behaviorism and psychological behaviorism is centrally important. For example, radical behaviorism did and does not call for study of emotion, personality, attitudes, intelligence, psychotherapy, the interrelationship of classical and operant conditioning, and many more.

This concerns an important heuristic function of the overarching theory. As another example, let us take the relationship of the biological level and the basic learning level. One result of the PB overarching theory treatment is a call for work to resolve the biological–behavioral opposition. PB's position is that the biological events that are important to behavior operate according to behavior principles. Simple to say, this position has broad implications. At the basic level PB calls for the study of the biology of the basic conditioning principles, of the emotional response, and of the mechanisms involved in the relationship between the emotion-eliciting and reinforcing functions of stimuli (see Staats, 1975, chap. 15). There is already research in this area and it needs to be included as an important part of a new basic field of learning/behavior. The biological–behavioral relationship posited in PB, however, also calls for research at each of its levels of study. For example, as has been indicated, at the abnormal behavior level of study it would be important to establish specifically how the biological defect of Down's syndrome affects the learning of the child. The same is true of any biological defect that leads to behavior disorder.

In addition to these types of uses, however, the overarching theory is a general guide for the development of the discipline, and it provides a general conception or worldview (philosophy) of human nature that can serve the various uses to which such general conceptions are put. For example, in its 1975 version psychological behaviorism included a chapter dealing with humanistic concepts and the humanistic perspective and also a chapter on the social sciences and humanities. With respect to the latter, cultural evolution was said to take place through learning principles, not the principles of biological evolution that are implied by the concept. As another example, the laws of marginal utility (supply and demand) of economics were analyzed in behavior principles. The analysis continued on to include Karl Marx's historical materialism and Charles Beard's Marxist *Economic interpretation of the Constitution of the United States* (1913). "[It] is proposed that there is a unity of science extending through the biological, behavioral, and social sciences and the humanities" (Staats, 1975, p. 584). In more recent times radical behaviorists have adopted similar interests (see Malagodi, 1986; Ulman, 1995). Interestingly Ulman, while rejecting psychological behaviorism (1990), takes the same position as psychological behaviorism with respect to constructing a worldview of human behavior that includes analysis of Marx's materialism (Ulman, 1979, 1983). Skinner (1953, 1971) never projected the use of reinforcement principles for this purpose. As indicated in PB the various social sciences and humanities (such as history and ethics) base themselves in a "psychology" that provides them with principles and concepts for analyzing their domains of phenomena. Anthropology in the past employed Freud's theory for that purpose as have other social theorists. It is suggested that PB could be widely employed as such a psychology in sociology, anthropology, political science, economics, and history to yield an extensive program of research and conceptual development. The result would be an important development toward unifying the social sciences.

Finally, as I have already mentioned, clinicians employ a worldview in dealing with their clients. How they interpret a particular case will depend upon the worldview they employ. For example, a psychoanalytic clinician will view a case of uncovered memories of childhood sexual molestation differently than a behavior therapist. I suggest that study would reveal that behavior therapists, moreover, have different incidences of occurrence of such cases in their practices *because* they have different worldviews. The point I wish to make is that different overarching theories in psychology should be compared and evaluated multidimensionally. Different overarching theories have different characteristics. Thus, for example, PB differs from radical behaviorism in its structure (multilevel versus two-level), in its philosophy of science (as in PB's concern with unifying psychology), in its general methodology (as in its multimethod research approach), in its agenda (as in behaviorizing psychology versus displacing psychology), in its goal of creating a detailed theory of human behavior versus the goal of creating a philosophy of human behavior, and so on. Such overarching characteristics have heuristic impact and differences are thus important.

The Level Theories

Psychological behaviorism says that psychology must concern itself with its fields as levels of study and thus construct conceptual frameworks for those fields. Any theory that claims to be general must address the various fields and have framework theories for them. PB states that each level of study requires a theoretical framework by which to guide some good part of the work of the field. The fact is, at least in some cases, theories do exist that are theories for a field. Thus, the various behaviorisms were taken to be theories of the field of learning (Hilgard, 1948), and theories of personality should act as level theories for the fields of personality and personality measurement. Because these things have not been recognized, the grand theories have not been constructed to include level theories, but they should be.

The level theories of PB, with varying degrees of completeness are intended to be theories of the relevant fields. The level theories should provide the principles, concepts, findings, methods, and exemplars that form a structure for the field. Thus, PB's theories of the three BBRs provide principles, concepts, and findings that are relevant for the fields of personality and psychological measurement. Since the level theory is a framework it is heuristic in calling for researchers and theorists to analyze additional areas of research that are relevant to the level theory. For example, PB's social interaction level has not addressed the topic of love (among various other phenomena), now of current interest in social psychology. The PB theory of social interaction, however, could be employed in the analysis of love research. The result would be unification of love research with the study of attitudes, attraction, group cohesiveness, and such (see Staats, 1975, chap. 7). Such a theory would also suggest new types of research. Thus several types of heuristic value are involved.

A level theory begins with the principles and concepts of the overarching theory and elaborates them by applying them to the phenomena, concepts, and principles of the field. In doing so the level theory grows by abstracting from the many elements of knowledge that have been generated in the field those that lend themselves to unified connection. Not every element of knowledge in a field will fit into the level theory. But those that do will gain significance in addition to that which they have as isolated endeavors. As indicated, the central heuristic value of the level theory is that it provides a beginning framework theory that perforce can only address a few of the field's phenomena. The incompleteness of the framework calls for analysis of the other phenomena in the field, in the construction of additional individual theories. This aspect of the level theory constitutes a very broad heuristic guide. Each analysis needs empirical validation, which is a measure of the value of the theory. Each success will elaborate the unified coverage of the framework theory; each failure will delimit or invalidate the framework theory.

The Individual Theories

The individual theories are engines for specific research. Developed in an explicit behavioral sense, the individual theories can yield new empirical expectations. I have attempted to exemplify how PB's individual theories—such as those of intelligence, emotion, interests, depression, language, and reading—have generated developments in the past. The newest such development involves the Peter Staats, Hamid Hekmat, and Arthur Staats (in press) PB theory of pain. The theory has already begun to generate research (Hekmat, Staats, & Staats, 1995; Staats, Staats, & Hekmat, in preparation) and to initiate conceptual questions (see Tait, in press).

The individual theories are also exemplars. They show generally how the PB concepts and principles can be employed to analyze additional behavioral phenomena. They provide models for entering into new types of investigation. Examples of new implications for development at the individual theory level will now be exemplified in PB's several levels of study.

The Philosophy of Science Level

John Watson began the interest in considering what behaviorism stood for as a science. The major second-generation behaviorists continued this interest, focusing on analysis of the definition of theoretical concepts. Such considerations were influenced by the philosophies of science called operationism and logical positivism. These behaviorists did not develop new general philosophies of science by which to characterize what psychology is like as a science, for example, what features it has that are like those of the advanced sciences, and how psychology differs from those sciences. The general practice has always been to look to specific developments of the older sciences for elements that would be helpful in developing psychology. After all, the founding idea of our discipline was that science methods would be applied to psychology's phenomena. Thus, as one example, psychologists became enthralled with attempting to apply Heisenberg's principle of uncertainty to understanding behavior phenomena, as they have with many other specific developments in physics, chemistry, and biology. In contrast, the philosophy of science of PB takes the position that the general features of the sciences are the same, but not specific developments, such as the uncertainty principle. Psychology's own products should be studied—within a general understanding of science as an empirical endeavor—for the purpose of understanding the characteristics of psychology. Specifying those characteristics provides a basis for advancement.

Unified positivism attempts to describe important aspects of science that have not been considered in traditional philosophy of science, namely with respect to the disunity–unity dimension of development. This philosophy then serves as a foundation for considering psychology's chaotic unrelatedness and the need for unification. This philosophy constitutes one of PB's levels of study and it is thus relevant to indicate that this philosophy has heuristic features. For one thing, analyzing psychology as a disunified science has raised this as an issue in the field. At the beginning the position was opposed (see Baars, 1984), but progressively other psychologists have begun to adopt and advance unified positivism. Various people have considered and built on unified positivism (see, for example, Bechtel, 1988; Darden, 1993; Rappard, 1993; Robinson & Woodward, 1989). Kimble has adopted the unified positivism program (1995, p. 30) and states that "the major problem facing psychology today" is that it "is a discipline divided" (Kimble, 1995, p. 30).

But the philosophy has additional heuristic characteristics. For example, it sets forth various unification endeavors—such as establishing the commonalities among the many concepts, principles, findings, methods, phenomena, and theories in psychology. That calls for many theoretical studies, of various types (see Staats, 1983). The philosophy also calls for the construction of unified theories, and various theories have been constructed in response (see Boneau, 1988; Gilgen, 1985, 1987; Kimble, 1994). But accepting the unified positivism goal does not automatically provide the solution to psychology's problem. Thus, the new unified theories are being constructed in the same way that the old theories were constructed that did not produce unification. The field generally needs to develop knowledge of how to construct unified and unifying theory. The science and profession must systematically consider what characteristics a unified theory must have, what the theory must address, how to construct such a theory, and what it must yield. In addition, the manner in which psychology *operates* with respect to making its knowledge compact and parsimonious (or the converse) must be studied. At present there is huge unrecognized redundancy, repetition, and lack of interrelating of relevant materials. Research areas are developed, go through a furious activity, and later are dropped because in being related to nothing else they have no general meaning. Unified positivism makes the search for relationships a primary endeavor. The philosophy of the science generally held in psychology does not consider the nature of disunified science, and psychology's singular goal of producing novelty does not engender work to remove disunity and produce unity. Within the unified positivism analysis of psychology there lie large directions for philosophical and scientific development (see Staats, 1983, 1991, 1994).

The Basic Learning/Behavior Theory Level

Psychological behaviorism's individual theories in the basic level of study have been heuristic in producing studies, for example, in the three-function principles, in the basic theory of emotion-motivation, in the conditioned sensory response concepts and principles, and in higher-order operant conditioning. Let me give an example of the heuristic value of the three-function learning theory, the centerpiece of PB's basic theory. The manner in which the theory calls for biological–behavioral research was described earlier. Three-function learning theory also calls for development of apparatus and studies by which to investigate with animals the interaction between classical and operant conditioning already explored with human subjects (Harms & Staats, 1978; Staats & Hammond, 1972; Staats, Minke, Martin, & Higa, 1972; Staats & Warren, 1974). In addition, there are many phenomena in basic animal learning that need to be studied within the theory's principles. For example, auto-shaping has briefly been analyzed in terms of three-function principles but a general theoretical treatment is called for, along with additional empirical study. The same is true of transfer of control studies and others, such as in the analysis of the learning of feeding skills in ring-tailed doves (see Balsam, Deich, & Hirose, 1992). A program of research on the animal level is needed to establish clearly the three-function learning principles and their derivatives (such as how deprivation–satiation and extinction affect the three functions) with diverse subjects involved in different types of behavior relevant to different areas.

The Human Learning/Cognitive Level

Although there are many works in psychology that are relevant to the human learning/cognitive level developed in Chapter 2, ordinarily these works are conducted in theory frameworks foreign to behavioral analysis. Thus many works in cognitive psychology provide information on the language-cognitive BBRs but they need analysis before their significance for behavior theory can be seen. Without that analysis those works are seen as antagonistic to a behavioral approach. With behaviorizing analyses behaviorism and cognitivism could be unified. PB analyses have shown this many times, for example, with word meaning (Staats, 1968a, pp. 138–144) and purpose (Staats, 1963b). As another example, Rumelhart (see Peterson, 1993), in cognitive neural network theory, has made an analysis of the child developing past-tense verb endings that is exactly like the analysis made two decades earlier in PB theory (see Staats, 1971b). Psycholinguistics and connectionism could and should be unified broadly with psychological behaviorism

These are only exemplars. The PB position projects a systematic program of theory with the purpose of analyzing the various studies of humans' cognitive characteristics. That is, cognitive psychology studies human cognitive characteristics such as memory, information processing, verbal learning, perception, themes, problem solving, language, and on and on. Cognitive psychology assumes that humans' cognitive characteristics are an inherent part of being human, presumably because of humans' biological nature. Radical behaviorism rejects this study as mentalism and washes its hands of the matter. The PB position is that humans' cognitive characteristics are the result of learned BBRs. What is necessary is an integration of the two types of study. It is important to study what humans' cognitive characteristics are, as has been the goal of cognitive psychology. When such characteristics have been isolated, however, it is necessary to analyze in behavioral terms what those cognitive characteristics consist of, how those characteristics are learned, and how they operate to affect behavior. PB analysis can provide those missing components.

A cognitivism–behaviorism unification would be a powerful development for psychology. The PB approach (see Staats, 1968a) projects that goal, within which there is a huge new direction of research endeavor, that is the "behaviorizing" of cognitive research, and the consequent "cognitivizing" of behaviorism. This is an important part of the PB call for a human learning/cognitive field of study which would inspire many empirical, methodological, and theoretical studies, and help unify the very unrelated elements of knowledge in cognitive psychology. The results would provide an enriched basis for the more advanced levels of study of human behavior.

The Child Development Level

In the traditional field of child development many studies have been conducted for the purpose of establishing what are considered to be the biologically determined principles of child development. Child developmentalists have studied many types of behavior that arise in children over time. Frequently concepts will be introduced to depict the mental developments that are presumed to be biologically based and that cause the behavior development. But analyses of these characteristics in behavioral terms are not made.

In contrast to radical behaviorism, the psychological behaviorism theory of child development considers the traditional field to have produced multitudes of important observations and studies of the behavioral development of children. However, while the field of child development assumes the development occurs because of biological/mental maturation, PB has made analyses and studies of various kinds of development in learning terms—such as handedness, walking, number concepts, writing, attention and attention span, work habits, reading, intelligence, and speaking and other aspects of language development. These PB works constitute exemplars of the relevance of PB theory and methods for the study of child development. This theory level suggests that every important behavior that has been studied and specified in the traditional field should be subjected to "behaviorizing" within the framework of PB learning-behavior and human learning/cognition principles. This should be done with behaviors ranging from the sensory-motor development traditionally studied, to the moral development of Kohlberg (1981), to the cognitive abilities that were the focus of Piaget's (Piaget & Inhelder, 1964) interest, to the early temperament characteristics studied in infants (Thomas & Chess, 1977, 1981), to the repertoires measured on intelligence and adjustment tests, and to the many language characteristics studied in developmental psycholinguistics. Whether or not, and how, learning is important in these and all cases of behavior development in children cannot be answered by the nature–nurture schism and the research it spawns. The answer will only be provided by many analyses of the behaviors involved and studies that provide specific experimental-longitudinal training to produce those behaviors.

The Social Psychology Level

Social psychology includes many phenomena and research areas and multitudes of studies, mostly descriptive, but does not provide unifying analyses and theories. As one example, description of how races differ and how sexes differ and the beliefs (folk theories) about the differences (see Martin & Parker, 1995) does not produce general understanding of those social phenomena. Such description is important but does not provide explanatory principles, principles that will relate the particular phenomenon to other phenomena, and explain the phenomena. PB work and that of other learning-oriented social psychologists (for example, Berkowitz & Knurek, 1969; Byrne, 1971; Doob, 1947; Lott & Lott, 1960; Miller & Dollard, 1941; Staats, 1968b; Staats & Staats, 1958) involve the analysis of social phenomena in terms of learning-behavior principles. Such analysis can provide explanation, and can have empirical implications. What has not been grasped by the field, however, is that making analyses of different phenomena in terms of a unified set of principles results in unifying those phenomena. Social psychology is a chaotic field, with many unrelated phenomena, that desperately needs unifying theory development. The behaviorizing work accomplished thus far, while impressive, is only a bare beginning in the development of a unified framework theory for the phenomena, concepts, principles, findings, and methods of social psychology. Systematic and detailed work is needed on any *framework* that projects a general program of advancement in unified analysis. In the PB view this must involve addressing the important social *behaviors.* Traditional interests have included such things as aggression and violent behavior, persuasion, conformity, helping and altruistic behavior, leadership behavior, attribution (judgment concerning causes of happenings), attitudes and prejudice, attraction, impression formation, social perception, love, values, group cohesion, and ingratiating behavior, to name a few. Cognitive psychology's many unrelated concepts by themselves do not, and cannot, provide the foundation for unifying social psychology phenomena.

The same is true of social *stimuli*. For example, traditional social psychology has studied personal perception (including stimulus factors), the physical attributes (stimuli) that affect social interaction (such as attraction and leadership), the reference group as an influence on behavior, the extent of agreement of the other person, propinquity and exposure to social stimuli, aggression and helping cues, social influence stimulus variables (such as status and power), density and crowding effects, and stimulus effects on person perception. The general category of interest is in the immediate stimulus circumstance that affects social behavior. These interests also need to be behaviorized—that is, the effects of stimulus attributes need analysis in behavioral terms—for this will provide a common language with which to related stimulus effects to consequent social behavior. Such work would result in considering the phenomena within a common framework, which would unify and make more powerful the field of study. Within these two types of concern lie many potential studies.

Finally, a general point relevant to all the fields can be made here. Social psychology is based on the implicit assumption that it can develop autonomously on its own level. Currently a pretense is made that its foundation is in basic cognitive psychology, but there is no meaningful relationship. Social psychology's many cognitive concepts are derived with the restricted perspectives of its many different areas of specific study. Without unification within the level of study, and without connection to other levels, social psychology is sentenced to perpetual unrelated diversity and triviality, as shown by the faddishness that has been described (Elms, 1975; Moscovici, 1972).

The Personality Theory Level of Study

The character of the PB theory of personality raises questions concerning the various theories of personality. For example, the PB theory has an evidential foundation that covers the various levels of study. What are the evidential bases of other personality theories? Is the evidence direct or indirect (such as verbal reports of behavior)? Is it broad and diversified, or is it of one type (such as the clinical interview, or psychometric study)? Does the theory justify the use of various methods, since methods developed in different approaches are usually considered antagonistic? Theories constructed on the basis of different types of evidence will have different characteristics and uses, so each theory must be considered in those terms.

In terms of theory construction, how precisely are the concepts and principles of the theory defined? How susceptible are the concepts and principles to empirical specification? How internally consistent is the theory?

How closely reasoned is the theory—for example, as it moves from its more basic principles to its more advanced principles and empirical (or applied) hypotheses? Are the basic principles assumptions or are they specified empirically? How explicit, specific, and closely related are the parts of the theory? If the theory has animal and human parts, as is true in behaviorism, how consistent is the theory in both parts with respect to systematicity and empirical specification? How general is the theory? Does it apply only to a subset of the phenomena in personality? Or does it aim to address the phenomena broadly? Is the theory related to other personality theories? Does it call for unification or does it reject the products of other approaches? Is the theory heuristic, narrowly or broadly, in a vague or specific manner? What are the theory's goals and its program for attaining them? How does the theory intend to relate to the rest of psychology? The personality field of study desperately needs to examine its many theories to see just what their characteristics are, to compare theories, and to develop knowledge of the field's contents and its needs.

This PB analysis calls for an extensive set of theory studies of the field's theories. Presently, there is a great deal of unrelated knowledge in the field of personality, and much redundancy. There is great need for theoretical work to "clean up the mess," to separate out what the common principles, concepts, methods, and findings are. Such commonality would represent consensual knowledge, which presently is absent in the field. And, especially, it is important to begin working to put the knowledge of the field in a consistent terminology of a general theory language. Elements that are in one theory and not the others need also to be analyzed for possible inclusion in the general theory. The elements that are at issue among the theories need to be considered in studies aiming at resolution. It is time to begin the huge labor of systematization to organize and integrate the knowledge of the field and to make it consensual where possible. And it is time to evaluate the personality theories for what they can contribute to this task. There is a large program of theory work to be done, and the issues that arise in such work will lead to empirical work as well. Without any general guiding framework the work of the field seems random, without a goal, as is characteristic of early science. The many works that have been done in the past (Elms, 1975; Moscovici, 1972) are just filed away in favor of going on to some new topic of study. This lack of organized endeavor, and the lack of progress that follows, must figure into the question of some personologists that the field has a future.

It is suggested that the PB theory of personality could be employed as the framework for an organized, generally meaningful program of theoretical and empirical research. PB in behaviorizing different traditional personality concepts—such as the defense mechanisms, the self-concept, interests, values, and intelligence—illustrates that it can serve as a theory with which to unify presently diverse elements in the field. Research has been derived from some of these analyses, showing that the analyses can be heuristic empirically as well as theoretically. There are many other concepts and phenomena in the field that need to be analyzed within the framework, along with the generation of questioning research. Each additional analysis, thus, would place the concept involved into a unified body of knowledge with advantages with respect to parsimony, generality, and theoretical and empirical power. Each analysis, however, will constitute a difficult theory task.

The PB personality theory also aims to analyze and resolve schisms in the field of personality in ways that call for development. For example, with respect to the nature–nurture schism PB considers important the traditional study of personality development in childhood, on the one hand, and on the other calls for analyzing in behavioral terms what is involved and how development is learned. PB is also heuristic theoretically in introducing new concepts and principles to the study of personality, As one example, the theory of the three BBRs calls for the exhaustive study of the BBRs that are learned in childhood, the conditions of learning involved, individual differences in the BBRs and the effects on behavior, and the measurement of the BBRs.

Psychological behaviorism also calls for new methodological considerations. Typically a personality theory will be based upon a particular method. Thus, the clinical interview is the method underlying the observations obtained in formulating theories such as those of Kelley, Rogers, Maslow, and Freud, while psychometric methods underlie the personality theories of Eysenck and Cattell. PB, however, employs methods of study ranging from those of the animal behavior laboratory through experimental-longitudinal study with children to psychometric and clinical methods. The multimethod approach of PB has been displayed in various studies (see Staats, Brewer, & Gross, 1970; Staats & Burns, 1981, 1982).

The Psychological Measurement Level of Study

The PB approach to psychological measurement calls for very large new directions of research. For example, psychological testing is a chaos of unrelated tests. Analysis of the tests in terms of the basic behavioral repertoires would have important products. What the various tests measure would be indicated in basic terms and principles in a manner that would interrelate the tests. Redundancy would be exposed. Traits would be defined in substantive terms. The result would be simplification and unification of the field and provide a basis for relating the field to the rest of psychology.

Moreover, PB analysis of each psychological test calls for empirical research that would provide a means of *behavioral validity*. For example, the analysis of the Strong Vocational Interest test led to research showing that its items are measures of the individual's emotional responding to life stimuli. The items also were shown to be reinforcers. And the interest test was shown to accurately predict choice behavior (see Staats, Gross, Guay, & Carlson, 1973), very explicit validations. Many such analyses of psychological tests, along with related empirical studies, will provide an understanding of what tests measure and *why* tests are effective predictors of behavior. Together such a body of research would be essential in the development of the theories of personality and personality measurement and advance greatly the uses of the tests involved. Such developments, although needed, are presently lacking in the field.

It should be added that PB analysis of a psychological test typically calls for research on the *learning* of the BBRs measured by the test. For example, the analysis of intelligence items for young children indicated the BBRs involved. How the BBRs are learned had already been studied, so it was possible to train children in the BBRs and then employ intelligence tests to measure the effects (Staats & Burns, 1981). The results suggested intelligence is learned and can be changed via learning. There are many studies to be conducted on the learning of the BBRs that are measured on tests.

Not only does PB provide a basis for studying existing tests, but elaboration of its analyses could also provide a framework for reconstructing our fund of psychological tests. For example, tests could be combined to remove overlap, to produce new tests that although fewer in number would cover the same concerns. In addition, elaborated PB theory would also provide a basis for producing new tests that would measure variables not now being considered. To illustrate, PB theory suggests that we need tests that better measure the child's development of the three major BBRs. For example, as suggested in the analysis of childhood autism, one problem lies in the child's aberrant development of the emotional-motivational repertoire. Autistic children generally do not develop the usual positive emotional response to their parents as well as to other objects and activities. We have tests for adults to measure such things as interests, values, preferences, and attitudes—which are parts of the emotional-motivational BBR. But we do not have a test that measures the child's development of emotional responses, for example, love for the parent—a most central aspect of the child's emotional-motivational development. The PB theory of personality suggests various new tests that need to be developed, again projections that call for a large program of development.

The field of psychological measurement is presently unconnected to other fields of psychology. The type of research being described would establish such connections, a most important aspect of unifying the psychometric and the experimental traditions in the study of the content of psychology. The research would also provide a means for unifying behavior therapy with psychometrics, as described in the previous chapter.

The Abnormal Psychology Level

The PB theory of abnormal behavior is set forth as a general theory to be employed in the analysis of all the behavior disorders. The framework calls for various types of studies. For example, to the extent there is biological determination of a behavior disorder, PB takes the position that biology should work its effects through behavioral channels, for it is the behavior of the individual that is disordered. Thus, PB calls for a coordination of bio-logical study with behavioral study. For one thing, PB calls for elucidating how any brain disturbance associated with behavioral disorder affects (1) the original learning of the BBRs; (2) the BBRs after they have been learned; or (3) the manner in which the disturbance affects how the individual can respond to or perceive the current environment. Let us take genetic study as an example. If there are genetic factors that cause behavior disorders PB states this occurs via behavioral mechanisms. Genetic factors could affect the nature of the individual's learning and thus the BBRs. Genetic factors could affect the functioning of BBRs already learned, or the manner in which the individual can respond to the present environment. For the genetic approach to be complete it must indicate the biological and behav-ioral mechanisms that produce disordered behavior. PB suggests the need to pursue the biological–behavioral interplay in any biologically oriented research on human behavior. This is a new conception that calls for a large program of new research to unify behavioral and biological approaches rather than placing them in opposition.

To continue, there are also many studies that have found organic condi-tions that are *associated* with behavior disorders—anatomical, genetic, phys-iological, and biochemical variations. These studies are interpreted to mean that different types of personality and behavior are *caused* by brain differences. The PB interpretation, however, is that size or function differ-ences in parts of the brain can occur because people have been exposed to different environmental conditions, have had different experiences and have learned different BBRs. The PB position has just received support from study showing that people who play string instruments and develop skills with the left hand grow brain tissue in the area that governs that hand (Taub, 1995). Basic support for that position was provided by early studies showing that experience affects the brain development of animals (Rosenzweig, 1984). Thus, as an example, in the PB view it is not enough to find that schizophrenics display some biochemical (or other) feature that is different than normals. PB calls for establishing whether that feature is the *result* of the different life circumstances and drug consumption of schizophrenics from normals, or whether the brain feature *produces* schizo-phrenic behavior. PB calls for interpreting all studies showing brain differ-ences associated with behavior disorder categories to involve the possibility that the causation is not from the brain to behavior but the reverse.

In addition, although this can only be touched upon here, the PB framework suggests that a field of experimental psychopathology be developed that exploits knowledge in the various levels of study applied to the analysis of behavior disorders. Let me illustrate. PB suggests schizophrenia involves disturbances in both the language-cognitive and emotional-motivational BBRs. Can experimental expectations relevant to schizophrenia be derived from the PB theories of language and emotion? As one possibility, do some schizophrenics have a verbal-labeling repertoire that is less well controlled by environmental stimuli than is usual? As another possibility, is the schizophrenic's verbal-emotional repertoire less veridical, less appropriate to environmental stimuli, than is usual? The PB theories of language and emotion provide a basis for projecting various studies of schizophrenia.

As another example, let us take depression. The PB analysis is that the depressed person experiences a continuing negative emotional state. That state should have pretty general effects on behavior. It would be expected, for example, that depressed individuals might respond to some language stimuli with a more negative emotional response than is normal. If this is the case it might be possible to construct a test for the measurement of depression that would be quick and easy to administer and that would disguise what was being measured. James Browning (a graduate student at the University of Hawaii) and I, following this PB analysis, recently presented a group of 242 words to about 100 college students, with instructions to rate them on a seven-point pleasant–unpleasant scale. We found that depressed subjects rated about 20 of those words significantly differently than nondepressed subjects. It may be possible to compose a test of depression that is based upon the simple rating of a small number of such words—a test that would take only moments to administer. This is, thus, an example.

In the PB view, unlike the radical behaviorism view, the traditional taxonomies of the behavior disorders (such as the *DSM-IV*) are essentially behaviorally based. They rest upon clinician's descriptions of symptoms (behavioral deficits and inappropriacies). PB's theories of certain behavior disorders have been formulated, and this constitutes a heuristic suggestion that the theory be used in creating additional theories of other behavior disorders. In the PB view a large program of research is needed in the analysis of the various behavior disorders in terms of the BBRs, how the BBRs are learned, the role of the current environment, how these produce the individual's aberrant behaviors, and the effects of the aberrant behaviors on the social environment. Each analysis of a behavior disorder in the PB theory will place the disorder into a unified framework. When various PB theories of the behavior disorders have been constructed the result will be a compact, unified, parsimonious understanding of the behavior disorders. The construction of a systematic theory of abnormal behavior has been begun (see Staats, 1989). Psychoanalytic theory for a time was considered to have the potentiality for providing a unified theory, but that hope faded. PB retains that goal along with new empirical, methodological, and theoretical projections.

The Psychological Behavior Therapy Level

Various examples of the heuristic value of PBT for the field of behavior therapy were made in the preceding chapter. Only one additional point will be made here; that behavior therapy (like the other levels) should rest on the various more basic levels of study and draw upon those levels in its own development. Research that is conducted on the behavior disorders, although at the abnormal behavior level of study, is very relevant for behavior therapy. That is true of research at the social interaction, child development, and the personality and personality measurement levels in addition to the more basic levels. To illustrate, PB analyses of psychological tests in terms of BBRs can provide a theory foundation for developing treatment programs. For example, the study of intelligence in PB showed that the BBRs of intelligence could be produced through training. Behavior therapy could elaborate the research and develop a general treatment program for intelligence deficits in children. And this applies to the various behavior disorders and problems of behavior.

PSYCHOLOGY HAS THE RAW THREADS BUT THEY MUST BE WOVEN INTO UNIFIED SCIENCE

Psychology has been conducted as a cottage industry, with every problem area, every method, every theory (large and small) developed as an independent element. The various fields of psychology are conducted as autonomous sciences, with little interaction. This produces rival methods, theories, philosophies, and numberless unrelated findings. The product is a chaos, without general meaning and direction, and with faddishness, lack of consensuality, and randomness—the features that make philosophers characterize psychology as a "would-be science" (Toulmin, 1972).

This characterization is anathema to experimental psychologists in the various fields whose goal is to make psychology a science, and who know that the work they do represents good science in method, in results, and in analysis. And perusal of psychology's journals supports that opinion. It is central that the important science developments of psychology be appreciated, as the PB philosophy of unified positivism recognized from the beginning.

> [P]resent-day . . . psychology . . . consists of unorganized striving in large part, and great separatism. It is in a prescientific state. . . . But the science . . . has

great basic constituents. It has an experimental methodology, . . . principles, sophistication in the logic of science, and a comprehensive subject matter that goes from the simple to the very complex. It is a fund of knowledge and technique that with the concentration of a guiding framework—and the participation of a large number of science's members—could enter into the first rank of science. It is a science on the verge of making it big. These possibilities are obscured by the elements of separateness and antagonism that characterize the field of psychology, and by the lack of comprehensive theory to unite the separate strivings. A common set of goals within a common theoretical framework could mobilize the immense strengths now hidden in the field. It is suggested that we must strive for a theoretical framework which has those qualities. The present [and] other works of the author constitute an attempt in that direction. (Staats, 1971b, pp. 234–235).

This early description of psychology outlined the special problem of psychology. It is a science when its specific works are considered. But it is a "would-be science" when its various works are considered together, because they show the unrelated diversity of the endeavor. Psychology has developed part of what is necessary to be a science; but psychology has not developed the other, crucial, part. Psychology also has not generally recognized that it is lacking that crucial part. Psychology thus continues with its singular focus on discovering the new and different phenomenon, theory, concept, method, apparatus, study area, therapy, or test—regardless of the fact that each new element that remains unrelated to the others simply makes the science more complex and diverse, more "would-be" in nature.

Psychology must come to realize that conducting full science demands weaving an ordered, related, compact, generally meaningful body of knowledge. It is important to find the new phenomenon, method, or theory element. But an important part of the value of the new element is how it contributes to the fabric of organized knowledge, not as a wild thread, but as part of a design. Psychology must devote resources to the weaving part of science, not just to the spinning of raw threads. The fields need to be woven together such that their efforts are additive. The same is true of individual theories. It has been customary for theories to be constructed dealing only with particular areas of study. Various theories of personality, for example, have been composed on the basis of constructing a test. But, as has been demonstrated here, a theory of personality must address and include knowledge from various levels of study. In general, whenever a theory has been formulated it is incumbent on psychology to establish the relationship of that theory, and the phenomena it addresses, to other relevant developments in the science. The same is true of every new area of research, and every finding. It is not enough to produce scientific products that remain isolated.

The approach that has been presented here has been constructed within this understanding of the nature of psychology and its need for unified development. This work provides a model of broad, unified theory. Because of its aims PB is not a simple theory. Even its basic principles are more complex than other general behavioristic analyses of human behavior (see Dollard & Miller, 1950; Skinner, 1953, 1957). The extent to which PB can be useful will in good part depend upon how expert the user becomes with the theory. Those who learn the theory well and then apply it to the analysis of all the behavior phenomena they confront—in professional work and in life—will become very expert in the theory, and they will find that they will be able to use it with a wide variety of phenomena, for generating theory and research, for clinical purposes, for analyzing others' research and theory, for raising children and dealing with other life situations, and as a worldview.

The age of traditional grand theory is over, as generally recognized (Koch, 1981). None of the second-generation behaviorisms succeeded in the task of serving as a theory framework for the direction of psychology. The sole survivor of that generation, Skinner's behaviorism, has become an isolated part of the larger discipline. Despite the general recognition of the importance of learning/behavior principles in the development and operation of human behavior, the behavioral tradition has not harvested the *general* promise of its principles. Moreover, no other specific theory—for example, that of Freud or Piaget—has shown the generality needed.

Cognitive psychology gains much of its support because its adherents *believe* that cognitive psychology constitutes a grand theory for psychology. But cognitive psychology only gives the impression that it is a comprehensive unified theory. Primarily the impression is given by cognitive psychology's general use of a few commonsense cognitive terms—such as the mind—and by its acceptance as *cognitive* all the concepts with a cognitive flavor that are generated in widely varying studies. Actually cognitive psychology is composed of a huge fund of theoretical, empirical, and methodological elements that have no real conceptual relationship. As of now the "cognitive" terms that are used by those studying basic learning/behavior phenomena, human learning/cognitive phenomena, child development phenomena, personality phenomena, personality measurement phenomena, abnormal psychology phenomena, and clinical psychology phenomena remain different, but derivationally related to each other and lacking meaningful bridging. Studies or advances made in the basic experimental study of information processing, for example, have no implications for study in social psychology, child development, personality, or any of the other fields. Psychologists in those fields do not even read the basic cognitive literature. To bridge the separation of the many cognitive terms and to establish a unified theory would demand close, detailed, systematic constructions. The different phenomena addressed would have to be related in terms of common concepts and principles in a closely reasoned, derivational way.

The complex, variegated, unrelated diversity that is cognitive psychology does not represent real scientific theory, and it does not yield the powerful, general products of scientific theory.

But it should be understood that the construction of grand theory in psychology has not failed because the goal is inappropriate. The failure has occurred for want of understanding of what psychology is as a science, what its works consist of, and thus what the task of constructing large unified theory demands. Psychological behaviorism's position is that it is time in the development of the science and profession of psychology to again invest important efforts into the creation of comprehensive, unified (grand) theory. However, this time the discipline must do so with a more sophisticated understanding of the *special* characteristics of psychology, thus of the needed theory-construction methodology, as well as of the nature of unified theory in psychology. This time the discipline needs more sophisticated standards, and a systematic program for assessing and relating the unified theories that are formulated as well as for working systematically on their development. Only through the goal of unification, and the investment in that large enterprise, will psychology enter the pantheon of sciences.

REFERENCES/BIBLIOGRAPHY

Abelson, R.P. (1973). The structure of belief systems. In R.C. Schank & K.M. Colby (Eds.), *Computer models of thought and language.* San Francisco: Freeman.

Abidin, R.R. (1983). *Parenting Stress Index manual.* Charlottesville, VA: Pediatric Psychology Press.

Achinstein, P. (1968). *Concepts of science.* Baltimore: Johns Hopkins University Press.

Adams, G.L. (1984). *Test Manual: Comprehensive Test of Adaptive Behavior.* Columbus, OH: Charles E. Merrill.

Adams, J.S., & Romney, A.K. (1959). A functional analysis of authority. *Psychological Review, 66,* 234–251.

Adamson, R. (1959). Inhibitory set in problem solving as related to reinforcement learning. *Journal of Experimental Psychology, 58,* 280–282.

Aiello, L.C. (1994). Thumbs up for our early ancestors. *Science, 265,* 1540–1541.

Alexander, A.B., Chai, H., Cree, T.L., Micklich, D.R., Renne, C.M., & Cardoso, R.A. (1973). The elimination of chronic cough by response suppression shaping. *Journal of Behavior Therapy and Experimental Psychiatry, 4,* 75–80.

Alker, H.A. (1972). Is personality situationally specific or intrapsychically consistent? *Journal of Personality, 40,* 1–16.

Allen, K.E., Hart, B., Buell, J.S., Harris, F.R., & Wolf, M.M. (1964). Effects of social reinforcement on isolate behavior of a nursery school child. *Child Development, 35,* 511–518.

Allen, M.G. (1976). Twin studies of affective illness. *Archives of General Psychiatry, 33,* 1476–1478.

Allen, V.L., & Wilder, D.A. (1980). Impact of group consensus and social support on stimulus meaning: Mediation of conformity by cognitive restructuring. *Journal of Personality and Social Psychology, 39,* 1116–1124.

Allport, G.W., Vernon, P.E., & Lindzey, G. (1951). *Study of values* (rev. ed.). Boston: Houghton-Mifflin.

Ambert, A. (1992). *The effect of children on parents.* Binghamton, NY: Haworth.

American Psychiatric Association. (1987). *Diagnostic and statistical manual of mental disorders* (3rd ed., rev.). Washington, DC: Author.

American Psychiatric Association. (1994). *Diagnostic and statistical manual of mental disorders* (4th ed.). Washington, DC: Author.

Ames, L.B., Gillespie, B.S., Haines, J., & Ilg, F.L. (1979). *The Gesell Institute's child from one to six: Evaluating the behavior of the preschool child.* New York: Harper & Row.

Amsel, A. (1958). The role of frustrative non-reward in non-continuous reward situations. *Psychological Bulletin, 55,* 102–119.

Amsel, A. (1967). Partial reinforcement effects on vigor and persistence: Advances in frustration theory derived from a number of within-subjects experiments. In K.W. Spence & J.A. Taylor (Eds.), *The psychology of learning and motivation.* New York: Academic Press.

Amsel, A. (1972). Behavioral habituation, counter-conditioning, and a general theory of persistence. In A. Black & W. Prokasy (Eds.), *Classical conditioning II: Current theory and research.* New York: Appleton–Century–Crofts.

Anderson, N.H., & Butzin, C.A. (1978). Integration theory applied to children's judgments of equity. *Developmental Psychology, 14,* 607–613.

Andronico, M.P., & Gueney, B., Jr. (1967). The potential application of a filial therapy to the school situation. *Journal of School Psychology, 6,* 2–7.

Annon, J.S. (1975). *The behavioral treatment of sexual problems, Vol. 2.* Honolulu, HI: Enabling Systems.

Appley, M.H. (1990) Time for reintegration? *Science Agenda, 3*(1), 12–13.

Ardila, R. (1983). La sintesis experimental del comportamiento. *Interamerican Psychologists, 58,* April.

Aronfreed, J. (1968). *Conduct and conscience: The socialization of internalized control over behavior.* New York: Academic Press.

Ashem, B., & Poser, E.G. (Eds.) (1973). *Behavior modification with children.* New York: Pergamon.

Atthowe, J.M., Jr., & Krasner, L. (1968). A preliminary report on the application of contingent reinforcement procedures (token economy) on a "chronic" psychiatric ward. *Journal of Abnormal Psychology, 73,* 37–43.

Axelrod, R. (Ed.) (1976). *The structure of decision.* Princeton, NJ: Princeton University Press.

Ayllon, T., & Azrin, N. (1968). *The token economy.* New York: Appleton–Century–Crofts.

Ayllon, T., & Haughton, E. (1962). Control of the behavior of schizophrenic patients by food. *Journal of the Experimental Analysis of Behavior, 5,* 343–352.

Ayllon, T., & Michael, J.L. (1959). The psychiatric nurse as a behavioral engineer. *Journal of the Experimental Analysis of Behavior, 2,* 323–334.

Azrin, N.H. (1975). Eliminating habitual vomiting in a retarded adult by positive practice and self correction. *Journal of Behavior Therapy and Experimental Psychiatry, 6,* 145–148.

Azrin, N.H., & Foxx, R.M. (1974). *Toilet training in less than a day.* New York: Simon & Schuster.

Azrin, N.H., & Lindsley, O.R. (1956). The reinforcement of cooperation between children. *Journal of Abnormal and Social Psychology, 52,* 100–102.

Azrin, N.H., & Wesolowski, M.D. (1974). Theft reversal: An overcorrection procedure for eliminating stealing by retarded persons. *Journal of Behavior Therapy and Experimental Psychiatry, 6,* 145–148.

Baars, B.J. (1984). View from a road not taken. *Contemporary Psychology, 29,* 804–805.

Baars, B.J. (1985a). The logic of unification. *Contemporary Psychology, 30,* 340.

Baars, B.J. (1985b). And once more 'round the mulberry bush. *Contemporary Psychology, 30,* 421.

Bachrach, A.J., Erwin, W.J., & Mohr, J.P. (1965). The control of eating behavior in an anorexic by operant conditioning techniques. In L.P. Ullmann & L. Krasner (Eds.), *Case studies in behavior modification.* New York: Holt, Rinehart & Winston.

Baekeland, F., & Lundwall, L. (1975). Dropping out of treatment: A critical review. *Psychological Bulletin, 82,* 738–783.

Bandura, A. (1961). Psychotherapy as a learning process. *Psychological Bulletin, 58,* 143–159.

Bandura, A. (1962). Social learning through imitation. In M.R. Jones (Ed.), *Nebraska symposium on motivation.* Lincoln: University of Nebraska Press.

Bandura, A. (1968). A social learning interpretation of psychological dysfunctions. In P. London & D. Rosenahn (Eds.), *Foundations of abnormal psychology.* New York: Holt, Rinehart, and Winston.

Bandura, A. (1969). *Principles of behavior modification.* New York: Holt, Rinehart, and Winston.

Bandura, A. (1971). *Psychological modeling.* Chicago: Aldine-Atherton.

Bandura, A. (1974). Behavior theory and the models of man. *American Psychologist, 29,* 859–869.

Bandura, A. (1977a). *Social learning theory.* Englewood Cliffs, NJ: Prentice-Hall.

Bandura, A. (1977b). Self-efficacy: Toward a unifying theory of behavioral change. *Psychological Review, 84,* 191–215.

Bandura, A. (1978). The self-system in reciprocal determinism. *American Psychologist, 33,* 344–358.

Bandura, A. (1986). *Social foundations of thought and action.* Englewood Cliffs, NJ: Prentice-Hall.

Bandura, A., Ross, D., & Ross, S.A. (1963). A comparative test of the status envy, social power, and the secondary reinforcement theories of identification learning. *Journal of Abnormal and Social Psychology, 67,* 527–534.

Bandura, A., & Walters, R. (1959). *Adolescent aggression.* New York: Ronald.

Bandura, A., & Walters, R. (1963). *Social learning and personality.* New York: Holt, Rinehart, and Winston.

Banham, K.M. (1975). *Manual for The Ring and Peg Tests of Behavior Development.* Munster, IN: Psychometric Affiliates.

Barber, T.X. (1976). *Pitfalls in human research: Ten pivotal points.* New York: Pergamon Press.

Barlow, D.H. (1988). *Anxiety and its disorders.* New York: Guilford.

Barlow, D.H., & Agras, W.S. (1973). Fading to increase heterosexual responsiveness in homosexuals. *Journal of Applied Behavior Analysis, 6,* 355–366.

Barnard, J.D., Christopherson, E.R., & Wolf, M.M. (1974). Supervising paraprofessional tutors in a remedial reading program. *Journal of Applied Behavior Analysis, 7,* 481.

Barnes, M.R. (1976). Token economy control of fluid overload in a patient receiving hemodialysis. *Journal of Behavior Therapy and Experimental Psychiatry, 7,* 305–306.

Baron, J. (1973). Phonemic stage not necessary in reading. *Quarterly Journal of Experimental Psychology, 25,* 241–246.

Baron, R.A. (1987). Outlines of a "grand theory." *Contemporary Psychology, 32,* 413–415.

Baron, R.M. (1971). Attitude change through discrepant action: A functional analysis. In A.G. Greenwald, T.C. Brock, & T.M. Ostrom (Eds.), *Psychological foundations of attitudes.* New York: Academic Press.

Barrett, B.H. (1962). Reduction in rate of multiple tics by free operant conditioning methods. *Journal of Nervous and Mental Diseases, 135,* 187–195.

Baum, A., Fisher, J.D., & Solomon, S.K. (1971). Type of information, familiarity, and the reduction of crowding stress. *Journal of Personality and Social Psychology, 40,* 11–23.

Baumeister, R.R., & Tice, D.M. (Eds.) (1994). Debate on how to teach personality. *Dialogue, 9*(2), 7–10.

Bayes, R. (1980). *Una introducción al metodo científico en psicologia.* Barcelona: Editorial Fontanella.

Beard, C.A. (1913). *An economic interpretation of the Constitution of the United States.* New York: Macmillan.

Bechtel, W. (1988). *Philosophy of science: An overview for cognitive science.* Hillsdale, NJ: Erlbaum.

Beck, A.T. (1967). *Depression: Clinical, experimental, and theoretical aspects.* New York: Harper & Row.

Beck, A.T. (1976). *Cognitive therapy and the emotional disorders.* New York: International Universities Press.

Beck, A.T., & Emery, G. (1985). *Anxiety disorders and phobias: A cognitive perspective.* New York: Basic Books.

Beck, A.T., Ward, C.H., Mendelson, M., Mock, J., & Erbaugh, J. (1961). An inventory for measuring depression. *Archives of General Psychiatry, 4,* 561–571.

Becker, W.C. (Ed.) (1971). *An empirical basis for change in education.* Chicago: Science Research Associates.

Begley, S. (1996). Beyond prozac. *Newsweek,* February 7, p. 40.

Bellack, A.S., & Mueser, K.T. (1994). Schizophrenia. In L.W. Craighead, W.E. Craighead, A.E. Kazdin, & M.J. Mahoney (Eds.), *Cognitive and behavioral interventions: An empirical approach to mental health problems.* Boston: Allyn & Bacon.

Bem, A.J., & Allen, A. (1974). On predicting some of the people some of the time: The search for cross-situational consistencies in behavior. *Psychological Review, 81,* 506–520.

Bem, D.J. (1965). An experimental analysis of self-persuasion. *Journal of Experimental Psychology, 1,* 199–218.

Bem, D.J. (1967). Self-perception: An alternative interpretation of cognitive dissonance phenomena. *Psychological Review, 74,* 183–200.

Bem, D.J. (1968). Attitudes as self-descriptions: Another look at the attitude-behavior link. In A.G. Greenwald, T.C. Brock, & T.M. Ostrom (Eds.), *Psychological foundations of attitudes.* New York: Academic Press.

Bender, L. (1938). A visual motor gestalt test and its clinical use. *Research Monograph of the American Orthopsychiatric Association,* No. 3.

Berger, S.M. (1962). Conditioning through vicarious instigation. *Psychological Review, 69,* 450–466.

Berkowitz, L. (1962). *Aggression: A social psychological analysis.* New York: McGraw-Hill.

Berkowitz, L. (1964). Aggressive cues in aggressive behavior and hostility catharsis. *Psychological Review, 71,* 104–122.

Berkowitz, L. (1970a). Theoretical and research approaches in experimental social psychology. In A.R. Gilgen (Ed.), *Contemporary Scientific Psychology.* New York: Academic Press.

Berkowitz, L. (1970b). Experimental investigations of hostility catharsis. *Journal of Consulting and Clinical Psychology, 35,* 1–7.

Berkowitz, L. (1973). Words and symbols as stimuli to aggressive responses. In J.F. Knutson (Ed.), *Control of aggression.* Chicago: Aldine.

Berkowitz, L. (1974). Some determinants of impulsive aggression: Role of mediated associations with reinforcements for aggression. *Psychological Review, 81,* 165–176.

Berkowitz, L., & Devine, P.G. (1989). Research traditions, analysis, and synthesis in social psychological theory. *Personality and Social Psychology Bulletin, 15,* 493–507.

Berkowitz, L., & Knurek, D.A. (1969). Label-mediated hostility generalization. *Journal of Personality and Social Psychology, 13,* 200–206.

Berkowitz, L., & LePage, A. (1967). Weapons as aggression-eliciting stimuli. *Journal of Personality and Social Psychology, 7,* 202–207.

Bevan, W. (1992). *The journey is everything: General-experimental psychology in the United States after a hundred years.* Baltimore: Johns Hopkins University Press.

Bieger, G.R. (1985). Metropolitan Readiness Tests. In D.J. Keyser & R.C. Sweetland (Eds.), *Test Critiques, Vol. II* (pp. 463–471). Kansas City, MO: Test Corporation of America.

Bierstedt, R. (1957). *The social order: An introduction to sociology.* New York: McGraw-Hill.

Bijou, S.W. (1955). A systematic approach to an experimental analysis of young children. *Child Development, 26,* 161–168.

Bijou, S.W. (1957). Methodology for an experimental analysis of child behavior. *Psychological Reports, 3,* 243–250.

Bijou, S.W. (1965). Experimental studies of child behavior, normal and deviant. In L. Krasner & L.P. Ullmann (Eds.), *Research in behavior modification.* New York: Holt, Rinehart, & Winston.

Bijou, S.W. (1976). *Child development: The basic stage of early childhood.* Englewood Cliffs, NJ: Prentice-Hall.

Bijou, S.W., & Baer, D.M. (1961). *Child development, Vol. 1.* New York: Appleton–Century–Crofts.

Bijou, S.W., Birnbrauer, J.S., Kidder, J.D., & Tague, C. (1967). Programmed instruction as an approach to teaching of reading, writing, and arithmetic in retarded children. In S.W. Bijou & D.M. Baer (Eds.), *Child development: Readings in experimental analysis.* New York: Appleton–Century–Crofts.

Bijou, S.W., Peterson, R.F., Harris, F.R., Allen, K.E., & Johnston, M.S. (1969). Methodology for experimental studies of young children in natural settings. *Psychological Record, 19,* 177–210.

Bindra, D. (1978). How adaptive behavior is produced: A perceptual-motivational alternative to response-reinforcement. *Behavioral and Brain Sciences, 1,* 41–91.

Bindra, D. (1984). Cognition: Its origin and future in psychology. In J.R. Royce & L.P. Mos (Eds.), *Annals of theoretical psychology.* New York: Plenum.

Birge, J.S. (1941). Verbal responses in transfer. Unpublished doctoral dissertation, Yale University, New Haven, CT.

Birnbrauer, J.S., Bijou, S.W., Wolf, M.M., & Kidder, J.D. (1965). Programmed instruction in the classroom. In L.P. Ullman & L. Krasner (Eds.), *Case studies in behavior modification.* New York: Holt, Rinehart, & Winston.

Black, J.A., & Champion, A.L. (1976). *Methods and issues in social research.* New York: John Wiley.

Blake, J., & Boysson-Bardies, B.D. (1992). Patterns in babbling: A cross-linguistic study. *Journal of Child Language, 19,* 51–73.

Blakely, E., & Schlinger, H. (1987). Rules: Function-altering, contingency-specifying stimuli. *Behavior Analyst, 10,* 183–187.

Blanchard, R.J., Flores, T., Magee, L., Weiss, S., & Blanchard, D.C. (1992). Pregrouping aggression and defense scores influences alcohol consumption for dominant and subordinate rats in visible burrow systems. *Aggressive Behavior, 18,* 459–467.

Blanchard, R.J., Hori, K., Tom, P., & Blanchard, D.C. (1987). Social structure and ethanol consumption in the laboratory rat. *Pharmocology, Biochemistry, and Behavior, 28,* 437–442.

Block, J. (1971). *Lives through time.* Berkeley, CA: Bancroft Books.

Block, J. (1977). Advancing the psychology of personality: Paradigmatic shift or improving the quality of research? In D. Magnusson & N. Endler (Eds.), *Personality at the crossroads.* Hillsdale, NJ: Erlbaum.

Blum, G.S., & Barbour, J.S. (1979). Selective inattention to anxiety-linked stimuli. *Journal of Experimental Psychology, 108,* 182–224.

Bolles, R.C. (1979). *Learning theory* (rev. ed.). New York: Holt, Rinehart, and Winston.

Bond, G.L., & Dykstra, R. (1967). The cooperative research program in first grade reading instruction. *Reading Research Quarterly, 6,* 5–11.

Boneau, C.A. (1988). Making psychology useful: A framework for understanding human action. *International Newsletter of Uninomic Psychology, 6,* 1–13.

Boodman, S. (May, 1995). What your baby really knows. *Redbook.*

Boring, E.G. (1950). *A history of experimental psychology* (2nd ed.). New York: Appleton.

Bouchard, T.J., Jr. (1984). Twins reared together and apart: What they tell us about human diversity. In S.W. Fox (Ed.), *Individuality and determinism.* New York: Plenum.

Bouchard, T.J., Jr., Lykken, D.T., McGue, M., Segal, N.L., & Tellegen, A. (1990). Sources of human psychological differences: The Minnesota study of twins reared apart. *Science, 250,* 223–228.

Boudin, H.M. (1972). Contingency contracting as a therapeutic tool in the deceleration of amphetamine use. *Behavior Therapy, 3,* 604–608.

Bower, B. (1994). *Science News, 145*(23), (June 4), 359.

Bowers, K.S. (1973). Situationism in psychology: An analysis and critique. *Psychological Review, 80,* 307–336.

Bozarth, M.A., & Wise, R.A. (1984). Anatomically distinct opiate receptor fields mediate reward and physical dependence. *Science, 224,* (9 February), 516–517.

Brackbill, Y., & Koltsova, M.M. (1967). Conditioning and learning. In Y. Brackbill (Ed.), *Infancy and early childhood.* New York: Free Press.

Brady, J.P., & Lind, D.L. (1961). Experimental analysis of hysterical blindness. *Archives of General Psychiatry, 4,* 331–339.

Braithwaite, R.B. (1955). *Scientific explanation.* London: Cambridge University Press.

Brehm, J.W., & Cohen, A.R. (1962). *Explorations in cognitive dissonance.* New York: John Wiley.

Breland, K., & Breland, M. (1961). The misbehavior of organisms. *American Psychologist, 16,* 681–684.

Broadbent, D.E. (1957). *Perception and communication.* New York: Pergamon Press.

Broadbent, D.E. (1970). Stimulus set and response set: Two kinds of selective attention. In D.I. Mostofsky (Ed.), *Attention: Contemporary theories and analysis.* New York: Appleton–Century–Crofts.

Broadbent, D.E., Cooper, P.J., & Broadbent, M.H.P. (1978). A comparison of hierarchical and matrix retrieval schemes in recall. *Journal of Experimental Psychology: Human Learning and Memory, 4,* 486–497.

Brogden, W.J. (1939). Sensory pre-conditioning. *Journal of Experimental Psychology, 25,* 323–332.

Brogden, W.J. (1947). Sensory preconditioning of human subjects. *Journal of Experimental Psychology, 37,* 527–540.

Brown, A.R. (Ed.). (1972). *Modifying children's behavior.* Springfield, IL: C.C. Brown.

Brown, J.F. (1936). *Psychology and the social order: An introduction to the dynamic study of social fields.* New York: McGraw-Hill.

Brown, P.L., & Jenkins, H.M. (1968). Autoshaping of the pigeon's key-peck. *Journal of the Experimental Analysis of Behavior, 11,* 1–8.

Brown, R., & Fraser, C. (1961, June). *The acquisition of syntax.* Paper delivered at the Second ONR-New York University Conference on Verbal Learning. Dobbs Ferry, NY.

Brown, R., & Lenneberg, E.H. (1954). A study in language and cognition. *Journal of Abnormal and Social Psychology, 49,* 454–462.

Browning, R.M., & Stover, D.O. (1971). *Behavior modification in child treatment.* Chicago: Aldine-Atherton.

Brownstein, A.J, & Shull, R.L. (1985). A rule for the use of the term "rule-governed behavior." *Behavior Analyst, 8,* 265–267.

Bruininks, R.H. (1978). *Bruininks-Oseretsky Test of Motor Proficiency examiner's manual.* Circle Pines, ME: American Guidance Service.

Bugelski, B.R., & Hersen, M. (1966). Conditioning acceptance or rejection of information. *Journal of Experimental Psychology, 71,* 619–623.

Bugental, J.F.T. (1967). The challenge that is man. In J.F.T. Bugental (Ed.), *Challenge of humanistic psychology.* New York: McGraw-Hill.

Burian, R.M. (1977). More than a marriage of convenience: On the inextricability of history and philosophy of science. *Philosophy of Science, 63,* 1–42.

Burns, C.E., Heiby, E.M., & Tharp, R.G. (1983). A verbal behavior analysis of auditory hallucinations. *Behavior Analyst, 6,* 133–143.

Burns, G.L. (1980). Indirect measurement and behavioral assessment: A case for social behaviorism. *Behavioral Assessment, 2,* 197–206.

Burns, G.L., & Staats, A.W. (1991). Rule-governed behavior: Unifying radical and paradigmatic behaviorism. *Journal of Verbal Behavior, 9,* 127–143.

Burns, G.L., & Staats, A.W. (1992). Rule-governed behavior: Unifying radical and paradigmatic behaviorism. *Journal of Verbal Behavior, 9,* 129–143.

Bushell, D., Wrobel, P.A., & Michaelis, M.L. (1968). Applying "group" contingencies to the classroom study behavior of preschool children. *Journal of Applied Behavior Analysis, 1,* 55–61.

Byrne, D. (1961). Interpersonal attraction and attitude similarity. *Journal of Abnormal and Social Psychology, 62,* 713–715.

Byrne, D. (1962). Response to attitude similarity–dissimilarity as a function of affiliation need. *Journal of Personality, 30,* 164–177.

Byrne, D. (1971). *The attraction paradigm.* New York: Academic Press.

Byrne, D. (1977). Social psychology and the study of sexual behavior. *Personality and Social Psychology Bulletin, 3,* 3–30.

Byrne, D. (1978). Separatism, integration or parallel play? *Personality and Social Psychology Bulletin, 4,* 498–499.

Byrne, D., Bond, M.H., & Diamond, M.J. (1969). Response to political candidates as a function of attitude similarity–dissimilarity. *Human Relations, 22,* 251–262.

Byrne, D., & Clore, G.L. (1970). A reinforcement model of evaluative responses. *Personality: An International Journal, 1,* 103–128.

Byrne, D., Ervin, C.R., & Lamberth, J. (1970). Continuity between experimental study of attraction and real-life computer dating. *Journal of Personality and Social Psychology, 16,* 157–165.

Byrne, D., & Griffitt, W. (1969). Similarity and awareness of similarity of personality characteristics as determinants of attraction. *Journal of Experimental Research in Personality, 3,* 179–186.

Byrne, D., Griffitt, W., & Clore, G.L., Jr. (1968). Attitudinal reinforcement effects as a function of stimulus homogeneity–heterogeneity. *Journal of Verbal Learning and Verbal Behavior, 7,* 962–964.

Byrne, D., & Nelson, D. (1965). Attraction as a linear function of proportion of positive reinforcements. *Journal of Personality and Social Psychology, 1,* 659–663.

Cameron, N. (1947). *The psychology of behavior disorders.* Boston: Houghton-Mifflin.

Cameron, N. (1963). *Personality development and psychopathology: A dynamic approach.* New York: Houghton-Mifflin.

Campbell, D.P. (1971). *Handbook for the Strong Vocational Interest Blank.* Stanford, CA: Stanford University Press.

Campbell, D.P. (1974). *Manual for the Strong-Campbell Vocational Interest Blank.* Stanford, CA: Stanford University Press.

Campbell, D.P., & Hansen, J.C. (1981). *Manual for the SVIB-SCII* (3rd edition). Stanford, CA: Stanford University Press.

Campion, J.E. (1972). Work sampling for personnel selection. *Journal of Applied Psychology, 56,* 40–44.

Carmichael, L. (1926). The development of behavior in vertebrates experimentally removed from the influence of external stimulation. *Psychological Review, 33,* 51–58.

Carriero, N.J. (1967). The conditioning of negative attitudes to unfamiliar items of information. *Journal of Verbal Learning and Verbal Behavior, 8,* 128–135.

Carrillo, J.M., Rojo, N., & Staats, A.W. (in press). Vulnerable personality in depression:Investigating commonality in the search for unification. *European Journal of Psychological Assessment.*

Carter, H.D. (1940). The development of vocational attitudes. *Journal of Consulting Psychology, 4,* 185–191.

Carver, C.S. (1979). A cybernetic model of self-attention processes. *Journal of Personality and Social Psychology, 37,* 1251–1281.

Casey, R.J. (1993). Children's emotional experience: Relations among expression, self-report, and understanding. *Developmental Psychology, 29,* 119–129.

Catania, A.C. (1989). Rules as classes of verbal behavior: A reply to Glenn. *Analysis of Verbal Behavior, 7,* 49–50.

Cattell, R.B. (1946). *The description and measurement of personality.* New York: Harcourt Brace Jovanovich.

Cattell, R.B. (1976). *Comprehensive personality and learning theory.* New York: Springer.

Chall, J. (1967). *Learning to read.* New York: McGraw-Hill.

Chandler, M.J., Paget, K.F., & Koch, D.A. (1978). The child's emystification of psychological defense mechanisms: A structural and developmental analysis. *Developmental Psychology, 14,* 197–205.

Chapman, C., & Risely, T.R. (1974). Anti-litter procedures in an urban high-density area. *Journal of Applied Behavior Analysis, 7,* 377–384.

Chawarski, M.C., & Sternberg, R.J. (1993). Negative priming in word recognition: A context effect. *Journal of Experimental Psychology: General, 122,* 195–206.

Chesney, M., & Tasto, D.L. (1975). The effectiveness of behavior modification with spasmodic and congestive dysmenorrhea. *Behavior Research and Therapy, 13,* 321–332.

Chiesa, M. (1994). *Radical behaviorism: The philosophy and the science.* Boston: Author's Cooperative.

Chomsky, N. (1959). Verbal behavior (a review of Skinner's book). *Language, 35,* 26–58.

Chomsky, N. (1968). Linguistic contributions to the study of mind. In N. Chomsky (Ed.), *Language and mind.* New York: Harcourt, Brace and World.

Cialdini, R.B., Darby, B.L., & Vincent, J.E. (1973). Transgression and altruism: A case for hedonism. *Journal of Experimental Social Psychology, 9,* 502–516.

Cialdini, R.B., & Kenrick, D.T. (1976). Altruism as hedonism: A social development perspective on the relationship of negative mood state and helping. *Journal of Personality and Social Psychology, 34,* 907–914.

Cofer, C.N., & Foley, J.P. (1942). Mediated generalization and the interpretation of verbal behavior: I. Prolegomena. *Psychological Bulletin, 49,* 513–540.

Cofer, C.N., & Musgrave, B.S. (Eds.). (1963). *Verbal behavior and learning.* New York: McGraw-Hill.

Cole, S., & Cole, J.R. (1967). Scientific output and recognition: A study in the operation of the regard system in science. *American Sociological Review, 32,* 377–390.

Coleman, D.E. (1967). The classical conditioning of attitudes toward selected educational concepts. *Dissertation Abstracts, 27,* 4125.

Coleman, J.C. (1950). *Abnormal psychology and modern life* (2nd. ed.). New York: Appleton.

Coleman, S.R., & Mehlman, S. (1992). An empirical update 1969–1989 of D.L. Kranz' thesis that the experimental analysis of behavior is isolated. *Behavior Analyst, 15,* 43–49.

Collette-Harris, M.A., & Minke, K.A. (1978). A behavioral experimental analysis of dyslexia. *Behavior Research and Therapy, 16,* 291–295.

Cooper, J.B. (1959). Emotion in prejudice. *Science, 130,* 314–318.

Cooper, J.B. (1969). Emotional response to statements congruent with prejudicial attitudes. *Journal of Social Psychology, 79,* 189–193.

Cooper, M.L., Thomson, C.L., & Baer, D.M. (1970). The experimental modification of teacher attending behavior. *Journal of Applied Behavior Analysis, 3,* 153–157.

Coopersmith, S. (1981). *Self-esteem inventories.* Palo Alto, CA: Consulting Psychologists Press.

Costa, L.D., Vaughan, H.G., Levita, E., & Farber, N. (1963). Purdue Pegboard as a predictor of the presence and absence of cerebral lesions. *Journal of Consulting Psychology, 27,* 133–137.

Craighead, L.W., Craighead, W.E., Kazdin, A.E., & Mahoney, M.J. (1994). *Cognitive and behavioral interventions: An empirical approach to mental health problems.* Boston: Allyn and Bacon.

Craighead, L.W., & Kirkley, B.G. (1994). Obesity and eating disorders. In L.W. Craighead, W.E. Craighead, A.E. Kazdin, & M.J. Mahoney (1994). *Cognitive and behavioral interventions: An empirical approach to mental health problems.* Boston: Allyn and Bacon.

Craik, F.I.M., & Tulving, E. (1975). Depth of processing and the retention of words in episodic memory. *Journal of Experimental Psychology: General, 104,* 268–294.

Craik, R.I.M., & Lockhart, R.S. (1972). Levels of processing: A framework for memory research. *Journal of Verbal Learning and Verbal Behavior, 11,* 671–684.

Crane, D.M. (1967). The gatekeepers of science: Some factors affecting the selection of articles for scientific journals. *American Sociologist, 2,* 195–201.

Cuber, J.F. (1955). *Sociology: A synopsis of principles.* New York: Appleton.

Cunningham, G.K. (1986). *Educational and psychological measurement.* New York: Macmillan.

Dahlstrom, W.G., & Welsh, G.S. (1960). *An MMPI handbook: A guide for use in clinical practice and research.* Minneapolis: University of Minnesota Press.

Danforth, J.S., Barkley, R.A., & Stokes, T.F. (1991). Observations of parent–child interactions with hyperactive children: Research and clinical implications. *Clinical Psychology Review, 11,* 703–727.

Darden, L. (1974). *Reasoning in scientific change: The field of genetics at its beginnings.* Ph.D. dissertation, University of Chicago.

Darden, L. (1976). Reasoning in scientific change. *Studies in the History and Philosophy of Science, 7,* 127–169.

Darden, L. (1986). Relations among fields in the evolutionary synthesis. In W. Bechtel (Ed.), *Integrating scientific disciplines.* Dordrecht, Netherlands: Martinus Nijhoff.

Darden, L. (1987). Hypothesis formation using interrelations: Interfield and inter-level theories. *International Newsletter of Uninomic Psychology, 4,* 2–10.

Darden, L. (1993). Comments on Woodward and Devonis: Interfield theories and strategies for theory change. In H.V. Rappard, P.J. van Strein, & L.P. Mos (Eds.), *Annals of theoretical psychology,* vol. 8, New York: Plenum.

Darden, L., & Maull, N. (1977). Interfield theories. *Philosophy of Science, 44,* 43–64.

Darley, J.G. (1960). The theoretical basis of interests. In W.L. Layton (Ed.), *The Strong Vocational Interest Blank: Research and uses.* Minneapolis: University of Minnesota Press.

Davenport, J.W. (1966). Higher-order conditioning of fear. *Psychonomic Science, 4,* 27–28.

Davidson, G.C., D'Zurilla, T.J., Goldfried, M.R., Paul, G.L., & Valins, S. (1968). In M.R. Goldfried (Chair), Cognitive processes in behavior modification. Symposium presented at the meetings of the American Psychological Association, San Francisco, August.

Davis, G.A. (1973). *The psychology of problem solving.* New York: Basic Books.

Davis, J.R., Wallace, C.J., Liberman, R.P., & Finch, B.E. (1976). The use of brief isolation to suppress delusional and hallucinatory speech. *Journal of Behavior Therapy and Experimental Psychiatry, 7,* 269–275.

Dawe, H.C. (1942). A study of the effect of an educational program upon language development and related mental functions in young children. *Journal of Experimental Education, 11,* 200–209.

Deese, J. (1969). Behavior and fact. *American Psychologist, 24,* 595–622.

de Groot, A.D. (in press). Unifying psychology: Its preconditions. In H.V. Rappard & P.J. van Strein (Eds.), *Current Issues in Theoretical Psychology.* Amsterdam: North Holland.

DeMonbreun, B., & Craighead, W.E. (1977). Distortion of perception and recall of positive and neutral feedback in depression. *Cognitive Therapy and Research, 1,* 311–329.

Dennis, W. (1940). Does culture appreciably affect patterns of infant behavior? *Journal of Social Psychology, 12,* 305–317.

Deutsch, J.A., & Deutsch, D. (1963). Attention: Some theoretical considerations. *Psychological Review, 70,* 80–90.

Dollard, J., Doob, L., Miller, N., Mowrer, O., & Sears, R. (1939). *Frustration and aggression.* New Haven, CT: Yale University Press.

Dollard, J., & Miller, N. (1950). *Personality and psychotherapy.* New York: McGraw-Hill.

Doob, L.W. (1947). The behavior of attitudes. *Psychological Review, 54,* 135–156.

Dorfman, D.D. (1978). The Cyril Burt question: New findings. *Science, 201,* 1177–1186.

Dougher, M.J. (1993). On the advantages and implications of a radical behavioral treatment of private events. *Behavior Therapist, 16,* 204–206.

Dougher, M.J. (1994). More on the differences between radical behavioral and rational emotive approaches to acceptance: A response to Robb. *Behavior Therapist, 17,* 249.

Dougher, M.J., & Hackbert, L. (1994). A behavior-analytic account of depression and a case report using acceptance-based procedures. *Behavior Analyst, 17,* 321–334.

Douglas, R.J. (1975). The development of hippocampal function. In R. Isaacson & K. Pribram (Eds.), *The hippocampus.* New York: Plenum.

Dow, M.G. (1994). In L.W. Craighead, W.E. Craighead, A.E. Kazdin, & M.J. Mahoney (Eds.), *Cognitive and behavioral interventions: An empirical approach to mental health problems.* Boston: Allyn and Bacon.

Dunham, P.J. (1978). Punishment of mice and men. *Contemporary Psychology, 23,* 5510–5552.

Dunnette, M.D. (1966). Fads, fashions, and folderol in psychology. *American Psychologist, 21,* 343–352.

Dupaul, G.J., Guevremont, D.C., & Barkley, R.A. (1994). Attention-deficit hyperactivity disorder. In L.W. Craighead, W.E. Craighead, A.E. Kazdin, & M.J. Mahoney (Eds.), *Cognitive and behavioral interventions: An empirical approach to mental health problems.* Boston: Allyn & Bacon.

Durkheim, E. (1927). *Les regles de la metode sociologique* (8th ed.). Paris: Alcan.

Dweck, C.S., Goetz, T.E., & Strauss, N.L. (1980). Sex differences in learned helplessness: KV. An experimental and naturalistic study of failure generalization and its mediators. *Journal of Personality and Social Psychology, 38,* 441–452.

D'Zurilla, T., & Goldfried, M. (1971). Problem solving and behavior modification. *Journal of Abnormal Psychology, 78,* 107–126.

Early, J.C. (1968). Attitude learning in children. *Journal of Educational Psychology, 59,* 176–180.

Edsall, J.T. (1975). *Scientific freedom and responsibility.* Washington, D.C.: American Association for the Advancement of Science.

Edwards, A. (1953). *Edwards Personal Preference Schedule.* New York: Psychological Corporation.

Egeland, J.A., Gerhard, D.S., Pauls, D.L. Sussex, J.N., Kidd, K.K., Allen, C.R., Hostetter, A.M., & Housman, D.E. (1987). Bipolar affective disorder linked to DNA markers on chromosome 11. *Nature, 325,* 783–787.

Eiduson, B.T. (1962). *Scientists: Their psychological world.* New York: Basic Books.

Eifert, G.H. (1983). Test of social behaviorism's conceptualization of self verbalizations: An analogue treatment of phobias. *International Newsletter of Social Behaviorism, 2,* 2–19.

Eifert, G.H. (1985). Rewards for fragmentation. *International Newsletter of Paradigmatic Psychology, 1,* 19–20.

Eifert, G.H., Evans, I.M., & McKendrick, V. (1990). Matching treatments to client problems not diagnostic labels: A case for paradigmatic behavior therapy. *Journal of Behavior Therapy and Experimental Psychiatry, 21,* 245–253.

Ekehammar, B. (1974). Interactionism in personality from a historical perspective. *Psychological Bulletin, 81,* 1026–1048.

Ekstrand, B.R., Sullivan, M.J., Parker, D.F., & West, J.N. (1971). Spontaneous recovery and sleep. *Journal of Experimental Psychology, 88,* 142–144.

Ekstrand, B.R., Wallace, W.P., & Underwood, B.J. (1966). A frequency theory of verbal-discrimination learning. *Psychological Review, 73,* 566–578.

Elbert, T., Pantev, C., Wienbruch, C., Rockstroh, B., & Taub, E. (1995). Increased cortical representation of the fingers of the left hand in string players. *Science, 270,* 305–307.

Elliott, R., & Tighe, T. (1968). Breaking the cigarette habit: Effects of a technique involving threatened loss of money. *Psychological Record, 18,* 505–513.

Ellis, A. (1962). *Reason and emotion in psychotherapy.* New York: Lyle Stuart.

Ellis, A., & Harper, R.A. (1975). *A new guide to rational living.* Los Angeles: Wilshire.

Ellson, D. (1941). Hallucinations produced by sensory conditioning. *Journal of Experimental Psychology, 28,* 1–20.

Elms, A.C. (1975). The crisis of confidence in social psychology. *American Psychologist, 30,* 967–976.

Endler, N.S., & Magnusson, D. (1976). Toward an interactional psychology of personality. *Psychological Bulletin, 83,* 956–974.

Engel, B.T., Nikoomanesh, P., & Shuster, M.M. (1974). Operant conditioning of rectosphincter responses in the treatment of fecal incontinence. *New England Journal of Medicine, 290,* 646–649.

Epstein, R. (1966). Aggression toward outgroup as a function of authoritarianism and imitation of aggressive models. *Journal of Personality and Social Psychology, 3*, 574–579.

Epstein, R. (1984). The case for praxis. *Behavior Analyst, 7*, 110–119.

Epstein, R. (1985). Further comments on praxis: Why the devotion to behaviorism? *Behavior Analyst, 8*, 269–271.

Epstein, R. (1991). Skinner, creativity, and the problem of spontaneous behavior. *Psychological Science, 2*, 362–370.

Epstein, S. (1979). The stability of behavior: I. On predicting most of the people much of the time. *Journal of Personality and Social Psychology, 37*, 1097–1126.

Erdelyi, M.H. (1974). A new look at the new look: Perceptual defense and vigilance. *Psychological Review, 81*, 1–25.

Eriksen, C.W., & Kuethe, J.L. (1956). Avoidance conditioning of verbal behavior without awareness: A paradigm of repression. *Journal of Abnormal and Social Psychology, 53*, 203–209.

Ervin-Tripp, S. (1971). An overview of theories of grammatical development. In D.I. Slobin (Ed.), *The ontogenesis of grammar.* New York: Academic Press.

Esper, E.A. (1964). *A history of psychology.* Philadelphia: Saunders.

Estes, W. (1975). The locus of inferential and perceptual processes in letter identification. *Journal of Experimental Psychology: General, 1*, 122–145.

Estes, W.K. (1974). Learning theory and intelligence. *American Psychologist, 29*, 740–749.

Estes, W.K. (1976). Intelligence and cognitive psychology. In L.B. Resnick (Ed.), *The nature of intelligence.* Hillsdale, NJ: Lawrence Erlbaum Associates.

Evans, I.M. (1986). Response structure and the triple-response mode concept. In R.O. Nelson & S.C. Hayes (Eds.), *Conceptual foundations of behavioral assessment.* New York: John Wiley.

Evans, P. (1978). A visit with Michael Argyle. *APA Monitor, 9*(8), 6–7.

Eysenck, H.J. (1952). The effects of psychotherapy: An evaluation. *Journal of Consulting Psychology, 16*, 319–324.

Eysenck, H.J. (Ed.) (1960a). *Behavior therapy and the neuroses.* London: Pergamon.

Eysenck, H.J. (1960b). *The scientific study of personality.* New York: Macmillan.

Eysenck, H.J. (1987). The growth of a unified scientific psychology: Ordeal by quackery. In A.W. Staats & L.P. Mos (Eds.), *Annals of theoretical psychology,* vol. 5. New York: Plenum.

Eysenck, H.J., & Rachman, S. (1965). *Causes and cures of neurosis.* London: Routledge & Kegan Paul.

Fallon, I. (1988). Behavioral family therapy: Systems, structures and strategies. In E. Street & W. Dryden (Eds.), *Family therapy in Britain.* Philadelphia: Open University.

Fargo, G.A., Behrns, C., & Nolen, P.A. (1970). *Behavior modification in the classroom.* New York: Wadsworth.

Feigl, H. (1970). The "orthodox" view of theories: Remarks in defense as well as critique. In M. Radner & S. Winokur (Eds.), *Minnesota studies in the philosophy of science, Vol. 4.* Minneapolis: University of Minnesota Press.

Feist, J. (1994). *Theories of personality.* New York: Harcourt Brace.

Fenichel, O. (1945). *The psychoanalytic theory of neurosis.* New York: Norton.

Fernandez-Ballesteros, R. (1979). *Los métodos en evaluación conductual.* Madrid: Cincel-Kapelusz.

Fernandez-Ballesteros, R. (1981). *Evaluación conductual.* Madrid: Piramide.

Fernandez-Ballesteros, R. (1983). El concepto de psicodiagnostico. En R. Fernandez-Ballesteros (Ed.), *Psicodiagnostico.* Madrid: UNED.

Fernandez-Ballesteros, R. (1988). Qué escriben los evaluadores conductuales. Unpublished manuscript, Madrid: Universidad Autonoma de Madrid.

Fernandez-Ballesteros, R. (1994). *Evaluación conductual hoy.* Madrid: Piramide.

Fernandez-Ballesteros, R., & Staats, A.W. (1992). Paradigmatic behavioral assessment, treatment and evaluation: Answering the crisis in behavioral assessment. *Advances in Behavior Research and Therapy, 14,* 1–18.

Ferster, C.B. (1961). Positive reinforcement and behavioral deficits of autistic children. *Child Development, 32,* 437–456.

Ferster, C.B. (1973). A functional analysis of depression. *American Psychologist, 28,* 857–870.

Ferster, C.B., & Skinner, B.F. (1957). *Schedules of reinforcement.* New York: Appleton-Century-Crofts.

Feyerabend, P. (1970a). Against method: Outline of an anarchistic theory of knowledge. In M. Radner & S. Winokur (Eds.), *Minnesota studies in the philosophy of science, Vol. 4.* Minneapolis: University of Minnesota Press.

Feyerabend, P. (1970b). Consolations for the specialist. In I. Lakatos & A. Musgrave (Eds.), *Criticism and the growth of knowledge.* London: Cambridge University Press.

Feyerabend, P. (1970c). Against method: Outline of an anarchistic theory of knowledge. In M. Radner & S. Winokur (Eds.), *Minnesota studies in the philosophy of science, Vol. 4.* Minneapolis: University of Minnesota Press.

Feyerabend, P.K. (1963). How to be a good empiricist—a plea for tolerance in matters epistemological. In B. Baumrin (Ed.), *Philosophy of science: The Delaware Seminar, Vol. I.* New York: John Wiley.

Feyerabend, P.K. (1965). Problems of empiricism. In R. Colodny (Ed.), *Beyond the edge of certainty.* Englewood Cliffs, NJ: Prentice-Hall.

Fiedler, F.E. (1967). *A theory of leadership.* New York: McGraw-Hill.

Finch, G. (1938). Hunger as a determinant of conditional and unconditional salivary response magnitude. *American Journal of Physiology, 123,* 379–382.

Finley, J.R., & Staats, A.W. (1967). Evaluative meaning words as reinforcing stimuli. *Journal of Verbal Learning and Verbal Behavior, 6,* 193–197.

Fishman, D. (1990). The quantitative, naturalistic case study: A unifying element for psychology. *International Newsletter of Uninomic Psychology, 9,* 1–10.

Fishman, D.B. (1986). Where the underlying boundaries are: Organizing psychology by paradigm analysis. *International Newsletter of Unification Psychology, 2,* 4–9.

Fishman, D.B. (1987). Unification in psychology: Epistemological prerequisites. *International Newsletter of Uninomic Psychology, 3,* 25–34.

Fishman, D.B., Rotgers, F., & Franks, C.M. (1988). *Paradigms in behavior therapy.* New York: Springer.

Flanery, R.C., & Balling, J.D. (1979). Developmental changes in hemispheric specialization for tactile spatial ability. *Developmental Psychology, 15,* 364–372.

Flavell, J.H. (1963). *The developmental psychology of Jean Piaget.* New York: Van Nostrand.

Foffman, E. (1959). *The presentation of self in everyday life.* Garden City, NY: Doubleday Anchor.

Fowler, R.D. (1990). Psychology: The core discipline. *American Psychologist, 45,* 1–6.

Fraisse, P. (1987). Unity and diversity in the behavioral and natural sciences. In A.W. Staats & L.P. Mos (Eds.), *Annals of theoretical psychology, vol. 5.* New York: Plenum.

Fraley, L.E., & Vargas, E.A. (1986). Separate disciplines: The study of behavior and the study of the psyche. *Behavior Analyst, 9,* 47–59.

Frank, P. (1950). *Modern science and its philosophy.* Cambridge, MA: Harvard University Press.

Franks, C.M. (1960). Alcohol, alcoholism and conditioning. In H.J. Eysenck (Ed.), *Behaviour therapy and the neuroses.* New York: Pergamon.

Franks, C.M. (1964). *Conditioning techniques in clinical practice and research.* New York: Springer.

Franks, C.M. (1969). *Behavior therapy: Appraisal and status.* New York: McGraw-Hill.

Franks, C.M. (1983). Review of industrial behavior modification and organizational behavior management. *Child and Family Behavior Therapy, 5,* 68–70.

Franks, C.M. (1988). Unifying psychology: With special reference to clinical psychology. *International Newsletter of Uninomic Psychology, 5,* 25–27.

Frederiksen, J., & Kroll, J. (1976). Spelling and sound: Approaches to the internal lexicon. *Journal of Experimental Psychology: Human Perception and Performance, 2,* 361–379.

Freund, K. (1967). A laboratory method for diagnosing predominance of homo- or hetero-erotic interest in male. *Behavior Research and Therapy, 5,* 209–228.

Gagne, R.M. (1965). Learning hierarchies. *Educational Psychologist, 6,* 1–9.

Gagne, R.M., & Fleishman, E.A. (1959). *Psychology and human performance.* New York: Holt.

Gambril, E.D. (1977). *Behavior modification.* San Francisco: Jossey-Bass.

Garcia, J., Ervin, F.R., & Koelling, R.A. (1966). Learning with prolonged delay of reinforcement. *Psychonomic Science, 5,* 121–122.

Garvey, W.D., & Griffith, B.C. (1971). Scientific communication: Its role in the conduct of research and creation of knowledge. *American Psychologist, 26,* 349–362.

Gaston, J. (1973). *Originality and competition in science.* Chicago: University of Chicago Press.

Geen, R.G., & Berkowitz, L. (1967). Some conditions facilitating the occurrence of aggression after the observation of violence. *Journal of Personality, 35,* 666–676.

Geer, J.H. (1968). A test of the classical conditioning model of emotion: The use of nonpainful aversive stimuli as unconditioned stimuli in a conditioning procedure. *Journal of Personality and Social Psychology, 2,* 148–156.

Gelfand, D.M. (1962). The influence of self-esteem on rate of verbal conditioning and social matching behavior. *Journal of Abnormal and Social Psychology, 65,* 259–265.

Gellner, E. (1956). Explanation in history. *Proceedings of the Aristotelian Society, 1956.*

Georgi, A. (1987). Taking on the problem of psychology's unity. *International Newsletter of Uninomic Psychology, 4,* 26–31.

Gergen, K.J. (1973). Social psychology as history. *Journal of Personality and Social Psychology, 26,* 309–320.

Gergen, K.J. (1984). The cognitive movement: A turn in the mobius strip. In J.R. Royce & L.P. Mos (Eds.), *Annals of theoretical psychology.* New York: Plenum.

Gergen, K.J. (1985). The social constructionist movement in modern psychology. *American Psychologist, 40,* 266–275.

Gesell, A. (1929). Behavior resemblance in identical infant twins. *Eugenical News, 14*(5).

Gesell, A., Halverson, H.M., Thomson, H., Ilg, F.L., Castner, B.M., Ames, L.B., & Amatruda, C.S. (1940). *The first five years of life.* New York: Harper.

Gesell, A., & Thompson, H. (1929). Learning and growth in identical infant twins: An experimental study by the method of co-twin control. *Genetic Psychology Monographs, 6,* 1–24.

Gesell, A., & Thompson, H. (assisted by C. Strunk). (1938). *The psychology of early growth.* New York: Macmillan.

Gewirtz, J.L., & Baer, D.M. (1958). Deprivation and satiation of social reinforcers as drive conditions. *Journal of Abnormal and Social Psychology, 57,* 165–172.

Giddens, A. (1976). *New rules of sociological method.* New York: Basic Books.

Giles, D.K., & Wolf, M.M. (1966). Toilet training institutionalized, severe retardates: An application of operant techniques. *American Journal of Mental Deficiency, 1970,* 766–780.

Gilgen, A.R. (1985). A strategy for constructing a systematic psychology. *International Newsletter of Uninomic Psychology, 1,* 10.

Gilgen, A.R. (1987). The psychological level of organization in nature and interdependencies among major psychological concepts. In A.W. Staats & L.P. Mos (Eds.), *Annals of theoretical psychology, vol. 5.* New York: Plenum.

Gilgen, A.R. (1987). The psychological level of organization in nature and the interdependencies among major psychological concepts. In A.W. Staats & L. Mos (Eds.), *Annals of theoretical psychology: on unification, Vol. 5.* New York: Plenum.

Gilmor, T.M., & Minton, H.L. (1974). Internal versus external attribution of task performance as a function of locus of control, initial confidence and success-failure outcome. *Journal of Personality, 42,* 159–174.

Glad, B. (1973). Psychobiography. In J. Knutson (Ed.), *Handbook of political psychology.* San Francisco: Jossey-Bass.

Glashow, S.L. (1980). Toward a unified theory: Threads in a tapestry. *Science, 210,* 1319–1323.

Glenn, S.S. (1987). Rules as environmental events. *Analysis of Verbal Behavior, 5,* 29–32.

Glenn, S.S. (1989). On rules and rule-governed behavior: A reply to Catania's reply. *Analysis of Verbal Behavior, 7,* 51–52.

Golden, C.J., Purish, A.D., & Hammeke, T.A. (1985). *The Luria-Nebraska Neuropsychological Battery: forms I and II (manual).* Los Angeles: Western Psychological Services.

Goldfried, M.R. (1976). Behavioral assessment. In I.B. Weiner (Ed.), *Clinical methods in psychology.* New York: John Wiley.

Goldfried, M.R. (1980). Toward the delineation of therapeutic change principles. *American Psychologist, 35,* 991–999.

Goldfried, M.R. (November, 1990). *Psychotherapy integration: A mid-life crisis for behavior therapy.* Invited address presented at the Association for the Advancement of Behavior Therapy Convention, San Francisco.

Goldfried, M.R., & Kent, R.N. (1972). Traditional versus behavioral assessment: A comparison of methodological and theoretical assumptions. *Psychological Bulletin, 77,* 409–420.

Goldfried, M.R., & Pomeranz, D.M. (1968). Role of assessment in behavior modification. *Psychological Reports, 23,* 75–87.

Goldfried, M.R., & Sprafkin, J. (1974). *Behavioral personality assessment.* Morristown, NJ: General Learning Press.

Goldstein, M.K., & Pennypacker, H.S. (1978). Call for papers: APA '79. *Division 25, Recorder, 14,* 1–19.

Golightly, C., & Byrne, D. (1964). Attitude statements as positive and negative reinforcements. *Science, 146,* 798–799.

Goodstein, L.D., & Brazis, K.L. (1970). Psychology of the scientist: XXX. Credibility of psychologists: An empirical study. *Psychological Reports, 27,* 835–838.

Gosling, J. (1986). Analysis and strategy in the search for unity: Epistemic principles for psychology. *International Newsletter of Uninomic Psychology, 2,* 13–19.

Graubard, P.S. (Ed.). (1969). *Children against schools.* New York: Follett.

Grauman, C.F., & Sommer, M. (1984). Schema and interference models in cognitive social psychology. In J.R. Royce & L.P. Mos (Eds.), *Annals of theoretical psychology, vol. 1.* New York: Plenum.

Greenough, W.T., & Green, E.J. (1981). Experience and the changing brain. In J.L. McGaugh, J.G. March, & S.B. Kiesler (Eds.), *Aging: Biology and behavior.* New York: Academic Press.

Greenspoon, J. (1951). The effect of verbal and nonverbal stimuli on the frequency of members of two verbal response classes. Unpublished doctoral dissertation, Indiana University.

Greenwald, A.G. (1968). On defining attitude and attitude theory. In A.G. Greenwald, T.C. Brock, & T.M. Ostrom (Eds.), *Psychological foundations of attitudes.* New York: Academic Press.

Gregory, R.J. (1992). *Psychological testing.* Boston: Allyn and Bacon.

Griffitt, W., & Jackson, T. (1970). The influence of information about ability and non-ability on personnel selection decisions. *Psychological Reports, 27,* 259–262.

Gross, P.R. (1992). The crisis in family therapy: Paradigmatic family therapy solutions. *Child & Family Behavior Therapy, 4,* 39–62.

Groth-Marnat, G. (1990). *Handbook of psychological assessment.* New York: Wiley-Interscience.

Guess, D. (1969). A functional analysis of receptive language and productive speech: Acquisition of the plural morpheme. *Journal of Applied Behavior Analysis, 2,* 55–64.

Guess, D., Sailor, W., Rutherford, G., & Baer, D.M. (1968). An experimental analysis of linguistic development: The productive use of the plural morpheme. *Journal of Applied Behavior Analysis, 1,* 225–235.

Guthrie, E.R. (1935). *The psychology of learning.* New York: Harper.

Hagstrom, W.O. (1965). *The scientific community.* New York: Basic Books.

Hagstrom, W.O. (1967). Competition and teamwork in science. Final Report to the National Science Foundation (in mimeo).

Hamilton, S.A. (1988). Behavioral formulation of verbal behavior in psychotherapy. *Clinical Psychology Review, 8,* 181–194.

Hansburg, H.D. (1972). *Adolescent Separation Anxiety Test.* Huntington, NY: Kreiger Publishing.

Hanson, N.R. (1958). *Patterns of discovery.* Cambridge: Cambridge University Press.

Hanson, N.R. (1967). Observation and interpretation. In S. Morgenbesser (Ed.), *Philosophy of science today.* New York: Basic Books.

Hanson, N.R. (1969). *Perception and discovery: An introduction to scientific inquiry.* San Francisco: Freeman, Cooper & Company.

Harbin, S.P., & Williams, J.E. (1966). Conditioning of color connotations. *Perceptual and Motor Skills, 22,* 217–218.

Harlow, H. (1969). William James and instinct theory. In R. MacCleod (Ed.), *William James: Unfinished business.* Washington, DC: American Psychological Association.

Harms, J.Y., & Staats, A.W. (1978). Food deprivation and conditioned reinforcing value of food words: Interaction of Pavlovian and instrumental conditioning. *Bulletin of the Psychonomic Society, 12*(4), 294–296.

Harrington, R.G. (1985). *Bruininks-Oseretsky Test of Motor Proficiency.* In D.J. Keyser & R.C. Sweetland (Eds.), *Test Critiques: Volume III.* Kansas City, MO: Test Corporation of America.

Harris, F.R., Johnston, M.K., Kelley, C.S., & Wolf, M.M. (1964). Effects of positive social reinforcement on regressed crawling of a nursery school child. *Journal of Educational Psychology, 55,* 35–41.

Harris, M.B. (Ed.) (1971). *Classroom uses of behavior modification.* New York: Charles E. Merrill.

Hart, B.M., Allen, K.E., Buell, J.S., Harris, F.R., & Wolf, M.M. (1964). Effects of social reinforcement on operant crying. *Journal of Experimental Child Psychology, 1,* 145–153.

Hart, B., & Risely, T.R. (1992). American parenting of language-learning children: Persisting differences in family–child interactions observed in natural home environments. *Developmental Psychology,* 1096–1105.

Hartman, D.P., Roper, B.L., & Bradford, D.C. (1979). Some relationships between behavioral and traditional assessment. *Journal of Behavioral Assessment, 1,* 3–21.

Hartshorne, H., & May, M.A. (1928). *Studies in the nature of character. Vol. 1. Studies in deceit.* New York: Macmillan.

Hartshorne, H., & May, M.A. (1929). *Studies in the nature of character. Vol. 2. Studies in service and self-control.* New York: Macmillan.

Hawkins, R.P., Peterson, R.F., Schweid, E., & Bijou, S.W. (1966). Behavior therapy in the home: Amelioration of problem parent–child relations with the parent in a therapeutic role. *Journal of Experimental Child Psychology, 4,* 99–107.

Hayes, L.J., & Hayes, S.C. (1989). The verbal action of the listener as a basis for rule-governance. In S.C. Hayes (Ed.). *Rule-governed behavior* (pp. 153–190). New York: Plenum.

Hayes, S.C. (1986). The case of the silent dog—verbal reports and the analysis of rules: A review of Ericsson and Simaon's protocol analysis: Verbal reports as data. *Journal of the Experimental Analysis of Behavior, 45,* 351–363.

Hayes, S.C. (1987). A contextual approach to therapeutic change. In N.S. Jacobson (Ed.), *Psychotherapists in clinical practice: Cognitive and behavioral perspectives* (pp. 327–387). New York: Guilford.

Hayes, S.C. (Ed.). (1989). *Rule-governed behavior.* New York: Plenum.

Hayes, S.C. (1993). Psychological behaviorism: Causal, courtship or commitment? Panel discussion, 27th annual convention of the Association for Behavior Advancement, Atlanta, GA.

Hayes, S.C. (1995). Why cognitions are not causes. *Behavior Therapist, 18,* 59–60.

Hayes, S.C., & Brownstein, A.J. (1986). Mentalism, behavior-behavior relations, and a behavior-analytic view of the purposes of science. *Behavior Analyst, 9,* 175–190.

Hayes, S.C., Hayes, L.J., & Reese, H.W. (1988). Finding the philosophical core: A review of Stephen C. Pepper's *World hypotheses. Journal of the Experimental Analysis of Behavior, 50,* 97–111.

Hayes, S.C., & Wilson, K.G. (1994). Acceptance and commitment therapy: Altering the verbal support for experiential avoidance. *Behavior Analyst, 17,* 289–303.

Hayes, S.C., Zettle, R.D., & Rosenfarb, I. (1989). Rule-following. In S.C. Hayes (Ed.), *Rule-governed behavior* (pp. 191–220). New York: Plenum.

Haynes, S.N., & O'Brien, W.H. (1990). Functional analysis in behavior therapy. *Clinical Psychology Review, 10,* 649–669.

Hearst, E. (1967). The behavior of Skinnerians. *Contemporary Psychology, 12,* 402–404.

Hebb, D.O. (1955). Drives and the C.N.S. (conceptual nervous system). *Psychological Review, 62,* 243–254.

Heiby, E.M. (1981). Depression and frequency of self-reinforcement. *Behavior Therapy, 12,* 549–555.

Heiby, E. (1985). Depression: Radical vs. paradigmatic behaviorism. Eleventh annual convention of the Association for Behavior Analysis, Columbus, OH.

Heiby, E.M. (1989). Multiple skill deficits in depression. *Behavior Change, 6,* 76–84.

Heiby, E.M., & Staats, A.W. (1990). Depression: Classification, explanation, and treatment. In G. H. Eifert & I.M. Evans (Ed.), *Unifying behavior therapy: Contributions of paradigmatic behaviorism.* New York: Springer.

Heider, F. (1958). *The psychology of interpersonal relations.* New York: John Wiley.

Hekmat, H. (1972). The role of imagination in semantic desensitization. *Behavior Therapy, 3,* 223–231.

Hekmat, H. (1973). Systematic versus semantic desensitization and implosive therapy: A comparative study. *Journal of Consulting and Clinical Psychology, 40,* 202–209.

Hekmat, H. (1974). Three techniques of reinforcement modification: A comparison. *Behavior Therapy, 5,* 541–548.

Hekmat, H. (1990). Semantic behavior therapy of anxiety disorders: An integrative approach. In G.H. Eifert & I.M. Evans (Eds.), *Unifying behavior therapy: Contributions of paradigmatic behaviorism.* New York: Springer.

Hekmat, H., Edelstein, M., & Cook, L. (1994). Managing worries with eye movement desensitization. Paper presented at the 28th Annual Meeting of the Association for Behavior Analysis, San Diego, CA.

Hekmat, H., Staats, A.W., & Staats, P.S. (1995). *Type A personality and responsiveness to pain intervention.* Paper presented at the 103rd Annual Meeting of the American Psychological Association, New York City, NY.

Hekmat, H., & Vanian, D. (1971). Behavior modification through covert semantic desensitization. *Journal of Consulting and Clinical Psychology, 36,* 248–251.

Hellige, J.B., Cox, J.J., & Litvac, L. (1979). Information processing in the cerebral hemispheres: Selective hemispheric activation and capacity limitation. *Journal of Experimental Psychology: General, 108,* 251–279.

Hempel, W.E., & Fleishman, I.A. (1955). A factor analysis of physical proficiency and manipulative skill. *Journal of Applied Psychology, 39,* 12–16.

Hermann, C.F. (1972). *International crises: Insights from behavioral research.* New York: Free Press.

Herrnstein, R.J., & Murray, C. (1994). *The Bell Curve: The reshaping of American life by differences in intelligence.* New York: Free Press.

Herry, M. (1984). Le principe du conditionnement instrumental d' ordre superieur. In A. Leduc (Ed.), *Recherches sur le behaviofisme paradigmatique ou social.* Brossard, Quebec: Behaviora.

Hersen, M., Eisler, R.M., Alford, G.S., & Agras, W.S. (1973). Effects of token economy on neurotic depression: An experimental analysis. *Behavior Therapy, 4,* 392–397.

Hersey, J. (1968). *Algiers Motel incident.* New York: Knopf.

Hilgard, E. (1948). *Theories of learning.* New York: Appleton.

Himmelfarb, S. (1972). Integration and attribution theories in personality impression formation. *Journal of Personality and Social Psychology, 23,* 309–313.

Hishinuma, E. (1987). Psychoanalytic and cognitive dissonance theories: Producing unification through the unifying theory review. In A.W. Staats & L.P. Mos (Eds.), *Annals of theoretical psychology.* New York: Plenum.

Hishinuma, E.S., & Staats, A.W. (in mimeo). Psychoanalytic and cognitive dissonance theory: Unifying theory and its methodology.

Hoffman, M.L. (1975). Moral internalization, parental power, and the nature of parent–child interaction. *Developmental Psychology, 11,* 228–239.

Holden, C. (1979). FDA tells senators of doctors who fake data in clinical drug trials. *Science, 206,* 423–433.

Holland, J.G. (1958). Human vigilance. *Science, 128,* 61–67.

Holland, J.G. (1960). Teaching machines: An application of principles from the laboratory. *Journal of the Experimental Analysis of Behavior, 3,* 275–287.

Holland, J.G., & Skinner, B.F. (1961). *The analysis of behavior: A program for self-instruction.* New York: McGraw-Hill.

Hollon, S.D., & Carter, M.M. (1994). Depression in adults. In L.W. Craighead, W.E. Craighead, A.E. Kazdin, & M.J. Mahoney (Eds.), *Cognitive and behavioral interventions: An empirical approach to mental health problems.* Boston: Allyn & Bacon.

Holmes, T.H., & Masuda, M. (1974). Life change and stress susceptibility. In R.S. Dohrenwend & B.P. Dohrenwend (Eds.), *Stressful life events: Their nature and effects* (pp. 45–72). New York: John Wiley.

Holmes, T.H., & Rahe, R.H. (1967). The social readjustment rating scale. *Journal of Psychosomatic Research, 11,* 213–218.

Holsti, O.R. (1976). Foreign policy formation viewed cognitively. In R. Axelrod (Ed.), *The structure of decision.* Princeton, NJ: Princeton University Press.

Holzman, A.D., & Levis, D.J. (1991). Differential aversive conditioning of an external (visual) and internal (imaginal) CS: Effects of transfer between and within CS modalities. *Journal of Mental Imagery, 15,* 77–90.

Homans, G.C. (1961). *Social behavior.* New York: Harcourt.

Hounshell, D.A. (1980). Edison and the pure science ideal in 19th-century America. *Science, 207,* 612–617.

Hovland, C.K., Janis, I.L., & Kelley, H.H. (1953). *Communication and persuasion.* New Haven, CT: Yale University Press.

Howell, N. (1979). Cultures under stress. *Science, 203,* 1235–1236.

Hudson, L. (1966). *Contrary imaginations.* New York: Schocken Books.

Hull, C.L. (1920). Quantitative aspects of the evolution of concepts. *Psychological Monographs*, No. 123.

Hull, C.L. (1930). Knowledge and purpose as habit mechanisms. *Psychological Review, 37*, 511–525.

Hull, C.L. (1939). Simple trial-and-error learning—an empirical investigation. *Journal of Comparative Psychology, 27*, 233–258.

Hull, C.L. (1943a). *Principles of behavior.* New York: Appleton–Century–Crofts.

Hull, C.L. (1943b). The problem of intervening variables in molar behavior theory. *Psychological Review, 50*, 273–291.

Hull, C.L. (1952). *A behavior system.* New Haven, CT: Yale University Press.

Hyland, M.E. (1985). Questions and answers: Do we know the questions. *International Newsletter of Uninomic Psychology, 1*, 22.

Insko, C.A., & Butzine, K.W. (1967). Rapport, awareness, and verbal reinforcement of attitude. *Journal of Personality and Social Psychology, 6*, 225–228.

Ireton, H., & Thewing, E. (1974). *Manual for the Minnesota Child Development Inventory.* Minneapolis: Behavior Science Systems.

Isaacs, W., Thomas, J., & Goldiamond, I. (1960). Application of operant conditioning to reinstate verbal behavior in psychotics. *Journal of Speech and Hearing Disorders, 25*, 8–12.

Iwata, B., Pace, G., Kalsher, M., Cowdery, G., & Cataldo, M. (1990). Experimental analysis and extinction of self-injurious behavior. *Journal of Applied Behavior Analysis, 23*, 11–27.

Jensen, A.R. (1969). How much can we boost I.Q. and scholastic achievement? *Harvard Educational Review, 39*(1), 1–123.

John, O.P. (1990). The "big five" factor taxonomy: Dimensions of personality in the natural language and in questionnaires. In L.A. Pervin (Ed.), *Handbook of personality: Theory and research.* New York: Guilford.

Jones, H.E. (1930). The galvanic skin reflex in infancy. *Child Development, 1*, 106–110.

Jones, R.J., & Azrin, N.H. (1973). An experimental application of a social reinforcement approach to the problems of job finding. *Journal of Applied Behavior Analysis, 6*, 345–354.

Judson, A.J., Cofer, C.N., & Gelfand, S. (1956). Reasoning as an associative process. II. "Direction" in problem solving as a function of prior reinforcement of relevant responses. *Psychological Reports, 2*, 501–507.

Kagan, J. & Snidman, N. (1991). Infant predictors of inhibited and uninhibited profiles. *Psychological Science, 2*, 40–44.

Kamil, A.C. (1969). Some parameters of the second-order conditioning of fear in rats. *Journal of Comparative and Physiological Psychology, 67*, 364–369.

Kamin, L.J. (1974). *The science and politics of IQ.* Potomac, MD: Erlbaum.

Kanfer, F.H., & Phillips, J.S. (1970). *Learning foundations of behavior therapy.* New York: John Wiley.

Kanfer, F.H., & Saslow, G. (1965). Behavioral analyses. *Archives of General Psychiatry, 12*, 529–538.

Kaye, H. (1967). Infant sucking behavior and its modification. In L.P. Lipsitt & C.C. Spiker (Eds.), *Advances in child development and behavior,* Vol. 3. New York: Academic Press.

Kazdin, A.E. (1994). Antisocial behavior and conduct disorder. In L.W. Craighead,

W.E. Craighead, A.E. Kazdin, & M.J. Mahoney (Eds.), *Cognitive and behavioral interventions: An empirical approach to mental health problems.* Boston: Allyn & Bacon.

Keefe, F.J., & Beckham, J.C. (1994). In L.W. Craighead, W.E. Craighead, A.E. Kazdin, & M.J. Mahoney (Eds.), *Cognitive and behavioral interventions: An empirical approach to mental health problems.* Boston: Allyn & Bacon.

Keller, F.S., & Schoenfeld, W.N. (1950). *Principles of psychology.* New York: Appleton.

Kelso, J.A. (1977). Motor control mechanisms underlying human movement reproduction. *Journal of Experimental Psychology: Human Perception and Performance, 3,* 529–543.

Kendler, H.H. (1987). A good divorce is better than a bad marriage. In A.W. Staats & L.P. Mos (Eds.), *Annals of theoretical psychology,* vol. 5. New York: Plenum.

Kety, S. (1975) Biochemistry of the major psychoses. In A. Freedman, H. Kaplan, & B. Sadock (Eds.), *Comprehensive textbook of psychiatry/II.* Baltimore: Williams & Wilkins.

Koch, S. (Ed.) (1959). *Psychology: A study of a science.* Vols. *1–7.* New York: McGraw-Hill.

Koch, S. (1981). The nature and limits of psychological knowledge: Lessons of a century qua "science." *American Psychologist, 36,* 257–269.

Kohlberg, L. (1981). *The philosophy of moral development.* New York: Harper & Row.

Kohlenberg, R.J., & Tsai, M. (1994). Improving cognitive therapy for depression with functional analytic psychotherapy: Theory and case study. *Behavior Analyst, 17,* 305–319.

Kolb, B., & Wishaw, I. (1984). *Fundamentals of neuropsychology.* San Francisco: Freeman.

Korn, Z. (1995). The pivotal role of self in two behavioral therapies. *Behavior Therapist, 18,* 135–137.

Krantz, D.L. (1985). Psychology: A community of gregarious isolates. Symposium paper presented at the 93rd Annual Convention of the American Psychological Association, Los Angeles, August, 23–27.

Krantz, D.L. (1987). Psychology's search for unity. *New Ideas in Psychology, 6,* 219–222.

Krasner, L. (1958). Studies of the conditioning of verbal behavior. *Psychological Bulletin, 55,* 148–170.

Krasner, L. (1962). The therapist as a social reinforcement machine. In H.H. Strupp & L. Luborsky (Eds.), *Research as psychotherapy.* Vol. II. Washington, DC: American Psychological Association.

Krasner, L., & Ullmann, L.P. (1965). *Research in behavior modification.* New York: Holt, Rinehart, & Winston.

Krasnogorski, N.I. (1907). The formation of artificial conditioned reflexes in young children. *Russkii Vrach. 36,* 1245–1246. (Translated and republished in Y. Brackbill & G.G. Thompson (Eds.), *Behavior in infancy and early childhood.* New York.

Kraus, S.J. (1995). Attitudes and the prediction of behavior: A meta-analysis of the empirical literature. *Journal of Personality and Social Psychology, 21,* 58–74.

Krech, D. (1970). Epilogue. In J.R. Royce (Ed.), *Toward unification in psychology.* Toronto: University of Toronto Press.

Kruglanski, A.W. (1976). On the paradigmatic objections to experimental psychology: A reply to Gadlin and Luyk. *American Psychologist, 31,* 655–663.

Kuhn, T.S. (1962). *The structure of scientific revolutions* (2nd ed.). Chicago: University of Chicago Press.

Kuhn, T.S. (1977). Second thoughts on paradigms. In F. Suppe (Ed.), *The structure of scientific theories*. Urbana, IL: University of Illinois Press.

Kunkel, J.H. (1987). Disunity in psychology: Implications for and from sociology and anthropology. In A.W. Staats & L.P. Mos (Eds.), *Annals of theoretical psychology*, vol. 5. New York: Plenum.

Laffal, J., Lenkoski, L.D., and Aineen, L. (1956). "Opposite speech" in a schizophrenic patient. *Journal of Abnormal and Social Psychology, 52,* 409–413.

Lambert, N.M., Windmiller, M., Cale, L., & Figueroa, R. (1975). *Manual for the AAMD Adaptive Behavior Scale: Public School Version* (1974 rev.). Washington, DC: American Association on Mental Deficiency.

Landy, D., & Sigall, H. (1974). Beauty is talent: Task evaluation as a function of the performer's physical attractiveness. *Journal of Personality and Social Psychology, 29,* 299–304.

Lang, P.J. (1994). The varieties of emotional experience: A meditation on James–Lange theory. *Psychological Review, 101,* 211–221.

Lang, P.J. (1995). The emotion probe: Studies of motivation and attention. *American Psychologist, 50,* 372–385.

Lanyon, R.I., & Barocas, V.S. (1975). Effects of contingent events on stuttering and fluency. *Journal of Consulting and Clinical Psychology, 43,* 786–793.

LaPiere, R.T. (1934). Attitudes vs. actions. *Social Forces, 13,* 230–237.

Larimer, M.E., & Marlatt, G.A. (1994). In L.W. Craighead, W.E. Craighead, A.E. Kazdin, & M.J. Mahoney (Eds.), *Cognitive and behavioral interventions: An empirical approach to mental health problems*. Boston: Allyn & Bacon.

Laski, K.E., Charlop, M.H., & Schreibman, L. (1988). Training parents to use the natural language paradigm to increase their autistic children's speech. *Journal of Applied Behavior Analysis, 21,* 391–400.

Leduc, A. (1980a). L'apprentissage et le changement des attitudes: L'approche interactioniste de Staats. *Canadian Journal of Education, 5,* 15–33.

Leduc, A. (1980b). L'apprentissage et le changement des attitudes envers soi-meme: Le concept de soi. *Canadian Journal of Education, 5,* 91–102.

Leduc, A. (Ed.). (1984). *Recherches sur le behaviorisme paradigmatique ou social*. Brossard, Quebec: Editions Behaviora.

Leduc, A. (1988a). A paradigmatic behavioral approach to the treatment of a "wild" child. *Child and Family Behavior Therapy, 9,* 1–16.

Leduc, A. (1988b). *L'histoire d'apprentissage d'une enfant "sauvage:" Si toutes et tous les Dominiques avaient la chance d'apprende*. Broussard, Quebec: Editions Behaviora.

Lefkowitz, M.M., Blake, R.R., & Mouton, J.S. (1955). Status factors in pedestrian violation of traffic signals. *Journal of Abnormal and Social Psychology, 51,* 704–706.

Leuba, C. (1940). Images as conditioned sensations. *Journal of Experimental Psychology, 26,* 345–351.

Levitt, A.G, & Utman, J.G.A. (1992). From babbling towards the sound systems of English and French: A longitudinal two-case study. *Journal of Child Language, 19,* 19–50.

Lewinsohn, P.M. (1974). A behavioral approach to depression. In R. Friedman & M. Katz (Eds.). *The psychology of depression: Contemporary theory and research* (pp. 157–185). New York: John Wiley.

Lewinsohn, P.M., Hoberman, H.M., Teri, L., & Hautzinger, M. (1985). An integrative theory of depression. In S. Reiss & R.R. Bootzin (Eds.), *Theoretical issues in behavior therapy*. New York: Academic Press.

Liebert, R.M., & Spiegler, M.D. (1994). *Personality: Strategies and Issues*. Pacific Grove, CA: Brooks/Cole.

Lindsley, O.R. (1956). Operant conditioning methods applied to research in chronic schizophrenia. *Psychiatric Research Reports, 5*, 118–153.

Linehan, M.M., & Schmidt, H., III. (1995). The dialetics of effective treatment of borderline personality disorder. *Theories of behavior therapy*. Washington, DC: American Psychological Association.

Lipsitt, L.P., & Kaye, H. (1964). Conditioned sucking in the human newborn. *Psychonomic Science, 1*, 29–30.

Loeb, A., Beck, A., Diggory, J., & Tuthill, R. (1967). Expectancy, level of aspiration, performance, and self-evaluation in depression. *Proceedings, 75th Annual Convention APA, 75*, 193–194.

Lohr, J.M., Kleinknecht, R.A., Conley, A.T., Cerro, S.D., Schmidt, J., & Sonntag, M. (1992). A methodological critique of the current status of eye movement desensitization. *Journal of Behavior Therapy and Experimental Psychiatry, 23*, 159–167.

LoPiccolo, J. (1994). Sexual dysfunction. In L.W. Craighead, W.E. Craighead, A.E. Kazdin, & M.J. Mahoney (Eds.), *Cognitive and behavioral interventions: An empirical approach to mental health problems*. Boston: Allyn & Bacon.

Lott, A.J., & Lott, B.E. (1969). Liked and disliked persons as reinforcing stimuli. *Journal of Personality and Social Psychology, 11*, 129–137.

Lott, B.E., & Lott, A.J. (1960). The formation of positive attitudes toward group members. *Journal of Abnormal and Social Psychology, 61*, 297–300.

Lovaas, O.I. (1961). Interaction between verbal and non-verbal behavior. *Child Development, 32*, 329–336.

Lovaas, O.I. (1964). Cue properties of words: The control of operant responding by rate and content of verbal operants. *Child Development, 35*, 245–256.

Lovaas, O.I. (1966). A behavior therapy approach to the treatment of childhood schizophrenia. In J.P. Hill (Ed.), *Minnesota symposium on child psychology*. Vol. 1. Minneapolis: University of Minnesota Press.

Lovaas, O.I. (1977). *The autistic child*. New York: Irvington.

Lovaas, O.I., Berberich, J.P., Perloff, B.F., & Schaeffer, B. (1966). Acquisition of imitative speech by schizophrenic children. *Science, 151*, 705–707.

Lovaas, O.I., Freitag, G., Nelson, K., & Whalen, C. (1967). The establishment of imitation and its use for the development of complex behavior in schizophrenic children. *Behaviour Research and Therapy, 5*, 171–181.

Lovaas, O.I., Schaeffer, B., & Simmons, J.Q. (1965). Experimental studies in childhood schizophrenia: Building social behavior in children by use of electric shock. *Journal of Experimental Research in Personality, 1*, 99–109.

Maas, J., Fawcett, J., & Dekirmenjian, W. (1972). Catecholamine metabolism, depression illness and drug response. *Archives of General Psychiatry, 26*, 252.

MacCorquodale, K., & Meehl, P.E. (1948). On the distinction between hypothetical constructs and intervening variables. *Psychological Review, 55*, 95–107.

Macher, B.A. (1985). Underpinnings of today's chaotic diversity. *International Newsletter of Uninomic Psychology, 1*, 17.

MacIntyre, R.B. (1985). Psychology's fragmentation and suggested remedies. *International Newsletter of Uninomic Psychology, 1,* 20–21.

Mackenzie, B.D. (1977). *Behaviourism and the limits of scientific method.* Atlantic Highlands, NJ: Humanities Press.

Mackenzie, H.S., Clark, M., Wolf, M.M., Kothera, R., & Benson, C. (1968). Behavior modification of children with learning disabilities using grades as tokens and allowances as back up reinforcers. *Exceptional Children, 34,* 745–753.

MacPherson, A., Bonem, M., Green, G., & Osborne, J.G. (1984). A citation analysis of the influence on research of Skinner's *Verbal behavior. Behavior Analyst, 7,* 157–167.

MacPhillamy, D., & Lewinsohn, P. (1971). *The Pleasant Events Schedule.* Eugene, OR: University of Oregon Press.

Maier, N.R.F. (1949). *Frustration—the study of behavior without a goal.* New York: McGraw-Hill.

Malagodi, E.F. (1986). Radicalizing behaviorism: A call for cultural analysis. *Behavior Analyst, 9,* 1–17.

Malatesta, V.J., AuBuchon, P.G., & Bruch, M. (1994). A historical timeline in psychiatric settings: Development of a clinical science. *Behavior Therapist, 17,* Summer, 165–168.

Maltzman, I., Raskin, D.C., Gould, J., & Johnson, O. (1965). Individual differences in the orienting reflex and semantic conditioning and generalization under different UCS intensities. Paper delivered at the Western Psychological Association Meetings, Honolulu, 1965.

Marshall, E. (1980). Psychotherapy works, but for whom? *Science, 207,* 506–508.

Martin, C.L., & Parker, S. (1995). Folk theories about sex and race differences. *Journal of Personality and Social Psychology, 21,* 45–56.

Marx, M.H. (1951). *Psychological theory.* New York: Macmillan.

Marx, M.H. (Ed.) (1963). *Theories in contemporary psychology.* New York: Macmillan.

Maslow, A.H. (1954). *Motivation and personality.* New York: Harper.

Masterman, M. (1970). The nature of a paradigm. In I. Lakatos & A. Musgrave (Eds.), *Criticism and the growth of knowledge.* Cambridge: Cambridge University Press.

Mausner, B. (1954). The effect of one partner's success in a relevant task on the interaction of observer pairs. *Journal of Abnormal and Social Psychology, 49,* 557–560.

May, M.A. (1948). Experimentally acquired drives. *Journal of Experimental Psychology, 38,* 66–77.

McCandless, B.R. (1940). The effect of enriched educational experiences on the growth of intelligence of very superior children. Unpublished master's thesis, University of Iowa.

McCaul, K.D., & Malott, J.M. (1984). Distraction and coping with pain. *Psychological Bulletin, 95,* 516–535.

McFall, R.M., & Twentyman, C.T. (1973). Four experiments on the relative contribution of rehearsal, modeling, and coaching to assertion training. *Journal of Abnormal Psychology, 81,* 199–218.

McNair, D.M., Morr, M., & Droppleman, L.F. (1971). *Profile of Mood States.* San Diego: EdITS; Educational and Industrial Testing Service, Inc.

Meichenbaum, D. (1977). *Cognitive-behavior modification*. New York: Plenum.

Meichenbaum, D.H., & Goodman, J. (1971). Training impulsive children to talk to themselves. *Journal of Abnormal Psychology, 77*, 115–120.

Mencken, H.L. (1927). Psychologists in a fog. *American Mercury, 11*, 382–383.

Merton, R.K. (1957). Priorities in scientific discovery. *American Sociological Review, 22*, 635–659.

Merton, R.K. (Edited and with an introduction by Norman W. Storer) (1973). *The sociology of science*. Chicago: University of Chicago Press.

Merzenich, M.M., Jenkins, W.M., Johnston, P., Schreiner, C., Miller, S.L., & Tallal, P. (1996). Temporal processing deficits of language-impaired children ameliorated by training. *Science, 271*, 77–81.

Messer, S.B. (1988). Philosophical obstacles to unification of psychology. *International Newsletter of Uninomic Psychology, 5*, 22–24.

Meyer, V., & Chesser, E. (1970). *Behavior therapy in clinical psychiatry*. Harmondsworth, UK: Penguin.

Michael, J. (1993). Establishing operations. *Behavior Analyst, 16*, 191–206.

Miller, N.E. (1948). Studies of fear as an acquired drive: I. Fear as motivation and fear-reduction as reinforcement in the learning of new responses. *Journal of Experimental Psychology, 38*, 89–101.

Miller, N.E., & Dollard, J. (1941). *Social learning and imitation*. New Haven, CT: Yale University Press.

Mills, M., & Melhuish, E. (1974). Recognition of mother's voice in early infancy. *Nature, 252*, 123–124.

Mischel, W. (1968). *Personality and assessment*. New York: John Wiley.

Mischel, W. (1972). Direct versus indirect personality assessment: Evidence and implications. *Journal of Consulting and Clinical Psychology, 38*, 319–324.

Mischel, W. (1973). Toward a cognitive social learning reconceptualization of personality. *Psychological Review, 80*, 252–283.

Mischel, W., & Shoda, Y. (1995). A cognitive-affective system theory of personality: Reconceptualizing situations, dispositions, dynamics, and invariance in personality structure. *Psychological Review, 102*, 246–268.

Moore, J. (1985). Some historical and conceptual relations among logical positivism, operationism, and behaviorism. *Behavior Analyst, 8*, 53–63.

Moran, D.R., & Whitman, T.L. (1985). The multiple effects of a play-oriented parent training program for mothers of developmentally delayed children. *Analysis and Intervention in Developmental Disabilities, 5*, 79–96.

Moran, D.R., & Whitman, T.L. (1991). Developing generalized teaching skills in mothers of autistic children. *Child & Family Behavior Therapy, 13*, 13–37.

Moscovici, S. (1972). Society and theory in social psychology. In J. Israel & H. Tajfel (Eds.), *The context of social psychology*. New York: Academic Press.

Mowrer, O.H. (1947). On the dual nature of learning—a reinterpretation of "conditioning" and "problem-solving." *Harvard Educational Review, 17*, 102–148.

Mowrer, O.H. (1950). *Learning theory and personality dynamics*. New York: Ronald.

Mowrer, O.H. (1952). The autism theory of speech development and some clinical applications. *Journal of Speech and Hearing Disorders, 17*, 263–268.

Mowrer, O.H. (1954). The psychologist looks at language. *American Psychologist, 9*, 660–694.

Mowrer, O.H. (1960). *Learning theory and the symbolic processes.* New York: John Wiley.

Murray, H.A. (1938). *Explorations in personality.* New York: Oxford University Press.

Myers, D.G. (1986). *Psychology.* New York: Worth.

Neurath, O., Carnap, R., & Morris, C. (Eds.). (1938). *International encyclopedia of unified science.* Chicago: University of Chicago Press.

Newcomb, T.M. (1929). *Consistency of certain extrovert-introvert patterns in 51 problem boys.* New York: Columbia University Teachers College, Bureau of Publications.

Newell, A. (1990). *Unified theories of cognition.* Cambridge, MA: Harvard University Press.

O'Leary, K.D., & Drabman, R. (1971). Token reinforcement programs in the classroom: A review. *Psychological Bulletin, 75,* 379–398.

O'Leary, K.D., O'Leary, S.G., & Becker, W.C. (1967). Modification of a deviant sibling interaction pattern in the home. *Behaviour Research and Therapy, 5,* 113–120.

Olds, J., & Milner, P. (1954). Positive reinforcement produced by electrical stimulation of the septal area and other regions of the rat brain. *Journal of Comparative and Physiological Psychology, 47,* 419–427.

Olweus, D. (1974). Personality factors and aggression: With special reference to violence within the peer group. In J. de Wit & W.W. Hartup (Eds.), *Determinants of origins of aggressive behavior* (pp. 535–565). The Hague, The Netherlands: Mouton.

Olweus, D. (1977). A critical analysis of the "modern" interactionist position. In D. Magnusson & N.S. Endler (Eds.), *Personality at the crossroads: Current issues in interactional psychology* (pp. 221–235). Hillsdale, NJ: Lawrence Erlbaum.

Osgood, C.E. (1953). *Method and theory in experimental psychology.* New York: Oxford University Press.

Osgood, C.E., & Sebeok, T.A. (Eds.). (1954). *Psycholinguistics: Supplement to the Journal of Abnormal and Social Psychology, 49,* 1–203.

Osgood, C.E., & Suci, G.L. (1957). Factor analysis of meaning. *Journal of Experimental Psychology, 50,* 325–338.

Osgood, C.E., Suci, G.J., & Tannenbaum, P.H. (1957). *The measurement of meaning.* Urbana, IL: University of Illinois Press.

Pandey, J., & Griffitt, W. (1974). Attraction and helping. *Bulletin of Psychonomic Science, 3,* 123–124.

Parish, T. (1974). The conditioning of racial attitudes in children. *Perceptual and Motor Skills, 39,* 704–714.

Parrott, L.J. (1987). Rule-governed behavior: An implicit analysis of reference. In S. Modgil & C. Modgil (Eds.), *B.F. Skinner: Consensus and controversy* (pp. 265–276). Barcombe, England: Palmer Press.

Patterson, G.R. (1959, April). Fathers as reinforcing agents. Paper presented at the annual meetings of Western Psychological Association, San Diego.

Patterson, G.R. (1963). Parents as dispensers of social disapproval. Unpublished manuscript, University of Oregon.

Patterson, G.R. (1965a). Responsiveness to social stimuli. In L.P. Ullmann & L. Krasner (Eds.), *Case studies in behavior modification.* New York: Holt, Rinehart, & Winston.

Patterson, G.R. (1965b). An application of conditioning techniques to the control of a hyperactive child. In L.P. Ullman & L. Krasner (Eds.), *Case studies in behavior modification.* New York: Holt, Rinehart, & Winston.

Patterson, G.R. (1967). Prediction of victimization from an instrumental conditioning procedure. *Journal of Consulting Psychology, 31,* 147–152.

Patterson, G.R. (1976). The aggressive child: Victim and architect of a coercive system. In L.A. Hamerlinck, L.C. Handy, & E.J. Mash (Eds.), *Behavior modification and families: Theory and research.* New York: Brunner/Mazel.

Patterson, G.R. (1985). Beyond technology: The next stage in developing an empirical base for parent training. In L. L'Abet (Ed.), *Handbook of family psychology and therapy.* Homewood, IL: Dorsey Press.

Peese, J. (1969). Behavior and fact. *American Psychologist, 24,* 515–522.

Pelechano, V. (1987). Behavioral intervention: An old aspiration with a new profile. In A.W. Staats & L.P. Mos (Eds.), *Annals of theoretical psychology, vol. 5.* New York: Plenum.

Pepper, S. (1942). *World hypotheses: A study in evidence.* Berkeley: University of California Press.

Pervin, L.A. (1980). *Personality, theory, assessment, and research.* New York: John Wiley.

Peters, C.C., & McElwee, A.R. (1944). Improving functioning intelligence by analytical training in a nursery school. *Elementary School Journal, 45,* 213–219.

Peterson, I. (1993, February 27). Neural networks for learning verbs. *Science News, 143*(9), 141.

Phillips, E.L. (1968). Achievement place: Token reinforcement procedures in a home-style rehabilitation setting for "pre-delinquent" boys. *Journal of Applied Behavior Analysis, 1,* 213–223.

Phillips, L.W. (1958). Mediated verbal similarity as a determinant of the generalization of a conditional GSR. *Journal of Experimental Psychology, 55,* 56–62.

Piaget, J. (1953). How children form mathematical concepts. *Scientific American, 189,* 74–79.

Piaget, J., & Inhelder, B. (1964). *The early growth of logic in the child.* London: Routledge and Kegan Paul.

Piaget, J., & Kamii, C. (Trans.). (1978). What is psychology? *American Psychologist, 33,* 648–652.

Piotrowski, M., & Keller, J.W. (1984, March). Attitudes towards assessment by members of the AABT. Paper presented at the Meetings of the Southeastern Psychological Association, New Orleans.

Plaud, J.J. (1995). Analysis of complex human behavior: A reply to Staats. *Behavior Analyst, 18,* 167–169.

Poppen, R.L. (1989). Some clinical implications of rule-governed behavior. In S.C. Hayes (Ed.), *Rule-governed behavior: Cognition, contingencies, and instructional control.* New York: Plenum.

Popper, K.R. (1972). *Objective knowledge.* Oxford: Clarendon Press.

Porier, G.W., & Lott, A.J. (1967). Galvanic skin responses and prejudice. *Journal of Personality and Social Psychology, 5,* 253–259.

Postman, L. (1971). Transfer, interference, and forgetting. In J.W. Kling & L. A. Riggs (Eds.), *Woodward and Schlossberg's experimental psychology* (3rd ed.). New York: Holt, Rinehart, and Winston.

Rankin, R.E., & Campbell, D.T. (1955). Galvanic skin responses to negro and white experimenters. *Journal of Abnormal and Social Psychology, 51,* 30–35.

Rappard, A.V. (1985). Theoretical psychology and the unity of psychology. *International Newsletter of Uninomic Psychology, 1,* 6.

Rappard, H.V. (1993). History and system. In H.V. Rappard, P.J. van Strein, L.P. Mos, & W.J. Baker (Eds.), *Annals of Theoretical Psychology, 8.* New York: Plenum.

Raven, B.H., & French, J.R.P., Jr. (1958). Group support, legitimate power, and social influence. *Journal of Personality, 26,* 400–409.

Ravetz, J.R. (1971). *Scientific knowledge and its social problems.* Oxford: Clarendon Press.

Raymond, M.J. (1960). Case of fetishism treated by aversion therapy. In H.J. Eysenck (Ed.), *Behaviour therapy and the neuroses.* New York: Pergamon.

Razran, G.H. (1939). A quantitative study of meaning by a conditioned salivary technique (semantic conditioning). *Science, 90,* 89–90.

Rehm, L.P. (1977). A self-control model of depression. *Behavior Therapy, 8,* 787–804.

Reitan, R.M., & Wolfson, D. (1985). *The Halsted-Reitan Neuropsychological Battery: Theory and clinical interpretation.* Tucson, AZ: Tucson Neuropsychology Press.

Rescorla, R.A., & Solomon, R.L. (1967). Two-process learning theory: Relationships between Pavlovian conditioning and instrumental learning. *Psychological Review, 74,* 151–182.

Rheingold, H.L., Gewirtz, J.L., & Ross, H.W. (1959). Social conditioning of vocalizations in the infant. *Journal of Comparative and Physiological Psychology, 52,* 68–73.

Rickert, V.I., Sottolano, D.C., Parrish, J.M., Riley, A.W., Hunt, F.M., & Pelco, L.E. (1988). Training parents to become better behavior managers: The need for a competency-based approach. *Behavior Modification, 12,* 475–496.

Ridenour, M. (1982). Infant walkers: Developmental tool or inherent danger. *Perceptual and Motor Skills, 55,* 1201–1202.

Risely, T.R., & Wolf, M.M. (1967). Establishing functional speech in echolalic children. *Behaviour Research and Therapy, 5,* 75–88.

Ritzer, G. (1981). Paradigm analysis in sociology: Clarifying the issues. *American Sociological Review, 46,* 245–248.

Robb, H.B., III (1994). Rational-emotive-behavioral and radical behavioral treatment of acceptance. *Behavior Therapist, 17,* 247–248.

Robinson, J.K., & Woodward, W.R. (1989). The convergence of behavioral biology and operant psychology: Toward an interlevel and interfield science. *Behavior Analyst, 12,* 121–141.

Rogers, C. (1951). *Client-centered therapy.* Boston: Houghton Mifflin.

Rolider, A., & Van Houten, R. (1985). Movement suppression time-out for undesirable behavior in psychotic and developmentally delayed children. *Journal of Applied Behavior Analysis, 18,* 275–288.

Rondal, J.A. (1985). *Adult–child interaction and the process of language interaction.* New York: Praeger.

Rose, G.D., & Staats, A.W. (1988). Depression and the frequency and strength of pleasant events: Exploration of the Staats-Heiby theory. *Behavior Research and Therapy, 26,* 489–494.

Rosen, W.D., Adamson, L.B., & Bakeman, R. (1992). An experimental investigation of infant social referencing: Mothers' messages and gender differences. *Developmental Psychology, 28,* 1172–1178.

Rosenzweig, M.R. (1984). Experience, memory, and the brain. *American Psychologist, 39,* 365–376.

Rosenzweig, M.R., Bennett, E.L., & Diamond, M.C. (1972, February). Brain changes in response to experience. *Scientific American,* 22–29.

Rotter, J. (1954). *Social learning and clinical psychology.* Englewood Cliffs, NJ: Prentice-Hall.

Roy, S. (1994). La genese de l'image sensorielle conditionnee. *Comportement humain, 8,* 80–113.

Royce, J.R. (1970). *Toward unification in psychology: The first Banff Conference on theoretical psychology.* Toronto: University of Toronto Press.

Royce, J.R. (1987). A strategy for developing unifying theory in psychology. In A.W. Staats & L.P. Mos (Eds.), *Annals of theoretical psychology, vol. 5.* New York: Plenum.

Ruff, H.A., Saltarelli, L.M., Capozzoli, M., & Dubiner, K. (1992). The differentiation of activity in infants' exploration of objects. *Developmental Psychology, 28,* 851–861.

Rushton, J.P., Jackson, D.N., & Paunonen, S.V. (1981). Personality: Nomothetic or ideographic? A response to Kendrick and Stringfield. *Psychological Review, 88,* 582–589.

Russell, W.A., & Storms, L.H. (1955). Implicit verbal chaining in paired-associate learning. *Journal of Experimental Psychology, 49,* 287–293.

Ryback, D., & Staats, A.W. (1970). Parents as behavior therapy-technicians in treating reading deficits (dyslexia). *Journal of Behavior Therapy and Experimental Psychiatry, 1,* 109–119.

Rychlak, J.F. (1988). Unification through understanding and tolerance of opposition. *International Newsletter of Uninomic Psychology, 5,* 13–15.

Sachs, D.H., & Byrne, D. (1970). Differential conditioning of evaluative responses to neutral stimuli through association with attitude statements. *Journal of Experimental Research in Personality, 4,* 181–185.

Sailor, W. (1971). Reinforcement and generalization of productive plural allomorphs in two related children. *Journal of Applied Behavior Analysis, 4,* 305–310.

Sailor, W., & Tamar, T. (1972). Stimulus factors in the training of prepositional usage in three autistic children. *Journal of Applied Behavior Analysis, 5,* 183–190.

Salzinger, K. (1969). The place of operant conditioning of verbal behavior in psychotherapy. In C.M. Franks (Ed.), *Behavior therapy: Appraisal and status.* New York: McGraw-Hill.

Samuels, S.J. (1966). Effect of experimentally learned word associations on the acquisition of reading responses. *Journal of Educational Psychology, 57,* 159–163.

Samuels, S.J. (1973). Effect of distinctive feature training on paired-associate learning. *Journal of Educational Psychology, 64,* 164–170.

Sanders, M., & Glynn, T. (1981). Training parents in behavioral self-management: An analysis of generalization and maintenance. *Journal of Applied Behavior Analysis, 14,* 104–111.

Sato, T., Sakado, K., & Sato, S. (1993). Is there any specific personality disorder or personality disorder cluster that worsens the short-term treatment outcome of major depression? *Acta Psychiatrica Scandinavica, 88,* 342–349.

Sawin, D.B., Langlois, J.H., & Ritter, J.M. (1995). Infant attractiveness predicts maternal behavior and attitutes. *Developmental Psychology, 31,* 464.

Scarr, S. (1982). Development is internally guided, not determined. *Contemporary Psychology, 27,* 852–853.

Scarr, S., & Weinberg, R.A. (1976). IQ scores of black children adopted by white families. *American Psychologist, 31,* 726–739.

Schacter, S. (1970). The assumption of identity and peripheralist-centralist controversies in motivation and emotion. In M.B. Arnold (Ed.), *Feelings and emotions.* New York: Academic Press.

Schaefer, C.E. (1971). *Manual for the creativity attitude survey.* Jacksonville, Ill.: Psychologists and Educators, Inc.

Schildkraut, J. (1970). *Neropsychopharmacology of the affective disorders.* Boston: Little, Brown.

Schlaug, G., Jancke, L., Huang, Y., & Steinmetz, H. (1995, Feb. 3). In vivo evidence of structural brain asymmetry in musicians. *Science, 267*(5198), 699–701.

Schlinger, H. (1990). A reply to behavior analysts writing about rules and rule-governed behavior. *The Analysis of Verbal Behavior, 8,* 77–82.

Schlinger, H., & Blakely, E. (1987). Function-altering effects of contingency-specifying stimuli. *Behavior Analyst, 10,* 41–45.

Schreibman, L. (1994). Autism. In L.W. Craighead, W.E. Craighead, A.E. Kazdin, & M.J. Mahoney (Eds.), *Cognitive and behavioral interventions: An empirical approach to mental health problems.* Boston: Allyn & Bacon.

Seligman, M.E.P. (1975). *Helplessness: On depression, development and death.* San Francisco: W.H. Freeman.

Seward, J.P., & Seward, G.H. (1940). Studies on reproductive activities of the guinea pig: IV. A comparison of sex drive in males and females. *Journal of Genetic Psychology, 57,* 429–440.

Shapere, D. (1971). The paradigm concept. *Science, 172,* 706–709.

Shapere, D. (1977). Scientific theories and their domains. In F. Suppe (Ed.), *The structure of scientific theories* (2nd ed.). Urbana: University of Illinois Press.

Shapere, D. (1979). *The character of scientific change.* Unpublished manuscript.

Shaver, K.G. (1987). *Principles of social psychology.* Hillsdale, NJ: Erlbaum.

Shaw, R. (1972). Towards continued disunity in psychology. *Contemporary Psychology, 17,* 75–76.

Shipley, W.C. (1933). An operant transfer of conditioning. *Psychological Bulletin, 30,* 541.

Sidman, M. (1960). *Tactics of scientific research.* New York: Basic Books.

Sidman, M., & Tailby, W. (1982). Conditional discrimination versus matching-to-sample: An expansion of the testing paradigm. *Journal of the Experimental Analysis of Behavior, 37,* 5–22.

Sigall, H., & Landy, D. (1973). Radiating beauty: Effects of having a physically attractive partner on person perception. *Journal of Personality and Social Psychology, 28,* 218–224.

Silva, F. (1993). *Psychometric foundations of behavioral assessment.* New York: Sage.

Silverstein, A. (1972). Secondary reinforcement in infants. *Journal of Experimental Child Psychology, 13,* 138–144.

Skinner, B.F. (1938). *The behavior of organisms.* New York: Appleton.

Skinner, B.F. (1945). The operational analysis of psychological terms. *Psychological Review, 52,* 270–277.

Skinner, B.F. (1948). *Walden two*. New York: Macmillan.

Skinner, B.F. (1950). Are theories of learning necessary? *Psychological Review, 57,* 193–196.

Skinner, B.F. (1953). *Science and human behavior.* New York: Macmillan.

Skinner, B.F. (1957). *Verbal behavior.* New York: Appleton–Century–Crofts.

Skinner, B.F. (1966a). Phylogeny and ontogeny of behavior. *Science, 153,* 1205–1213.

Skinner, B.F. (1966b). An operant analysis of problem-solving. In B. Kleinmuntz (Ed.), *Problem solving research, method and theory* (pp. 225–257). New York: Appleton–Century–Crofts.

Skinner, B.F. (1969). *Contingencies of reinforcement.* New York: Appleton–Century–Crofts.

Skinner, B.F. (1971). *Beyond freedom and dignity.* New York: Alfred A. Knopf.

Skinner, B.F. (1974). *About behaviorism.* New York: Alfred A. Knopf.

Skinner, B.F. (1975). The steep and thorny way to a science of behavior. *American Psychologist, 30,* 42–49.

Skinner, B.F. (1988). The cuckoos. *The ABA Newsletter, 11*(3), 9.

Slobin, D.I. (Ed.). (1971). *The ontogenesis of grammar.* New York: Academic Press.

Smith, M.B. (1968). The revolution in mental health care: A bold new approach? *Trans-Action, 5,* 19–23.

Snider, J.G., & Osgood, C.E. (1969). *Semantic differential technique.* Chicago: Aldine.

Solomon, R.L., & Wynne, L.C. (1954). Traumatic avoidance learning: The principle of anxiety conservation and partial irreversibility. *Psychological Review, 61,* 353–385.

Spelt, D.K. (1948). The conditioning of the human fetus in utero. *Journal of Experimental Psychology, 38,* 375–376.

Spence, K.W. (1936). The nature of discrimination learning in animals. *Psychological Review, 43,* 427–449.

Spence, K.W. (1944). The nature of theory construction in contemporary psychology. *Psychological Review, 51,* 47–68.

Spence, K.W. (1948). The methods and postulates of "behaviorism." *Psychological Review, 55,* 67–78.

Spielberger, C., Gorsuch, R., & Lushene, R. (1970). *Manual for the State-Trait Anxiety Inventory.* Palo Alto, CA: Consulting Psychologists Press.

Spielberger, C.D. (1980). *Preliminary professional manual for the Test Anxiety Inventory.* TAI, Palo Alto, CA: Consulting Psychologists Press.

Staats, A.W. (1956). A behavioristic study of verbal and instrumental response hierarchies and their relationship to human problem solving. Unpublished doctoral dissertation, University of California, Los Angeles.

Staats, A.W. (1957a). Learning theory and "opposite speech." *Journal of Abnormal and Social Psychology, 55,* 268–269.

Staats, A.W. (1957b). Verbal and instrumental response hierarchies and their relationship to problem-solving. *American Journal of Psychology, 70,* 442–446.

Staats, A.W. (1961). Verbal habit families, concepts, and the operant conditioning of word classes. *Psychological Review, 68,* 190–204.

Staats, A.W. (with contributions by C.K. Staats). (1963a). *Complex human behavior.* New York: Holt, Rinehart & Winston.

Staats, A.W. (1963b). Comments on Professor Russell's paper. In C.N. Cofer & B.S. Musgrave (Eds.), *Verbal behavior and learning.* New York: McGraw-Hill.

Staats, A.W. (Ed.) (1964). *Human learning.* New York: Holt, Rinehart & Winston.

Staats, A.W. (1968a). *Learning, language, and cognition.* New York: Holt, Rinehart, & Winston.

Staats, A.W. (1968b). Social behaviorism and human motivation: Principles of the attitude-reinforcer-discriminative system. In A.G. Greenwald, T.C. Brock, & T.M. Ostrom (Eds.), *Psychological foundations of attitudes.* New York: Academic Press.

Staats, A.W. (1969). Experimental demand characteristics and the classical conditioning of attitudes. *Journal of Personality and Social Psychology, 11,* 187–192.

Staats, A.W. (1970a). Intelligence, biology or learning? Competing conceptions with social consequences. In H.C. Haywood (Ed.), *Social-cultural aspects of mental retardation.* New York: Appleton–Century–Crofts.

Staats, A.W. (1970b). A learning-behavior theory: A basis for unity in behavioral-social science. In A.R. Gilgen (Ed.), *Contemporary scientific psychology.* New York: Academic Press.

Staats, A.W. (1970c). Reinforcer systems in the solution of human problems. In G.A. Fargo, C. Behrns, & P. Nolen (Eds.), *Behavior modification in the classroom.* Belmont, CA: Wadsworth.

Staats, A.W. (1971a). *Child learning, intelligence and personality.* New York: Harper & Row.

Staats, A.W. (1971b). Linguistic-mentalistic theory versus an explanatory S-R learning theory of language development. In D.I. Slobin (Ed.), *The ontogenesis of grammar.* New York: Academic Press.

Staats, A.W. (1972). Language behavior therapy: A derivative from social behaviorism. *Behavior Therapy, 3,* 165–192.

Staats, A.W. (1975). *Social behaviorism.* Homewood, IL: Dorsey Press.

Staats, A.W. (1977). Social behaviorism's assessment conception: Behavioral interaction principles, tripartite personality repertoires and abnormal psychology. Initiated symposium paper at the annual meetings of the Association for the Advancement of Behavior Therapy, Atlanta, December.

Staats, A.W. (1979a). El conductismo social: un fundamento de la modificacion del comportamiento. *Revista Latinoamericana de Psicologia, 11,* 9–46.

Staats, A.W. (1979b). The three-function learning theory of social behaviorism: A third generation, unified theory. *Aprendizaje y Comportamiento, 2,* 13–38.

Staats, A.W. (1979c). About social behaviorism and social learning theory. In mimeo.

Staats, A.W. (1980). "Behavioral interaction" and "interactional psychology" theories of personality: Similarities, differences, and the need for unification. *British Journal of Psychology, 71,* 205–220.

Staats, A.W. (1981). Social behaviorism, unified theory, unified theory construction methods, and the zeitgeist of separatism. *American Psychologist, 36,* 239–256.

Staats, A.W. (1983a). *Psychology's crisis of disunity: Philosophy and methods for a unified science.* New York: Praeger.

Staats, A.W. (1983b). Paradigmatic behaviorism: Unified theory for social-personality psychology. In L. Berkowitz (Ed.), *Advances in experimental social psychology,* vol. 16. New York: Academic.

Staats, A.W. (1984). Unified positivism: Philosophy for the revolution to unity. In A.W. Staats & L.P. Mos (Eds.), *Annals of theoretical psychology, vol. 5.* New York: Plenum.

Staats, A.W. (1985). Disunity's prisoner, blind to a new approach to unification. *Contemporary Psychology, 30,* 339–340.

Staats, A.W. (1986a). Behaviorism with a personality: The paradigmatic behavioral assessment approach. In R.O. Nelson & S.C. Hayes (Eds.), *Conceptual foundations of behavioral assessment.* New York: Guilford Press.

Staats, A.W. (1986b). Left and right paths for behaviorism's development. *Behavior Analyst, 9,* 231–237.

Staats, A.W. (1987). Unified positivism: Philosophy for a unification psychology. In A.W. Staats & L. Mos (Eds.), *Annals of theoretical psychology,* Vol. 4. New York: Plenum.

Staats, A.W. (1988). Paradigmatic behaviorism, unified positivism, and paradigmatic behavior therapy. In D. Fishman, R. Rotgers, & C. Franks (Eds.), *Paradigms in behavior therapy.* New York: Springer.

Staats, A.W. (1989). *Personality and abnormal behavior.* Copyrighted book manuscript.

Staats, A.W. (1990). Paradigmatic behavior therapy: A unified heuristic theory for the third generation. In G.H. Eifert & I.M. Evans (Eds.), *Unifying behavior therapy: Contributions of paradigmatic behaviorism.* New York: Springer.

Staats, A.W. (1991). Unified positivism and unification psychology: Fad or new field? *American Psychologist, 46,* 899–912.

Staats, A.W. (1993a). Psychological behaviorism: An overarching theory and a theory-construction methodology. *The General Psychologist, 48,* 58–59.

Staats, A.W. (1993b). Personality theory, abnormal psychology, and psychological measurement: A psychological behaviorism. *Behavior Modification, 17,* 8–42.

Staats, A.W. (1993c). Why do we need another behaviorism (such as paradigmatic behaviorism)? *Behavior Therapist, 6,* 64–68.

Staats, A.W. (1994). Psychological behaviorism and behaviorizing psychology. *Behavior Analyst, 17,* 93–114.

Staats, A.W. (1995a). Paradigmatic behaviorism and paradigmatic behavior therapy. In W. O'Donohue & L. Krasner (Eds.), *Theories of behavior therapy.* Washington, DC: American Psychological Association.

Staats, A.W. (1995b). Good news and bad news in behavior therapy: And a look at Craighead, Craighead, Kazdin, and Mahoney's new text *Cognitive and behavioral interventions. Child and Family Behavior Therapy, 17,* 27–47.

Staats, A.W., Brewer, B.A., & Gross, M.C. (1970). Learning and cognitive development: Representative samples, cumulative-hierarchical learning, and experimental-longitudinal methods. *Monographs of the Society for Research in Child Development, 35*(8, Whole No. 141).

Staats, A.W., & Burns, G.L. (1981). Intelligence and child development: What intelligence is and how it is learned and functions. *Genetic Psychology Monographs, 104,* 237–301.

Staats, A.W., & Burns, G.L. (1982a). Emotional personality repertoire as cause of behavior: Specification of personality and interaction principles. *Journal of Personality and Social Psychology, 43,* 873–881.

Staats, A.W., & Burns, G.L. (1982b). Personality specification and interaction theory. *Journal of Personality and Social Psychology, 43,* 873–881.

Staats, A.W., & Butterfield, W.H. (1965). Treatment of nonreading in a culturally-deprived juvenile delinquent: An application of reinforcement principles. *Child Development, 36,* 925–942.

Staats, A.W., & Eifert, G.H. (1990). A paradigmatic behaviorism theory of emotions: A basis for unification. *Clinical Psychology Review, 10,* 1–40.

Staats, A.W., & Fernandez-Ballesteros, R. (1987). The self-report in personality measurement: A paradigmatic behaviorism approach to psychodiagnostics. *Evaluacion Psicologica/Psychological Assessment, 3,* 151–190.

Staats, A.W., Finley, J.R., Minke, K.A., & Wolf, M.M. (1964). Reinforcement variables in the control of unit reading responses. *Journal of the Experimental Analysis of Behavior, 7,* 139–149.

Staats, A.W., Finley, J.R., Osborne, J.G., Quinn, W.D., & Minke, K.A. (1963). The use of chain schedules in the study of reinforcement variables in a reading task. Technical Report No. 25, Arizona State University, Office of Naval Research Contract 2305 (00).

Staats, A.W., Gross, M.C., Guay, P.F., & Carlson, C.C. (1973). Personality and social systems and attitude-reinforcer-discriminative theory: Interest (attitude) formation, function, and measurement. *Journal of Personality and Social Psychology, 26,* 251–261.

Staats, A.W., & Hammond, O.W. (1972). Natural words as physiological conditioned stimuli: Food-word-elicited salivation and deprivation effects. *Journal of Experimental Psychology, 96,* 206–208.

Staats, A.W., & Heiby, E.M. (1985). Paradigmatic behaviorism's theory of depression. In S. Reiss & R. Bootzin (Eds.), *Theoretical issues in behavior therapy.* New York: Academic Press.

Staats, A.W., & Higa, W.R. (1970). Effects of affect-loaded labels on interpersonal attitudes across ethnic groups. Unpublished manuscript.

Staats, A.W., Higa, W.R., & Reid, I.E. (1970). *Names as reinforcers: The social value of social stimuli.* Technical Report No. 9. University of Hawaii, Contract N00014-67-L-0387-0007, with the office of Naval Research.

Staats, A.W., & Lohr, J.M. (1979). Images, language, emotions and personality: Social behaviorism's theory. *Journal of Mental Imagery, 3,* 85–106.

Staats, A.W., Minke, K.A., & Butts, P. (1970). A token-reinforcement remedial reading program administered by black instructional technicians to backward black children. *Behavior Therapy, 1,* 331–353.

Staats, A.W., Minke, K.A., Finley, J.R., Wolf, M.M., & Brooks, L.O. (1964). A reinforcer system and experimental procedure for the laboratory study of reading acquisition. *Child Development, 35,* 209–231.

Staats, A.W., Minke, K.A., Goodwin, W., & Landeen, J. (1967). Cognitive behavior modification: "Motivated learning" reading treatment with sub-professional therapy technicians. *Behavior Research and Therapy, 5,* 283–299.

Staats, A.W., Minke, K.A., Martin, C.H., & Higa, W.R. (1972). Deprivation–satiation and strength of attitude conditioning: A test of attitude-reinforcer-directive theory. *Journal of Personality and Social Psychology, 24,* 178–185.

Staats, A.W., & Staats, C.K. (1958). Attitudes established by classical conditioning. *Journal of Abnormal and Social Psychology, 57,* 37–40.

Staats, A.W., & Staats, C.K. (1959). Effect of number of trials on the language conditioning of meaning. *Journal of General Psychology, 61,* 211–223.

Staats, A.W., & Staats, C.K. (1962). A comparison of the development of speech and reading behavior with implications for research. *Child Development, 33,* 831–846.

Staats, A.W., Staats, C.K., & Crawford, H.L. (1962). First-order conditioning of a GSR and the parallel conditioning of meaning. *Journal of General Psychology, 67,* 159–167.

Staats, A.W., Staats, C.K., & Finley, J.R. (1966). Operant conditioning of serially ordered verbal responses. *Journal of General Psychology, 74,* 145–155.

Staats, A.W., Staats, C.K., & Heard, W.G. (1961). Denotative meaning established by classical conditioning. *Journal of Experimental Psychology, 61,* 300–303.

Staats, A.W., Staats, C.K., & Minke, K.A. (1966). Operant conditioning of a class of word associates. *Journal of General Psychology, 74,* 157–164.

Staats, A.W., Staats, C.K., Schutz, R.E., & Wolf, M.M. (1962). The conditioning of reading responses using "extrinsic" reinforcers. *Journal of the Experimental Analysis of Behavior, 5,* 33–40.

Staats, A.W., & Warren, D.R. (1974). Motivation and three-function learning: Food deprivation and approach-avoidance to food words. *Journal of Experimental Psychology, 103,* 1191–1199.

Staats, C.K., & Staats, A.W. (1957). Meaning established by classical conditioning. *Journal of Experimental Psychology, 54,* 74–80.

Staats, P.S., Hekmat, H., & Staats, A.W. (in press). The psychological behaviorism theory of pain: A basis for unity. *Pain Forum.*

Staats, P.S., Staats, A.W., & Hekmat, H. (in press). *The placebo-suggestion and pain: Negative as well as positive.*

Stanovich, K.E., West, R.F., & Harrison, M.R. (1995). Knowledge growth and maintenance across the life span: The role of print exposure. *Developmental Psychology, 31,* 811–823.

Sternberg, R.J. (1977). *Intelligence, information processing, and analogical reasoning: The componential analysis of human abilities.* Hillsdale, NJ: Erlbaum.

Sternberger, L.G., & Burns, G.L. (1991). Obsessive-compulsive disorder: Symptoms and diagnosis in a college sample. *Behavior Therapy, 22,* 569–576.

Stevens, S.S. (1939). Psychology and the science of science. *Psychological Bulletin, 36,* 221–263.

Street, E., & Dryden, W. (1988). *Family therapy in Britain.* Philadelphia: Open University.

Street, L.L., & Barlow, D.H. (1994). Anxiety disorders. In L.W. Craighead, W.E. Craighead, A.E. Kazdin, & M.J. Mahoney (Eds.), *Cognitive and behavioral interventions: An empirical approach to mental health problems.* Boston: Allyn & Bacon.

Strickland, G.P., Hoepfner, R., & Klein, S.P. (1976). *Attitude to school questionnaire manual.* Hollywood, CA: Monitor.

Strong, E.K., Jr. (1952). *Vocational Interest Blank for Men: Manual.* Stanford, CA: Stanford University Press.

Strong, E.K., Jr., Hansen, J.C., & Campbell, D.P. (1985). *Strong interest inventory.* Palo Alto, CA: Stanford University Press.

Suinn, R., & Richardson, F. (1971). Anxiety management training: A nonspecific behavior therapy program for anxiety control. *Behavior Therapy, 2,* 498–510.

Sulzer-Azeroff, B., & Mayer, G.R. (1986). *Achieving educational excellence and behavioral strategies.* New York: Holt, Rinehart, & Winston.

Suomi, S. (1990). In *Discovering Psychology*, Program 5 [PBS video series]. Washington, DC: Annenberg/CPB Project.

Super, D.E., & Crites, J.O. (1962). *Appraising vocational fitness.* New York: Harper and Brothers.

Suppe, F. (1977). *The structure of scientific theories.* Urbana: University of Illinois Press.

Susman, R.L. (1988). Hand of *Paranthropus robustus* from Member 1 Swartkrans: Fossil evidence for tool behavior. *Science, 240,* 781–784.

Tait, R.C. (in press). Integrative theories of pain: Unity at what price? *Pain Forum.*

Terman, L.M., & Merrill, M.A. (1937). *Measuring intelligence.* Boston: Houghton-Mifflin.

Thomas, A., & Chess, S. (1977). *Temperament and development.* New York: Brunner-Mazel.

Thomas, A., & Chess, S. (1981). The role of temperament in the contributions of individuals to their development. In R.M. Lerner & N.A. Bush-Rossnagel (Eds.), *Individuals as producers of their own development.* New York: Academic Press.

Thorne, F.C. (1950). *Principles of personality counseling.* Brandon, VT: Journal of Clinical Psychology.

Tolman, E.C. (1932). *Purposive behavior in animals and man.* New York: Century.

Tolman, E.C. (1936). An operational analysis of "demands." *Erkenntnis, 6,* 383–390.

Tolman, E.C. (1948). Cognitive maps in rats and men. *Psychological Review, 55,* 189–208.

Tolman, E.C. (1951). The intervening variable. In M.H. Marx (Ed.), *Psychological theory.* New York: Macmillan.

Tolman, E.C. (1959). Principles of purposive behavior. In S. Koch (Ed.), *Psychology: A study of a science. Vol. 2.* New York: McGraw-Hill.

Tolman, E.C., Honzik, C.H., & Robinson, E.W. (1930). The effect of degrees of hunger upon the order of elimination of long and short blinds. *University of California Publications in Psychology, 4,* 189–202.

Toulmin, S. (1972). *Human understanding.* Princeton, NJ: Princeton University Press.

Trapold, M.A., & Winokur, S.W. (1967). Transfer from classical conditioning and extinction to acquisition, extinction, and stimulus generalization of a positively reinforced instrumental response. *Journal of Experimental Psychology, 73,* 517–525.

Tronick, E.Z., Morelli, G.A., & Ivey, P.K. (1992). The Efe forager infant and toddlers patterns of social relationships: Multiple and simultaneous. *Developmental Psychology, 28,* 568–577.

Tryon, W.W. (1974). A reply to Staats' language behavior therapy: A derivative of social behaviorism. *Behavior Therapy, 5,* 273–276.

Tryon, W.W. (1990). Why paradigmatic behaviorism should be retitled psychological behaviorism. *Behavior Therapist, 13,* 127–128.

Tryon, W.W. (1995). Neural networks: II. Unified learning theory and behavioral psychotherapy. *Clinical Psychology Review, 13,* 353–371.

Tryon, W.W., & Briones, R.G. (1985). Higher-order semantic counterconditioning of Filipino women's evaluation of heterosexual behaviors. *Journal of Behavior Therapy and Experimental Psychiatry, 16,* 125–131.

Turner, J.A., & Clancey, S. (1988). Chronic low back pain: Relationship to pain and disability. *Pain, 12,* 23–46.

Ullmann, L.P., & Krasner, L. (1965). *Case studies in behavior modification.* New York: Holt, Rinehart & Winston.

Ullmann, L.P., & Krasner, L. (1968). *A psychological approach to abnormal behavior.* Englewood Cliffs, NJ: Prentice-Hall.

Ulman, J. (1979). A critique of Skinnerism: Materialism minus the dialectic. *Behaviorists for Social Action Journal, 1*(2), 1–8.

Ulman, J. (1983). Toward a united front: A class analysis of social and political action. *Behaviorists for Social Action Journal, 4*(1), 17–24.

Ulman, J.D. (1990). Paradigmatic behaviorism: Hierarchically schematized eclecticism. *TIBA Newsletter, 2,* 6–7.

Underwood, B.J., & Schulz, R.W. (1960). *Meaningfulness and verbal learning.* Philadelphia: J.B. Lippincott.

Uzgiris, I.C., & Hunt, J. McV. (1975). *Assessment in infancy: Ordinal scales of psychological development.* Urbana: University of Illinois Press.

Van Buren, A. (January 11, 1980). Dear Abby. *Honolulu Star-Bulletin,* p. B3.

Vargas, E.A. (1988). Verbally-governed and event-governed behavior. *Analysis of Verbal Behavior, 6,* 11–22.

Vaughan, M.E. (1987). Rule-governed behavior and higher mental processes. In S. Modgil & C. Modgil (Eds.), *B.F. Skinner: Consensus and controversy* (pp. 257–264). Barcombe, UK: Palmer Press.

Vaughan, M.E. (1989). Rule-governed behavior in behavior analysis: A theoretical and experimental history. In S.C. Hayes (Ed.), *Rule-governed behavior* (pp. 97–118). New York: Plenum.

Viney, W. (1989). The cyclops and the twelve-eyed toad: William James and the unity–disunity problem in psychology. *American Psychologist, 44,* 1261–1265.

Wachtel, P.L. (1984). Toward the integration of individual psychodynamic theories and family systems theories. In A.W. Staats & L.P. Mos (Eds.), *Annals of theoretical psychology, vol. 5.* New York: Plenum.

Wachtel, P.L. (1985). Need for theory. *International Newsletter of Uninomic Psychology, 1,* 15.

Wade, N. (1982). Editorial notebook. *New York Times,* April 30, 30A.

Wahler, R.G., & Foxx, J.J. (1980). Solitary toy play and time out: A family treatment package for children with aggressive and oppositional behavior. *Journal of Applied Behavior Analysis, 13,* 23–29.

Walker, D., Greenwood, C.R., & Terry, B. (1994). Management of classroom disruptive behavior and academic performance. In L.W. Craighead, W.E. Craighead, A.E. Kazdin, & M.J. Mahoney (Eds.), *Cognitive and behavioral interventions: An empirical approach to mental health problems.* Boston: Allyn & Bacon.

Walster, E., Aronson, V., Abrahams, D., & Rottman, L. (1966). The importance of physical attractiveness in dating behavior. *Journal of Personality and Social Psychology, 4,* 508–516.

Walton, D. (1960). The application of learning theory to the treatment of a case of neurodermatitis. In H.J. Eysenck (Ed.), *Behaviour therapy and the neuroses.* New York: Pergamon.

Wanchisen, B.A. (1990). Forgetting the lessons of history. *Behavior Analyst, 13,* 31–38.

Wapner, S., & Demick, J. (1989). A holistic, developmental systems approach to person-environment functioning. *International Newsletter of Uninomic Psychology, 8,* 15–30.

Watson, J.B. (1930). *Behaviorism.* (Rev. ed.). Chicago: University of Chicago Press.

Watson, J.B., & Raynor, R. (1920). Conditioned emotional reactions. *Journal of Experimental Psychology, 3,* 1–14.

Wechsler, D. (1955). *Manual for the Wechsler Adult Intelligence Scale.* New York: Psychological Corporation.

Wechsler, D. (1958). *The measurement and appraisal of adult intelligence* (4th ed.). Baltimore: Williams and Wilkins.

Wechsler, D. (1967). *Wechsler Preschool and Primary Scale of Intelligence.* New York: Psychological Corporation.

Weigl, R.H. (1978). Personality and behavior revisited. *Contemporary Psychology, 23,* 553–554.

Weiss, A.R., & Evans, I.M. (1978). Process studies in language conditioning: I. Counterconditioning of anxiety by "calm" words. *Journal of Behavior Therapy and Experimental Psychiatry, 9,* 115–119.

Weiss, R.L. (1968). Operant conditioning techniques in psychological assessment. In P. McReynolds (Ed.), *Advances in psychological assessment.* Palo Alto, CA: Science and Behavior Books.

Wells, K.C. (1994). Parent and family management training. In L.W. Craighead, W.E. Craighead, A.E. Kazdin, & M.J. Mahoney (Eds.), *Cognitive and behavioral interventions: An empirical approach to mental health problems.* Boston: Allyn & Bacon.

Wener, A., & Rehm, I. (1975). Depressive affect: A test of behavioral hypotheses. *Journal of Abnormal Psychology, 84,* 221–227.

Wentworth, N., & Haith, M.M. (1992). Event-specific expectations of 2- and 3-month-old infants. *Developmental Psychology, 28,* 842–850.

Wertheimer, M. (1972). *Fundamental issues in psychology.* New York: Holt, Rinehart & Winston.

Wertheimer, M. (1988). Obstacles to the integration of competing theories in psychology. *Philosophical Psychology, 1,* 131–137.

Westie, F.R., & DeFleur, M.L. (1959). Autonomic responses and their relationship to race attitudes. *Journal of Abnormal and Social Psychology, 58,* 340–347.

White, R. (in collaboration with Fallaci, D.). (1967). The dead body and the living brain. *Look, 24,* Nov. 28.

Whitman, T.L. (1994). Mental retardation. In L.W. Craighead, W.E. Craighead, A.E. Kazdin, & M.J. Mahoney (Eds.), *Cognitive and behavioral interventions: An empirical approach to mental health problems.* Boston: Allyn & Bacon.

Wierson, M., & Forehand, R. (1994). Parent behavioral training for child noncompliance: Rationale, concepts, and effectiveness. *Current Directions, 3,* 146–150.

Williams, C.D. (1959). The elimination of tantrum behavior by extinction procedures. *Journal of Abnormal and Social Psychology, 59,* 269.

Wittig, A.F. (1985). Reflections on unity-disunity by a general psychologist. *International Newsletter of Uninomic Psychology, 1,* 13.

Wolf, M.M., Phillips, E.L., Fixsen, D.I., Braukmann, C.J., Kirigin, K.A., Willner, A.G., & Schumaker, J.B. (1976). Achievement place: The teaching-family model. *Child Care Quarterly, 5,* 92–101.

Wolf, M.M., Risely, T., & Mees, H. (1964). Application of operant conditioning procedures to the behavior problems of an autistic child. *Behavior Research and Therapy, 1,* 305–312.

Woll, S. (1978). The best of both worlds? A critique of cognitive social learning. Unpublished manuscript.

Wolpe, J. (1958). *Psychotherapy by reciprocal inhibition.* Stanford, CA: Stanford University Press.

Wolpe, J. (1969). *The practice of behavior therapy.* London: Pergamon.

Wolpe, J., & Lang, P.J. (1964). A fear survey schedule for use in behavior modification. *Behaviour Research and Therapy, 2,* 27–30.

Woodward, W.R., & Devonis, D. (1993). Toward a new understanding of scientific change: Applying interfield theory to the history of psychology. In H.V. Rappard, P.J. van Strien, & L.P. Mos (Eds.), *Annals of theoretical psychology, vol. 8.* New York: Plenum.

Worchel, S., Cooper, J., & Goethals, G.R. (1988). *Understanding social psychology* (4th ed.). Chicago: Dorsey Press.

Yela, M. (1987). Toward a unified psychological science: The meaning of behavior. In A.W. Staats & L.P. Mos (Eds.), *Annals of theoretical psychology, vol. 5.* New York: Plenum.

Young, P.T. (1936). *Motivation of behavior.* New York: John Wiley.

Zanna, M.P., Kiesler, C.A., & Pilkonis, P.A. (1970). Positive and negative attitudinal affect established by classical conditioning. *Journal of Personality and Social Psychology, 14,* 321–328.

Zeiberger, J., Sampen, S., & Sloane, H. (1968). Modification of a child's problem behaviors in the home with the mother as therapist. *Journal of Applied Behavior Analysis, 1,* 47–53.

Zelaso, P.R., Zelaso, N.A., & Kolb, S. (1972). "Walking" in the newborn. *Science, 176,* 314–315.

Zettle, R.D., & Hayes, S.C. (1982). Rule-governed behavior: A potential theoretical framework for cognitive-behavior therapy. In P.C. Kendall (Ed.), *Advances in cognitive-behavioral research and therapy* (Vol. I., pp. 73–118). New York: Academic Press.

Zimbardo, P.G. (1992). *Psychology and life.* New York: Harper Collins.

Zimmerman, D.W. (1957). Durable secondary reinforcement: Method and theory. *Psychological Review, 64,* 373–383.

Zuckerman, M., & Lubin, B. (1965). *Manual for the multiple affect adjective check list.* San Diego: Educational and Industrial Testing Service.

Index

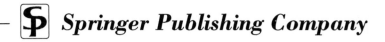 **Springer Publishing Company**

GENDER, IDENTITY, AND SELF-ESTEEM
A New Look at Adult Development

Deborah Y. Anderson, PhD
Christopher L. Hayes, PhD

Based on findings from their original research, Drs. Anderson and Hayes explore how men and women shape, form, and integrate their identities and sense of self-worth within the framework of the influential life-ties of family, work, friends, and education, among others.

Gender-balanced personal stories bring the text to life and help illustrate the major findings of their research. This text is of special interest to professors and students of courses in adult development, life-span development, gender studies, and family studies.

Contents:

- Prologue
- Reexamination of Adult Development
- Family of Origin
- Education
- Friends and Mentors
- Intimate Relationships
- Children
- Work
- Conclusion
- Appendices

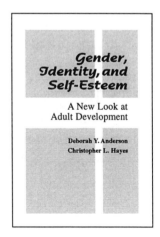

1996   320pp (est)   0-8261-9410-9   hardcover

536 Broadway, New York, NY 10012-3955 • (212) 431-4370 • Fax (212) 941-7842

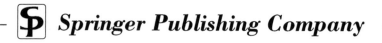

Springer Publishing Company

SELF-ESTEEM
Research, Theory, and Practice
Chris Mruk, PhD

Low self-esteem is frequently an underlying factor in a range of psychological disorders, including depression, suicide, and certain personality disorders. The recent explosion of research and literature on self-esteem only emphasizes the need for a comprehensive examination of what we know and do not know about

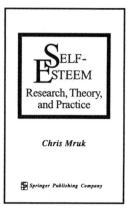

this complicated issue. Dr. Mruk provides a thorough analysis of the vast literature, from which he derives the most practical and effective methods available for the enhancement of self-esteem. His recommendations are based on both qualitative and quantitative findings, and take into account both individual and societal factors.

Contents:

- The Meaning and Structure of Self-Esteem
- Self-Esteem Research Problems and Issues
- Self-Esteem Research Findings — A Consensus
- Major Self-Esteem Theories and Programs
- A Phenomenological Theory of Self-Esteem
- Enhancing Self-Esteem Phenomenologically
- Appendix

Behavioral Science Book Service Selection
1994   240pp   0-8261-8750-1   hard

536 Broadway, New York, NY 10012-3955 • (212) 431-4370 • Fax (212) 941-7842

P *Springer Publishing Company*

DIFFERENTIATING NORMAL AND ABNORMAL PERSONALITY

Stephen Strack, PhD, and
Maurice Lorr, PhD, Editors

In this volume, the editors break from the traditional categorical definitions of personality, and explore the interface between normality and pathology in terms of a dimensional continuum. This text contains original contributions by theorists and researchers who have pursued integrative normal-abnormal approaches, representing the vanguard of thought in the field of personality today.

Partial Contents:

I: Theoretical Perspectives. Psychopathology From the Perspective of the Five-Factor Model, *R. R. McCrae* • Personality: A Cattellian Perspective, *S.E. Krug*

II: Methodology. Cluster Analysis: Aims, Methods, and Problems, *M. Lorr* • Multidimensional Scaling Models of Personality Responding, *M.L. Davison* • Revealing Structure in the Data: Principles of Exploratory Factor Analysis, *L.R. Goldberg & J.M. Digman*

III: Measurement. The Personality Psychopathology Five (PSY-5), *A. R. Harkness and J. L. McNulty* • Evaluating Normal and Abnormal Personality Using the Same Set of Constructs, E. Helmes & D.N. Jackson • The MMPI and MMPI-2: Fifty Years of Differentiating Normal and Abnormal Personality, *Y.S. Ben-Porath*

1994   464pp   0-8261-8550-9   hardcover

536 Broadway, New York, NY 10012-3955 • (212) 431-4370 • Fax (212) 941-7842

Springer Publishing Company

THE PRACTICE OF RATIONAL EMOTIVE BEHAVIOR THERAPY
Albert Ellis, PhD, and **Windy Dryden,** PhD

This volume systematically reviews the practice of Rational Emotive Behavior Therapy and, using an array of actual case examples, shows how it can be used by therapists in a variety of clinical settings. The book includes an explanation of REBT as a general treatment model and addresses different treatment modalities, including individual, couples, family, and sex therapy.

The new edition modernizes the pioneering theories of Albert Ellis and contains a complete updating of references over the past ten years. It features a new chapter on teaching the principles of unconditional self-acceptance in a structured group setting. This volume is an essential reference for clinical and counseling psychologists as well as other helping professionals providing therapy.

Partial Contents:
- The General Theory of REBT
- The Basic Practice of REBT
- A Case Illustration of the Basic Practice of REBT: The Case of Jane
- Rational Emotive Behavior Marathons and Intensives
- Teaching the Principles of Unconditioned Self-Acceptance in a Structured Group Setting
- The Rational Emotive Behavioral Approach to Sex Therapy
- The Use of Hypnosis with REBT

288pp(est)   0-8261-5471-9   1996   softcover

536 Broadway, New York, NY 10012-3955 • (212) 431-4370 • Fax (212) 941-7842